Bioethical Responsibilities in Twenty-First Century Crises

Revolutionary Bioethics

Series Editor: Rachel Haliburton, University of Sudbury

Revolutionary Bioethics is a new series composed of scholarly monographs and edited collections organized around specific topics that explore bioethical theory and practice through the frameworks provided by feminist ethics, narrative ethics, and virtue ethics, challenging the assumptions of mainstream bioethics in the process. Contemporary mainstream bioethics has become ideological and repetitive, a defender of activities that bioethics was originally created to critique, and an apologist for unethical practices and policies in medicine that it once saw itself as fighting against. Taking its title from recent work being done on MacIntyre's neo-Aristotelian ethics, Revolutionary Bioethics is organized around the idea that bioethics needs to reform both its theory and practice, and its goal is to begin the conversation about what a transformed bioethics—one that is unafraid to explore new theoretical approaches, and to examine and critique current bioethical practices—might look like.

Titles in the series

Bioethical Responsibilities in Twenty-First Century Crises, edited by Elizabeth Lanphier and Larry R. Churchill

Redescribing Bioethics: How the Field Constructs Its Argument, by Tod S. Chambers

Righting Health Policy: Bioethics, Political Philosophy, and the Normative Justification of Health Law and Policy, by D. Robert MacDougall

Caregiving, Carebots, and Contagion, by Michael C. Brannigan

Engineering Perfection: Solidarity, Disability, and Well-being, by Elyse Purcell

Physician-Assisted Suicide and Euthanasia: Before, During, and After the Third Reich, Edited by Sheldon Rubenfeld and Daniel P. Sulmasy, with Astrid Ley

Bioethical Responsibilities in Twenty-First Century Crises

Edited by
Elizabeth Lanphier and Larry R. Churchill

BLOOMSBURY ACADEMIC
NEW YORK • LONDON • OXFORD • NEW DELHI • SYDNEY

BLOOMSBURY ACADEMIC
Bloomsbury Publishing Inc, 1359 Broadway, New York, NY 10018, USA
Bloomsbury Publishing Plc, 50 Bedford Square, London, WC1B 3DP, UK
Bloomsbury Publishing Ireland, 29 Earlsfort Terrace, Dublin 2, D02 AY28, Ireland

First published in the United States of America 2018

A catalog record for this book is available from the Library of Congress.

ISBN: HB: 978-1-6669-5938-3
ePDF: 979-8-216-20132-8
eBook: 978-1-9787-6637-2

Series: Revolutionary Bioethics

Typeset by Deanta Global Publishing Services, Chennai, India

For product safety related questions contact productsafety@bloomsbury.com.

Contents

Introduction

Elizabeth Lanphier and Larry R. Churchill

A great deal of important and urgent work lies ahead for bioethics. This book explores areas, methods, and collaborations needed for the present and future of bioethics. By so doing, it also advocates for renewal and change in the field.

Perhaps the greatest difference bioethics had made over its first five decades is in acknowledging and promoting a deeper understanding of the humanity of those involved with healthcare and its practices. This deeper understanding extends to the range of roles involved in healthcare delivery—centrally, patients, and the doctors, nurses, other allied health professionals, and family and lay caregivers who care for them. But it also extends to scientists developing novel biomedical innovations and the patients and research subjects who volunteer to participate in biomedical research.

Yet despite this progress, bioethics must claim additional areas and methods as its proper purview to meet its responsibilities in the twenty-first century. Prominent among these responsibilities is a richer sense of the human situation—our complexity, our arrogance, and tendencies to overreach, as well as our benevolence and compassion, our significant and often disparate vulnerabilities, and our hopes and aspirations. Additionally, bioethics has contributed, and must continue to contribute, to policy changes regarding respecting self-determination in healthcare while recognizing the impact of environments and systems on health, and the need for structural and policy approaches to addressing them. This includes efforts to appreciate differences within and among populations that impact health, health research, and decision-making about both. And it requires ongoing work to (re)conceptualize and pursue justice in healthcare policies and practices.

Accompanying the recognition of these responsibilities is an enrichment of methods relevant to an evolving and future-oriented bioethics. Moving from its dominating identity as a field with a medico-centric preoccupation with doctors and patients, researchers and subjects, bioethics has recently and increasingly resurrected its other founding focus. Central to bioethics, a term broader than "medical ethics" or "healthcare ethics," is an understanding of life ("bios") as a whole, inclusive of the planet we and other beings inhabit. On this view, efforts to forge a future in which all of bios—not just human health—is the ethical focus of bioethics.

This bios-centered bioethics was initiated by Van Rensselaer Potter, whose 1973 book *Bioethics: Bridge to the Future* has been rediscovered by contemporary bioethics scholars with appreciation for its prescience about global warming, the degrading of the natural world, and issues of sustainability of economic and population growth.

In addition, bioethics has increasingly contributed insights, informed by the multidisciplinary nature of the field and its own ethical frameworks, into broader matters of justice, like social and structural racism, that impact health and well-being. The global Covid-19 pandemic has also been instrumental in opening the eyes of bioethicists (and the world) to generally neglected contributors to health, including what public health and public policy scholars term the social determinants of health and disease, or sometimes the political determinants of health.

As various chapters in this volume identify and explicate, bioethics, with its core commitment to justice, needs to grow its focus and tools. Bioethics must attend to the ways in which structural inequities and intersectional oppression (i.e., when factors like race, age, gender, disability, and more overlap and compound) impact medical care and healthcare access, as well as health policy, and research priorities and participation. But it must also address how these impact contributions to and vulnerability from climate change, or the impact social and political choices have on our health and well-being.

Expanding the scope of what falls within "bios" and deepening sensibilities regarding ethical thinking brings the need for new and renewed methods for bioethics. In this landscape, collaboration becomes not only acceptable for the field, but a necessity for bioethics to do its work. This includes collaboration among scholars and methodologies, but also between scholars and communities impacted by bioethical innovation. This is to say, bioethics is accountable to, and in conversation with, everyone inhabiting our planet now and in the future. The reign of conceptual analysis or casuistry as the primary or sole methods of bioethics is gone. An exciting new era of interdisciplinary theoretical, applied, and visionary work is well underway. With new methods come not only new applications for the existing framework of bioethics but new ways for bioethics to understand itself as a field.

This volume is an effort to capture some of the most impactful work in this present era of bioethics, by established and emerging voices looking to the future. Although we've noted the truly global reach of the "bios" in bioethics, given the particularities of not only healthcare systems but also political systems, this collection focuses on perspectives primarily from North America. It also reflects many of the unique social realities and structures of the United States.

However, our conviction is that as a field bioethics can greatly increase and expand its impact, in ways our contributors have delineated in their chapters, beyond the national borders in which the work is created. The scholarship may reflect and address the local histories and idiosyncrasies of health and politics in which these chapters were written, but we trust that they offer critical thinking that can and needs to be adapted to and built upon in new contexts. And like bioethics contributions of the past, these new bioethics chapters also express renewed and enriched understandings of ourselves, our values, and our place in the world.

The chapters within the collection are grouped under four thematic headings. However, we hope readers find, as we do, many thematic connections not only within but across these themes.

Bringing Current Practice into the Future

This section starts and ends with two chapters arguing for an expanded agenda for bioethics. Both offer examples of methods for bioethics work that will propel it into the future in a more effective way. Lisa S. Parker details the need for attention to identity-forming feelings and how bioethics can help inform public understanding of the process of scientific investigation. Howard A. Brody renews a call for better community dialogue in research and illustrates the shortcoming of "precision medicine" for providing truly personal care for patients. In between these chapters falls Arthur W. Frank's contribution on the essential role of dialogue as both the medium and goal of bioethical engagement, while Gregory E. Kaebnick brings his editorial expertise to bear on the complexity of bioethics communication in a pluralist democratic society. Advocacy is never far from the focus for any of these authors.

Witnessing Difference and Responding to Vulnerability

Several chapters point to areas of bioethics work that are undeveloped or underdeveloped, particularly regarding underappreciated differences and vulnerabilities that impact bioethics and health. Nancy M. P. King offers an analysis of the persistence and pervasiveness of "othering" generally, and in healthcare and bioethics particularly, and calls for greater awareness of the implicit or tacit forms of this common phenomenon. Takunda Matose and Elizabeth Lanphier examine the health and well-being of incarcerated persons and argue that bioethics has undertheorized how its core concepts and normative approaches interact with carceral contexts. These authors contend that carceral settings are sites in which to apply bioethical theory and can generate new bioethical theory and practice. Larry R. Churchill and David Schenck work toward a phenomenology of aging, arguing that this near-universal life experience is understudied in bioethics and can be a source of insight for investigating other vulnerable social groups, as well as better care for the aging. The final chapter in this section could fit with many of this volume's themes, but we are placing it here to underline the innovation of Virgina Brown's reading of the *Belmont Report* and its commitment to social justice for marginalized groups. She argues that interpreting the call for social justice must be rethought to better address intersectional forms of injustice. Doing so enables bioethics to better realize justice as one of its central pillars.

Bioethics Response to Global Warming

While many chapters in this collection make connections to climate and the environment, the chapters in this section tackle global warming and climate change as particularly bioethical problems. Travis N. Rieder lays out helpful distinctions between policy matters and individual actions toward mitigating climate risk. These distinctions also relate to responsibilities for advocacy in bioethics and conceptualizing the relationship between individual and shared responsibility to address structural harm that can apply widely to health and health systems. Stephen M. Gardiner and Paul Tubig argue for a new area of bioethics work understood as focusing on "planetary health," parsing what this emerging concept ought to mean, and considering its acceptability and usefulness for both professionals and the public. Cheryl C. Macpherson and Katharine Wright explore strategies for getting attention to, and deeper consideration for, the problems of environmental degradation in bioethics and healthcare. In the final chapter of this section, Nancy Tuana makes the case for a linkage between bioethics and geoethics to recognize and overcome what the author has termed "environmental indifference" through an ecointersectional approach. Each of these chapters shows that climate change is a matter for individual, population, and planetary health that requires bioethical attention, scholarship, and advocacy.

New Tools and Visions for Bioethics

All the chapters in this volume contain insights for new or renewed methods and directions for bioethics. But the four concluding chapters in particular foreground new tools and visions for the field. Marion Danis and Hollen N. Reischer probe the knotty psychological problems of adapting to change, and how clinical ethics in particular can better address change. As a coda to the previous section, they connect this adaption to change to the work of bioethics to address adaption and climate change.

Gail E. Henderson argues from both the history of social epidemiology and the current lapses in bioethical analysis that collaboration and long-term partnership with those who study the social determinants of disease and health are essential for future bioethics work. Bioethics narrowly attuned to individual clinical decisions and patient care has its place, but public health ethics and social determinants of health and disease profoundly impact the lives and well-being of populations.

Johnathan Flowers makes a striking claim that the citational norms of established bioethical discourse disenfranchise disability studies by mistaking it for simple advocacy rather than as sound scholarship that challenges the status quo bioethics. This same bias, he contends, affects queer studies and Black bioethics, which are rebellions against existing norms and demand the very reshaping of how bioethics ought to be done. In the final chapter of the collection, Leah Lomotey-Nakon offers a far-reaching critique and correction of both past and current bioethics scholarship, arguing for a visionary speculative bioethics building on Afrofuturism and visionary speculative fiction. This approach is a new tool that also connects with previously lost threads of bioethics increasingly in need of resurrection.

Our hope is that bioethics students and scholars will critically engage with these chapters and extend and develop them to bring bioethics into a new flourishing that will meet the field's responsibilities for the current century.

Bringing Current Practice into the Future

1

Bioethics in the Current Climate

Attending to Identity-Forming Feelings and Knowledge Production

Lisa S. Parker

Fifteen years ago, when I was asked to write a chapter on bioethics and social activism, I argued that bioethicists engage in social activism when they engage in reasoned argument about matters of justice and well-being, and when they provide resources for others to do the same (Parker 2007). Embracing norms of rational deliberation, bioethics contributes to deliberative democratic processes. It both "informs the debate" and demonstrates and teaches how fair, respectful debate should proceed. Bioethics should also, I argued, examine how the norms and processes of rational deliberation, as well as material conditions and social structures, exclude some people and discount some perspectives. By investigating and giving voice to perspectives and interests otherwise excluded, bioethics serves justice and promotes the well-being of those materially and structurally vulnerable. In this way, I argued, bioethics engages in activism.

Today, whether those practices can count as activism is no longer my concern. In light of so many things affecting health and well-being—the now endemic Covid-19 pandemic and failures of public health infrastructure . . . shootings at stores, schools, parades, and traffic stops, and in neighborhoods and houses of worship . . . deaths of despair . . . disparities of health and healthcare, widening wealth and education gaps . . . being incarcerated, being unhoused . . . the climate, refugees, and economies in crisis . . . war abroad, insurrection at home . . . poisonous nationalism, persistent racism—in light of all this, the real question is whether reasoned argument still matters. Lurking behind and complicating so many of these urgent issues are the factors that have led to the proclamation of a post-truth epoch, "in which objective facts are less influential in shaping political debate or public opinion than appeals to emotion and personal belief" (OED 2023). Perhaps the pressing question for bioethics is whether reasoned argument can still persuade.

I believe that arguments do still matter and that they can persuade. I believe this with a type and degree of confidence familiar in bioethics. At least in discussing particular clinical ethics cases, we often state with substantial confidence that some claims or courses of action are worse or less well justified than others, even if we do not have the same degree of confidence that one alternative is irrefutably best and highly likely to lead to good outcomes. In this case, the alternative of abandoning reasoned argument is worse. Most of the alternatives to reasoned argument—manipulation, might-making-right, violence, creating or joining a cult of personality, authoritarianism—have historically been demonstrated to be worse than continuing to engage in reasoned argument. Indeed, abandonment of reasoned argument—and its strictures of logic and reliance on facts—is a cause or a prime perpetuator of the events, profound failures, and exigent needs of our time, as listed in the previous paragraph.

This isn't a "knock down argument" in support of reasoned argument, but a modest claim: we have reason to keep at it, to keep making reasoned arguments and appealing to the best, most carefully vetted empirical evidence available. It is the best that we can do. In this chapter, I sketch three suggestions for bioethics that might help us do it better, more persuasively.

The first two are prompted by my work on ethical issues related to genetic/genomic medicine and research. First, I suggest that bioethics' arguments and empirical research need to pay more attention to the roles that feelings and emotions play in a broad range of health-relevant behaviors. Second, I suggest that bioethics should advocate for taking a longer view and for empirical research—in bioethics and in general—that has a longer time horizon and broader scope. Though they emerge from a domain seemingly distant from the many threats to health and well-being I recounted, these suggestions may help bioethics contribute to addressing such threats, in large part by understanding people's resistance to addressing them. Third, I conclude by indicating how bioethics may employ insights from feminist epistemology to help people deal with the evolving nature of scientific understanding and other knowledge claims without declaring the end of truth and objectivity, or feeling an overwhelming threat to their way of life.

Feelings, Behavior, and Bioethics

Ethical, legal, and social implications (ELSI) researchers have been concerned with people's responses to learning personal predictive genetic information since the ELSI Research Program was created and the human genome was mapped. Initially, there was concern that people would respond fatalistically: either not bothering to reduce their health risks or despairing and even committing suicide if testing revealed a high risk or near certainty of developing serious disease. Those feared responses have generally not materialized (Sabatello and Juengst 2019).

Instead, with the exception of people who are specifically motivated by history or circumstance to seek genetic risk information, the response to this information may turn out to be "meh." Members of "cancer families," those at risk of rare diseases, or those wanting prenatal or preconception testing may seek and use genetic information. But thus far, widespread and effective use of whole genome sequencing to prevent or treat common complex conditions—genomics' Holy Grail of providing a crystal ball and road map to health—seems unlikely. One reason, as sociologist Jenny Reardon heard from a representative interviewee, is a feeling that genetics "is not important. And it is not important because there is *so much else wrong*" (Reardon 2017, 64). That "so much else" includes economic and other practical challenges, racism and other structural injustices, and immediate serious health concerns.

Even those well-situated to make use of genomic information to promote their health often do not. The Personal Genome Sequencing Outcomes (PeopleSeq) Consortium is a large-scale longitudinal study of the medical, behavioral, and economic outcomes of returning genomic sequencing information to healthy individuals. Its participants are not the less affluent people in the US Black Belt interviewed by Reardon, for whom "so much else" is persistently, structurally wrong. Like most studies of nondiagnostic genomic sequencing, PeopleSeq participants are predominantly white, affluent, and highly educated. Yet in a substudy of PeopleSeq participants, 90 percent reported making no changes in their health-related behaviors (Zoltick et al. 2019). This lack of effect on health behaviors is consistent with other studies, including those finding that genetic information may affect intentions to change behavior, but not health behaviors themselves (Gray et al. 2014).

Ethics has examined the information-action disconnect for millennia, from ancient attention to *akrasia* to discussions of first- and second-order preferences, to decision theory and insights of behavioral economics. Empirical bioethics should expand from studying people's preferences, beliefs, and understanding, to learn how their emotions, feelings, and affect-inflected beliefs relate to their health and health-related behaviors. Empirical bioethics might profitably examine more thoroughly what motivates behavior change and delve more broadly and deeply to understand emotions and motivations more fully. More attention to feelings and behavior will be necessary if preventive health-related innovations are to be adopted. The role of feeling and emotion in health-related decision-making warrants their study by bioethicists, as well as psychologists, behavioral economists, and other social scientists.

Beyond such empirical inquiry, bioethics should provide normative analysis of these affective aspects of health-related decisions and behaviors. It is the bringing of empirical findings and normative analysis to bear on each other that is the hallmark of bioethics, as distinct from social science or ethical theory (Parker et al. 2019). What should be made of the fact that despite not changing their health behaviors, 58 percent of PeopleSeq participants nevertheless considered sequencing to be empowering? Undergoing genomic sequencing "made them feel like they had more control over their health" (Zoltick et al. 2019, 7). Bioethics should consider what is an ethically appropriate response to sequencing's feeding a sense of control in the absence of the resources or will to exercise that power. Such consideration might explore the long-term effects of the trend to individualize health risks and distract attention from shared environmental risks and social responsibility (Tabery 2023). These might include erosion of support for public health initiatives for which people fail to see individual benefit or that require self-sacrifice, as well as increased self-blame and stigma regarding ill health.

It might consider the effects of fueling people's beliefs that they have control, and that having control is in itself valuable. The prospect of people using high-tech tools to perfect themselves and their children may not be as corrosive as the way that the illusion of control renders the reality of dependency ever more threatening to people's self-identities and widens the divide between those with and without disabilities (Sandel 2007; Tronto 1993). Valorizing control may further erode trust in health-related institutions that remain incapable of preventing or treating some conditions, while simultaneously warranting people's postponement of difficult discussions—within families and within society—about using resources to try to stave off inevitable death (Gawande 2014).

In coupling empirical study of the feeling-motivation-behavior connection with normative analysis, bioethics should expand both the range of feelings and the range of health-relevant behaviors to which it attends. Beyond studying, for example, how nudges may influence health behaviors and whether weak paternalist policies may be justified, bioethics might encourage more investigation of how fear—not only of disease, but also of losing face, or losing a sense of place, stability, or entitlement—affects health and health behaviors. Indeed, we need to study how a range of feelings—like fear, hope, entitlement, neglect, betrayal, anger, despair, belonging, empowerment—affect health and health-relevant behaviors. Moreover, health-relevant behaviors include not only diet, exercise, and health surveillance but also taking umbrage at being given health recommendations and stridently rejecting them (or acquiescing and feeling like an outcast or sissy for doing so). Health-relevant behaviors include substance use, family planning, voting, seeking education and employment, and so on. Bioethics might point out that health-relevant behaviors include even further upstream behaviors such as encouraging democratic deliberation, enabling or restricting voting, and facilitating shifting alliances of interests or permanently pitting groups against each other.

The health relevance of voting is likely obvious, given past and recent legislation and court decisions that affect health, most obviously at the beginning and end of life. Indeed, elected officials legislate, regulate, and allocate funds to activities that affect people's health across the lifespan, from providing for clean air and water to food and pharmaceutical safety, to medical research and medical assistance (including Medicaid and Medicare, HRSA-funded health centers, and health insurance exchanges). What hurdles or facilitators are enacted to discourage/encourage voting (ID requirements, mail-in ballots, or ballot drop-off boxes), by what process electoral districts are drawn, and whose vote is allowed—these upstream political actions obviously affect the outcomes of elections. Further upstream are the cultural contexts and social interactions that ultimately shape the beliefs, values, fears, affinities, and disaffections that inform people's political views and voting patterns, which ultimately affect people's prospects for health and healthcare in turn affecting people's prospects for health and well-being through the actions of those elected.

But these value- and affect-inflected views and behaviors also affect health more directly. In the face of substantial uncertainty, such as uncertainty surrounding the novel coronavirus, deep suspicion of the intent and worldview of "the other side," or even of the whole political enterprise, led people to trust familiar celebrities as much or more than scientists (Liu et al. 2020; Vaduganathan et al. 2020). Disappointment in difficult and incompletely efficacious treatment for acute and chronic conditions, especially coupled with suspicion of expertise and mainstream science, leads people to seek alternative therapies—for example, laetrile for cancer, supplements to cure lupus, or hydroxychloroquine for Covid-19 (Kravitz 2020; Métraux 2024; Milazzo and Horneber 2015). Decades of overselling the practical and immediate benefits of medical science to attract federal funding and shareholder investments have helped to create the gap between expectations and reality that people find discouraging and frightening. Those who feel that they always get the short end of the societal stick may feel tricked yet again and be particularly disappointed in healthcare realities. Those with their own political and economic interests can weaponize that disappointment against what then become sociopolitical targets: science, public health infrastructure, and claims of expertise. Alternative treatments that are both ineffective and potentially dangerous can be touted by people who establish their celebrity by bucking mainstream expertise, and most importantly, who appeal to people's feelings and provide anecdotes not data to support their claims.

While not all bioethical inquiries can or should take such a broad view as to examine the problem of "dying of whiteness" in the United States (Metzl 2019) or the multiple causes of our "inflamed" population (Marya and Patel 2021), bioethicists need to pay increased attention to feelings and their role in decisions and behavior. This is necessary if bioethical arguments are to support the efforts of science, healthcare, and public health to promote the well-being of those less well-off and address unjust disparities in health. It is important to attend not only to "the usual" feelings prompted by serious illness—fear, regret, hope, anger—but also to feelings of group loyalty and self-identity, security and stability, absence/presence of threat, and sense of place and order (Graham et al. 2011).

Moreover, it may be insufficient for bioethical analysis to regard these feelings and affect-inflected interests as signaling mere interests: they may play particular and especially important constitutive roles in some people's conception of the good and indeed their self-identity. They may thus play outsized roles with regard to some health-relevant behaviors and attempts to change them. In this way, bioethics might contribute to understanding not only why people don't change their individual health behaviors, but also why people—individually and collectively—don't undertake to address the "so much else wrong" that, for example, makes acting on genetic risk information seem a "luxury"—for example, the lack of emergency healthcare, safe drinking water, safe neighborhoods, and feelings of social respect, as well as the persistence of unemployment, racism, and threats to valued ways of life.

Coupling cognitive and social sciences with ethical, political, and critical theory, bioethics could illuminate connections among feelings, reasoned arguments, and health-relevant behaviors, both up and downstream from interventions like supplying genetic risk information or offering vaccination.

In the Fullness of Time

Attempting to understand how health-related behaviors are affected not only by information and reason, but by feelings, especially identity-related or constituting feelings, will require that bioethics take a longer time horizon for at least some of its empirical studies. This is especially true if bioethicists are to collaborate with behavioral scientists to engage in intervention research focused on feelings in an attempt to alter health-relevant behaviors.

Bioethics should also advocate for adopting longer time horizons in much of public health, medical, and health systems research, as well as its own empirical bioethics studies. As an example, consider the Electronic Medical Records and Genomics (eMERGE) Network. In its fourth 5-year phase, it includes embedded ELSI research to examine the psychosocial and healthcare utilization impact of returning Genome Informed Risk Assessments (GIRA) to eMERGE participants. Investigators report, however, that "the limited time frame of each phase (4–5 years) due to the constraints of National Institutes of Health (NIH) funding mechanisms . . . curtails the ability to assess outcomes effectively . . . [including] the medical and psychosocial outcomes of providing genetic information to participants" (Clayton et al. 2023, 1026–7), Many recipients' responses may be assessed only six or so months post-return, as the five-year study phase draws to an end.

It is possible that psychological sequelae or health services utilization prompted by the GIRA will be most intense in the period immediately following return. It is also noted, however, that the "emotional impact of learning about increased risk for future illness may intensify as individuals approach the typical age of onset or show initial signs of disease," or when family events (e.g., marriages, births, and even reunions) make risks that run in families more relevant or topical (Gray et al. 2014, 731). Qualitative research finds, for example, that some young women at increased risk for breast and ovarian cancer feel like "damaged goods" and worry about rejection by partners or about being considered unworthy by potential in-laws (Grubs et al. 2014, 244). Others report that their increased risk gave their lives "an underlying BRCA [breast cancer] vibe" and affected everything from career choice to clothes shopping with friends (Grubs et al. 2014, 244). From the perspective of concern about the physical and psychological well-being of participants and their families, or about the utility and cost-effectiveness of such risk assessment, it is indeed the fullness of time, not the immediate aftermath of return that is truly of health-related and ethical interest.

Moreover, the normative import of subtle psychological effects can only be considered if participants are asked about those subtle effects that may emerge or have an impact in the longer term (Hamilton and Hurley 2010). In the genomics context, the appropriate time to measure psychological responses to receipt of information remains unknown, while studies examine only short- and intermediate-term behavior change and healthcare resource utilization (Gray et al. 2014). "These time constraints limit what can be learned from translational research efforts. If the study cannot adequately achieve the goal of assessing the impact of returning genomic information, the studies cannot fully meet their obligation to the participants who enrolled in the research, as well as those who fund it," which is itself a bioethical concern (Clayton et al. 2023, 1027). Bioethicists (including those attached to eMERGE) should (and do) advocate for changes in funding structures to address "the lack of long-term follow-up [that] is a limitation of much government-funded research," and "weigh the costs of follow-up against the value of learning about the long-term benefits of preventive measures and early detection in real-world healthcare" (Clayton et al. 2023, 1027).

Potential benefits of taking a longer and broader, more systemic view are not limited to ELSI research on genomics. To take another example, the effects of racism on health and on people's interactions with healthcare and research systems are well established (De La Vega and Fullerton 2018; McCall et al. 2019; Williams et al. 2010). Developing evidence-based interventions to address the impact of racism on health, healthcare utilization, and research participation would require prospective studies conducted over a longer term and examining the structural interconnection of multiple types of health-affecting factors. In genomic and other health research, in addition to calling for greater diversity among populations studied, more nuanced instruments and scales, and more emphasis on social and intrafamilial impact (Roberts 2019), bioethics should articulate the ethical warrant for accruing data not over a short interval or at a somewhat arbitrary time point, but instead in longer-term studies in order to understand behaviors, attitudes, costs, benefits, and other outcomes that are potentially more lasting and impactful.

Similarly, the appropriate time horizon for empirical bioethics studies needs to be determined in relation to the research question. A longer time horizon would be needed to investigate more complex questions (e.g., those involving systemic problems) or to test interventions for their effect on complex psychosocial responses or a network of responses (as within a family or healthcare organization). It takes more time to study actual behaviors in response to an intervention than to collect data on stated intentions or responses to hypothetical scenarios. Given differences among intention, behavior, and sustained behavior change, if *sustained* behavior change were the outcome of interest, that would require a still longer time horizon; how long might be extrapolated from prior research on other sustained behavior change. In bioethics, as in other research, it is important to have sound justification for choosing secondary endpoints or for generalizing from data at one time slice to the time period about which we really care.

Normative bioethical analysis should seek to ensure that the chosen time frame of a research study does not serve the interests of those with a financial or reputational interest in the research at the expense of the population(s) whose interests the research findings are supposed to serve. Bioethics might consider, for example, whether studies of psychological sequelae across a relatively short interval are inappropriately reassuring. In the short term, providing genomic risk information seems to do little damage, but a longer time horizon might demonstrate a disturbing failure of it to do much good beyond satisfying curiosity and instilling largely unjustified feelings of empowerment. If those outcomes are persistent over time, normative bioethical analysis might express ethical concern about the allocation of resources, about contradictions between people's responses and actions, or about the long-term effect of feeling empowered or in control of one's health without good reason. Similarly, bioethics might engage in empirical and normative analysis to determine whether the ethically salutary effects of community-engaged research (CER) are long-lasting: Is community-based infrastructure developed during the collaboration sustained post-study, in a particular study community, or generally in CER?

A study's ethical goals and its hypothesis or question should guide the study's time horizon, rather than arbitrary or exogenous factors. Enabling a longer time horizon for empirical bioethics studies would necessitate the restructuring of research funding streams or development of new ones, and perhaps incorporating more bioethics research into existing longitudinal studies (with sufficient time for the ethical question to be addressed). For example, eMERGE investigators note that despite the "laudable goal" of having results of embedded ELSI research inform the implementation of the primary discovery and translational studies, "the pressure to start enrolling in the main study quickly meant that processes were largely in place" before the yearlong ELSI studies' results could be analyzed (Clayton et al. 2023, 1022). In many areas of research, there would need to be increased resources to lay the groundwork for the long-term community-engaged collaborations or organizational restructuring (or development) that addressing some ethical concerns often requires. Amid calls to develop an evidence base for assessing the success of community engagement (Lavery 2018), a project of the Navrongo Health Research Centre (a division of the Ghana Health Service) is cited as a success story (Tindana et al. 2007). The project began with "community entry," a process of entering the community and consulting with community leaders *before* initiating *any* research activity. Community leaders served as local consultants at every research stage. What was, in effect, a pilot project grew into the Ghana Community-Based Health Planning and Services Initiative with nation-wide scope (Nyonator et al. 2005). To implement such a slow-entry groundwork-laying approach in the United States, there would need to be increased recognition within academia of the importance of this community-engaged groundwork and collaboration (Bell and Lewis 2023; Shephard 2018).

Adopting longer time horizons for empirical bioethics research might have positive effects even beyond the value of being able to answer questions of ethical import about the longer-term impact of health interventions. If we accept that research results and papers will emerge more slowly, over a longer time frame, there may be benefits for the field of bioethics and its practitioners. Embracing a slower, less "productive" pace, and insights from *The Slow Professor: Challenging the Culture of Speed in the Academy*, might help to address the burnout made so evident and exacerbated by the pandemic (Berg and Seeber 2016). Sometimes writing shorter, narrowly focused commentaries creates lively intellectual discussion and quickly advances understanding; sometimes it primarily contributes to the churn. Each contributes something more that colleagues must read to stay on top of things and on top of their game.

As a corollary to avowing the value of longer time horizons in some of our research, the field of bioethics might take up some of the conversations happening in higher education about its corporatization, its emphasis on productivity, courses as commodities, learning as outcomes, learning outcomes as quality assurance, faculty members' research "output," and assessment, not of their research or scholarship, but of their "productivity." We should recognize that the acceptance of productivity as the norm—as a chief measure of worth and a descriptor of everyday (and academic) life—distracts bioethics from focusing on deeper, broader questions. We focus on the implications of emerging technologies, not the deeper implications of their emergence or the implications of failing to face the finitude of human life and our overtaxing the planet. In countless conversations, but seldom in print, ELSI scholars worry that ELSI research/scholarship is more apologist and handmaiden for the current preoccupation with genomics than a critic of it, with relatively rare exceptions (Tabery 2023). The concern is not new or restricted to ELSI of genetics/genomics; in the mid-1990s, there was worry that "bioethics may have lost its critical capacity . . . that bioethics has stopped asking the big questions, instead of debating whether a technology . . . should be used at all, we end up debating merely how it should be used," and how to ensure equitable access to it (Wolf 1996). Reducing the speed and volume of bioethics' output might encourage bioethics to refocus on the "bigger questions." There is value not just in doing some empirical research with a longer time horizon, but also in doing some of our normative analysis more slowly and with a longer view.

This space is not the place to explore more fully how the practices, approaches, and content of bioethics are affected by the business models of universities (or their being remodeled as businesses). But being able to take a longer view in research likely requires remonstrance against pressures to produce results within shorter funding periods or while the tenure clock is ticking (if bioethicists are fortunate enough to have the security and intellectual liberty afforded by tenure). Recognizing the value of conducting bioethics research on a longer time horizon would require adjustment of academia's metrics.

Of course, we need not completely reject using impact factors and citation counts to quantify impact in the short-term in order to also evaluate quality and impact less quantitatively with longer backward- and forward-looking horizons in view. By insisting on the rejection of that false dichotomy, we model the insight from feminist epistemology that we have been socialized to organize differences (e.g., quantitative/qualitative, focused/wide-ranging) in terms of hierarchies, basically hierarchies ranging from good to bad (Young 1990).

Feminist epistemology also helps us to recognize that bias, interests, and perspective-taking are endemic in the production and reception of knowledge, as well as the evaluation of knowledge claims and, in turn, bodies of research. Relying on the quantification of quality through impact factors in a marketplace of ideas may disguise, but does not avoid, the cronyism and bias to which qualitative assessments are susceptible. In different ways, different evaluation and reward structures obscure some bias and render other bias more transparent, but none eliminate it.

Employ Insights of Feminist Epistemology and Extoll the Virtue of Modesty

Knowledge Production: Participants Are Moral Equals, Their Claims Are Not Necessarily Equivalent

Feminist epistemology emphasizes that knowledge production is a social activity (e.g., Longino 1990). Specifically, it is an activity requiring critical interactions among people with different perspectives, interests, and skills of inquiry, who share a commitment to cooperating to develop better justified understandings. The outcomes of this process are more objective—and more worthy of being relied upon as true—the more they have been subjected to, and refined as a result of, criticism from different points of view (e.g., Longino 2001). Objectivity is not a characteristic or a stance; it is procedural. Objective results are the results of procedures of discovery and criticism in which biases, values, and interests are made explicit, while claims are assessed from all available points of view. Employing different methods of discovery and criticism, as well as bringing different theories to bear on evidence, is part of what it means to employ all points of view to make, assess, and refine knowledge claims.

Knowledge production is an ongoing process; knowledge is the outcome of that process at a point in time but is subject to ongoing examination, criticism, and revision. The history of the etiology of peptic ulcer is an instructive example, as Radomski, Šešelja, and Naumann (2021) note it "is characterized by a premature abandonment of the bacterial hypothesis, which subsequently had its comeback, leading to the discovery of Helicobacter pylori—the major cause of the disease" (1). The article by Radomski et al., recounting the shift in etiological explanation from bacteria to excess acid to bacteria, is also instructive because it demonstrates how new methods in doing history—namely, digital textual analysis—reveal a change in understanding of the cause of the change in etiological attribution (i.e., no longer attributing the initial shift from bacterial explanation to the publication of a flawed large-scale study). This demonstrates that both medical science and humanities or social science research experience evolution.

While participants in the process of knowledge production are equals, some of their initial claims will not emerge from the process of knowledge production as worthy pretenders to the status of knowledge. People are equals; however, their claims are not of equivalent epistemic value. While participants' points of view are putatively worthy of respect, when their points of view are constituted by adherence to knowledge claims that are subsequently refined or refuted, maintaining those points of view is not justified or worthy of respect as grounds for subsequent knowledge claims. The people who hold such points of view, however, remain moral equals and are worthy of respect at least insofar as they participate in the knowledge production process, that is, reasoned argument, civil discourse, and/or scientific inquiry. Those who lapse into bullying, manipulation, violence, or deception warrant censure for their pernicious impact on both people's well-being and the knowledge production process. Knowledge production—through empirical inquiry or through reasoned argument—is thus tied to democratic values and processes.

If it could help to rescue truth and knowledge from the clutches of (perhaps willful) misunderstanding of feminist epistemological insights, bioethics could make important contributions to discussions of—and attempts to address—pressing public health concerns. Exposing the interests that support declaring the death of objectivity and the equivalence of all opinions may have some persuasive effect, particularly if the declarants' unjustified claims are also tested by realities and others' truth claims about those realities. Further, bioethics should also consider the feelings fed and relied upon to employ the alleged death of objectivity in service of those interests.

The declaration of an era of mere opinion, and worse, of indisputably equivalent opinions does not just lead to "a corrosive cynicism about science" or corrode public regard for science and claims of truth (Anderson 2020). It "substitutes social validation for scientific validation: if *a lot of people are saying* it . . . then it is true enough" (Muirhead and Rosenblum 2019, 3). In trying to advocate the importance of employing the best science in the interest of public health, for example, bioethics would be well served to recognize that the rejection of science is not just a matter of rejecting reason, but of embracing a feeling and being embraced by affectively constituted communities.

Bioethicists, scientists, and public health experts should attend to—and perhaps create substitutes for—the feelings of identity, community, belongingness, and purpose that frequently accompany current rejections of science. Traditionally, only the experts enjoyed the affective benefits of community and identity associated with embracing science; the rest of us were just the "general public." By cocreating or embracing a group identity, individuals can gain standing and a sense of personal dignity that may otherwise seem to be ignored. "When it isn't acting as a violent outlet for the narcissism of the age, [identity politics] can serve as its antidote, binding people into imagined collectives capable of taking action to secure their interests and assert their personhood" (Yang 2018, 16). Yet because a sense of belonging, self-identity, and personal dignity are not mere interests among many, the value and pressures of group affiliation may lead some individuals to act contrary to their other interests, ignoring evidence and arguments pertinent to those interests, while instead giving priority to the interests served by their group affiliation.

Groups themselves, in a more or less organized manner, may promote their interests *qua* group at the expense of their members' interests. Employing processes of feminist epistemology, bioethics might expose the narcissism and self-interest of groups and especially group leaders and demonstrate how those interests are used to construct a worldview or "alternative facts" that neither hold up to scrutiny nor benefit group members' other interests (Lozada 2020). This is not so different from bioethics' familiar illumination of how patients and professionals, for example, bring not just different values and priorities, but also different understandings of the facts to medical decision-making (Brock 1993). The stakes may seem higher, however, and the emotional entrenchment in their worldviews may seem stronger than was the paternalistic worldview of doctors who knew best back in the 1970s. However, in comparison to those paternalistic physicians, people who are today rejecting science and facts may not actually be more deeply invested in their identity-constituting groups, beliefs, and feelings. Instead, it may be that their feelings, their reasons for being so invested, are simply more foreign to most bioethicists than were the feelings of investment in professional identity (and paternalism) of our physician colleagues. Or, if those denying science are more emotionally invested in maintaining their anti-science perspectives, it may be that in comparison to physicians who have multiple bases of self-respect (in the Rawlsian sense), members of these affectively constituted communities feel they are accorded less social regard.

Bioethics might also help communities and healthcare institutions craft alternatives to the affective benefits of being in, for example, an anti-vax community or other identity-forming communities not conducive to health. The Baltimore Community Health Workers who were the subject of artist LaToya Roby Frazier's award-winning installation, *More Than Conquerors: A Monument for Community Health Workers of Baltimore, Maryland 2021–2022*, seem to constitute such a science-embracing community and helped to expand that community through their Covid-19 vaccination campaign (Akers 2023). Or bioethicists might find ways to collaborate with existing groups—even identity groups—to learn what gaps or needs science and public health might fill: if guns are kept in nightstands, what alternate storage would serve the needs of accessibility at night and a feeling of near-to-hand security, while increasing accident prevention? Bioethicists might work with identity and interest groups to encourage their participation in public discussion, while demanding that they support their claims with data and arguments; feminist political theory calls upon "claimants to justify their demands before others who explicitly stand in different social locations" (Young 1990, 190). Further, bioethicists might exhort identity and interest groups to demonstrate that their interests are compatible with substantive conceptions of justice.

In addition, because individuals and groups living in a free society will subscribe to conflicting moral doctrines and worldviews, bioethicists might encourage (and ultimately demand) that interest and identity groups recognize and shape their doctrines or worldviews to be compatible with what Rawls refers to as "reasonable pluralism"—conflicting moral doctrines will be "reasonable" insofar as they "leave their adherents willing to cooperate with those with whom they have moral disagreements" (Ainslie 2002, 1; Rawls 1993, xvi–xviii). Bioethicists should be well-equipped to point out when those advocating particular positions are being "reasonable" or "unreasonable" in this particular Rawlsian sense that is critical to reasoned deliberation, democracy, and the pursuit of health and well-being within a pluralistic society.

Bioethicists should guide people and shape perspectives in the direction of reasonability. They might also label and explain why people or positions are unreasonable, in hopes that the desirability of cooperation may eventually come to the fore, particularly if those in disagreement also have some shared interests. Bioethicists might point out, for example, where the Heritage Foundation's *Mandate for Leadership: The Conservative Promise* (2023) reflects perspectives or interests that overlap with those holding differing political, ethical, or religious commitments, as well as where its claims are not backed by a substantial body of evidence, or its normative foundation seems dogmatic. Failing to acknowledge where there are slivers of similar perspective or partially shared goals leaves those in different camps with no common ground to cross to engage in rapprochement. Members of the 2023 US Congress who were unwilling to compromise and unwilling to cooperate with those with whom they shared some, but not all interests and objectives, may be considered unreasonable in this sense (at least insofar as they were acting on a worldview, and not being merely strategic).

Knowledge Production: The Scientific and Ethical Value of Openness to Correction

Preparing the public for the ongoingness of knowledge production, for the fact that it is always a work in progress, is a contribution bioethics might make. Embracing insights from feminist epistemology, bioethics should help make transparent the processes of science, particularly those in medicine, epidemiology, and the development of drugs and biologics. Most importantly, it should help explain the evolving nature of scientific understanding. Bioethics should encourage more modesty in the production and use of scientific knowledge. It has long encouraged clinicians to accept the limits of the best of their abilities and the state of the art. Similarly, bioethics may play a role in restoring modesty's status as a virtue among both scientists and the public receiving scientific knowledge claims. Recognizing that people don't merely receive knowledge like empty vessels, but actively construct what they know, bioethics can help the public accept the value of claims that are limited, qualified, and subject to revision.

Recent frustration with evolving understanding and constantly changing recommendations during the Covid-19 pandemic is more intense and perhaps materially consequential, but not different in kind from the exasperation people feel when trying to choose healthfully between butter and margarine, or to decide whether drinking coffee or taking an aspirin is good for them. Each of these changes is an opportunity for bioethics to explain not just that this is science at work. It should also elucidate why evolving understanding is both scientifically and ethically a good thing. In short, we obviously don't yet understand everything; we haven't yet solved all the world's problems. There is room for change in our best-to-date accounts of the world, its people, and its processes. We should hope that our understanding of the world is evolving. Such evolution is a good thing.

Of course, we hope that our understanding is evolving in the direction of truth, accurate accounts of the way things actually are. Science tests proposed explanations and often demonstrates that they are wrong. When scientists admit what they don't know or what they were previously wrong about, they exhibit the virtues of modesty and honesty. Evolution in scientific understanding reflects not only improved understanding, but also that those who were "right" yesterday deferred to—or at least were forced by the system of knowledge production to listen to—other knowledge producers (i.e., other scientists and research participants). Ongoing change not only evidences the possibility of epistemic and material improvement, but also affirms a fundamental ethical value: the equal moral worth of those participating in the knowledge-making enterprise.

It is thus critical for bioethics' elucidation of the evolving nature of knowledge to proceed respectfully in a way that demonstrates the equal moral worth of its interlocutors—here, science-disputing members of the public. Bioethicists should always ask "why" or "how do you know" of each other, scientists, and policymakers, not just science-disputing celebrities or members of the public. *Always* inquiring "why" or "how do you know" demonstrates equal respect. Showing our work and demanding that others do the same demonstrates the process of knowledge production, its norms of fairness, and its reliance on evidentiary standards.

At the same time, bioethics may appropriately question whether all information reported should be regarded with the imprimatur of even a temporary truth status. Reputable science reporting, like that of *The New York Times*, increasingly distinguishes correlation and causation, and notes when findings are preliminary, from a small study, or in need of replication. It has progressed substantially from the days of reporting the discovery of "the gene for ____," only to qualify the headline many inches or days later. Yet, it is noted that "even *The New York Times* may have inadvertently contributed to the initial [hydroxychloroquine] prescribing stampede by covering the science before it was peer-reviewed, even though they clearly stated the shortcomings of the research" (Kravitz 2020). Thus, bioethics might nevertheless question whether some results are ready for mainstream reporting at all, and whether universities and corporations benefit more from zealous media relations than the public benefits from breaking scientific news (Caulfield and Condit 2012). Bioethics could help create a climate of nuance and sympathetic skepticism, a wait-and-see attitude, rather than either enthusiastic embrace of each new finding or wholesale rejection of science as snake oil. Unfortunately, the public has been schooled to expect speed and certainty. Science and society are not well served by those expectations. This may be another reason for bioethicists to slow our rate of productivity and reject the constant "churn" of intellectual output, soundbites, and tweets: we can show our work, and by our mode of work, model virtues of multi-perspectival, long-term analysis.

Of course, when people are ill or afraid of catching a new virus, they want clear answers and ideally a quick fix. Having been sold on fast fashion, the desirability of immediate gratification, and products and procedures that erase marks of the passage of time, people cannot be blamed for wanting certainty and fast results in more important domains. Acknowledging not just the lack of certainty, but the length and arduousness of many roads to recovery, is necessary to respect people with honesty and to educate them and their neighbors about medicine and public health. It's also important to acknowledge when a cure will not fully restore, and recovery is likely not a return to the previous normal. Grandma may make it out of the hospital, but not make it home; or she may return home, but not live there as she did before.

The need for action in the present in the face of the possibility of progress (aka revision) means determining when evidence and understanding are good enough to act. It means recognizing that mistakes will be made and will be made in good faith. Part of acting in good faith involves adopting personal and epistemic modesty and admitting the fallibility of a field, its practices, and practitioners. Taking more time to generate and validate findings—perhaps not while advising the populace during a pandemic, but when implementing interventions like reporting polygenic risk scores—may help people contextualize and appropriately accept findings of both types. A better understanding of science—including how it interacts with social needs and values—may help people differentiate between early pronouncements during a public health emergency that are appropriately revised with flip-flopping speed and the evolutionary changes in understanding that are the mark of normal scientific progress.

Conclusion

It is my hope that these suggestions may help bioethics address challenges facing the field and the current climate in which we find ourselves. Paying more attention to the effect of feelings, including feelings of self-identity, may help us understand and influence medical decision-making and health-related behaviors. Taking a broader view of "health-related behaviors" may expand the purview of bioethical analysis in useful ways. Adopting a longer time horizon for some empirical bioethics research may enable it to answer questions about people's behaviors, responses, social interactions, and needs that are of substantial bioethical importance. It should be part of bioethics' agenda to encourage the development of funding sources and fundamental changes in reward structures to enable health-related research of all types to take a sufficiently long time horizon to address important questions, including complex questions implicating social structures and interconnected health-related factors.

It should also be part of bioethics' agenda to help prepare the public to accept evolving knowledge and to participate in the ongoing process of knowledge production. Doing so may require increased understanding of people's feelings, especially their feelings of belonging to communities that constitute an important part of their identities. This will be especially challenging, but especially important, when a constitutive part of such a community is its rejection of the processes of knowledge production. Yet we must try. Engaging in such empirical inquiries and reasoned arguments demonstrates a way of living. Here, living and reasoning well is not the best revenge. It provides an alternative that in the fullness of time may attract currently disaffected participants. Bioethics may provide resources to investigate and address sources of such disaffection.

Bibliography

Ainslie, Donald C. 2002. "Bioethics and the Problem of Pluralism." *Social Philosophy and Policy*, 19 (2): 1–28.

Akers, Torey. 2023. "Baltimore Museum of Art acquires LaToya Ruby Frazier Installation Honouring Community Healthcare Workers." *The Art Newspaper*, June 26, 2023. https://www.theartnewspaper.com/2023/06/26/latoya-ruby-frazier-community-healthcare-workers-installation-acquired-baltimore-museum-art.

Anderson, Elizabeth. 2020. "Feminist Epistemology and Philosophy of Science." In Edward N. Zalta (ed.), *The Stanford Encyclopedia of Philosophy*, Spring 2020 ed., .

https://plato.stanford.edu/archives/spr2020/entries/feminism-epistemology/ (accessed June 1, 2022).

Bell, Marissa, and Neil Lewis Jr. 2023. "Universities Claim to Value Community-engaged Scholarship: So Why Do They Discourage It?" *Public Understanding of Science*, 32 (3): 304–21.

Berg, Maggie, and Barbara Karolina Seeber. 2016. *The Slow Professor: Challenging the Culture of Speed in the Academy*. University of Toronto Press.

Brock, Dan W. 1993. "The Ideal of Shared Decision Making between Physicians and Patients." In *Life and Death : Philosophical Essays in Biomedical Ethics*. Cambridge University Press.

Caulfield, Timothy, and Celeste M. Condit. 2012. "Science and the Sources of Hype." *Community Genetics*, 15 (3/4): 209–17.

Clayton, Ellen Wright, Maureen E. Smith, Katherine C. Anderson, Wendy K. Chung, et al. 2023. "Studying the Impact of Translational Genomic Research: Lessons from eMERGE." *American Journal of Human Genetics*, 110 (7): 1021–33.

De La Vega, Francisco M., and Carlos D. Bustamante. 2018. "Polygenic Risk Scores: A Biased Prediction?" *Genome Medicine*, 10 (1): 100.

Gawande, Atul. 2014. *Being Mortal : Medicine and What Matters in the End*. Metropolitan Books.

Graham, Jesse, Brian A. Nosek, Jonathan Haidt, Ravi Iyer, Spassena Koleva, and Peter H Ditto. 2011. "Mapping the Moral Domain." *Journal of Personality and Social Psychology*, 101 (2): 366–85.

Gray, Stacy W., Yolanda Martins, Lindsay Z. Feuerman, et al. 2014. "Social and Behavioral Research in Genomic Sequencing: Approaches from the Clinical Sequencing Exploratory Research Consortium Outcomes and Measures Working Group." *Genetics in Medicine*, 16 (10): 727–35.

Grubs Robin E., Lisa S. Parker, and Rebekkah J. Hamilton. 2014. "Subtle Psychosocial Sequelae of Genetic Test Results." *Current Genetic Medicine Reports*, 2: 242–9.

Hamilton, Rebekah, and Karen E. Hurley. 2010. "Conditions and Consequences of a BRCA Mutation in Young, Single Women of Childbearing Age." *Oncology Nursing Forum*, 37 (5): 627–34.

The Heritage Foundation. 2023. *Project* 2025: Mandate *for Leadership: The Conservative Promise*. https://s3.documentcloud.org/documents/24088042/project-2025s-mandate-for-leadership-the-conservative-promise.pdf.

Kravitz, Richard L. 2020. "When Trump Pushed Hydroxychloroquine to Treat COVID-19, Hundreds of Thousands of Prescriptions Followed Despite Little Evidence That It Worked." *The Conversation*, July 9, 2020. https://theconversation.com/when-trump-pushed-hydroxychloroquine-to-treat-covid-19-hundreds-of-thousands-of-prescriptions-followed-despite-little-evidence-that-it-worked-140156.

Lavery, James V. 2018. "Building an Evidence Base for Stakeholder Engagement." *Science (American Association for the Advancement of Science)*, 361 (6402): 554–56.

Liu, Michael, Theodore L. Caputi, Mark Dredze, Aaron S. Kesselheim, and John W. Ayers. 2020. "Internet Searches for Unproven COVID-19 Therapies in the United States." *JAMA Internal Medicine*, 180 (8): 1116–18.

Longino, Helen. 1990. *Science as Social Knowledge*. Princeton University Press.

Longino, Helen. 2001. *The Fate of Knowledge*. Princeton University Press.

Lozada, Carlos. 2020. *What Were We Thinking: A Brief Intellectual History of the Trump Era*. Simon & Schuster.
Marya, Rupa, and Raj Patel. 2021. *Inflamed: Deep Medicine and the Anatomy of Injustice*. Farrar, Straus and Giroux.
McCall, Maura K., Mary Connolly, Bethany Nugent, Yvette P. Conley, Catherine M. Bender, and Margaret Q. Rosenzweig. 2019. "Symptom Experience, Management, and Outcomes According to Race and Social Determinants Including Genomics, Epigenomics, and Metabolomics (SEMOARS + GEM): An Explanatory Model for Breast Cancer Treatment Disparity." *Journal of Cancer Education*, 35 (3): 428–40.
Métraux, Julia. 2024. "Meet the Influencer Who 'Reverses' Lupus—With Smoothies." *Mother Jones*, March 26, 2024. https://www.motherjones.com/food/2024/03/brooke-goldner-goodbye-lupus-smoothies-social-media-influencer/.
Metzl, Jonathan. 2019. *Dying of Whiteness: How the Politics of Racial Resentment Is Killing America's Heartland*. Basic Books.
Milazzo, Stefania, and Markus Horneber. 2015. "Laetrile Treatment for Cancer." *Cochrane Database of Systematic Reviews*, 2015 (4): CD005476.
Muirhead, Russell, and Nancy L. Rosenblum. 2019. *A Lot of People Are Saying: The New Conspiracism and the Assault on Democracy*. Princeton University Press.
Nyonator, Frank K., J. Koku Awoonor-Williams, James F. Phillips, Tanya C. Jones, and Robert A. Miller. 2005. "The Ghana Community-based Health Planning and Services Initiative for Scaling Up Service Delivery Innovation." *Health Policy and Planning*, 20 (1): 25–34.
Oxford English Dictionary. 2023. "Post-truth (adj.), sense 2," July 2023.
Parker, Lisa S. 2007. "Bioethics as Activism." In Lisa A. Eckenwiler and Felicia Cohn (eds.), *The Ethics of Bioethics: Mapping the Moral Landscape*, 144–60. Johns Hopkins University Press.
Parker, Lisa S., Pamela L. Sankar, Joy Boyer, J. D. Jean McEwen, and David Kaufman. 2019. "Normative and Conceptual ELSI Research: What It Is, and Why It's Important." *Genetics in Medicine*, 21 (2): 505–9.
Radomski, Bartosz Michał, Dunja Šešelja, and Kim Naumann. 2021. "Rethinking the History of Peptic Ulcer Disease and Its Relevance for Network Epistemology." *History and Philosophy of the Life Sciences*, 43 (4): Article 113.
Rawls, John. 1993. *Political Liberalism*. Columbia University Press.
Reardon, Jenny. 2017. *The Postgenomic Condition: Ethics, Justice, and Knowledge after the Genome*. University of Chicago Press.
Roberts, J. Scott. 2019. "Assessing the Psychological Impact of Genetic Susceptibility Testing." *The Hastings Center Report*, 49 (S1): S38–43.
Sabatello, Maya, and Eric Juengst. 2019. "Genomic Essentialism: Its Provenance and Trajectory as an Anticipatory Ethical Concern." *Hastings Center Report*, 49 (S1): S10–18.
Sandel Michael J. 2007. T*he Case Against Perfection: Ethics in the Age of Genetic Engineering*. Harvard University Press.
Shephard, Kerry, Kim Brown, Tess Guiney, and Lynley Deaker. 2018. "Valuing and Evaluating Community-engaged Scholarship." *Tertiary Education and Management*, 24: 83–94.
Tabery, James. 2023. *Tyranny of the Gene: Personalized Medicine and Its Threat to Public Health*. Knopf Doubleday Publishing Group.

Tindana, Paulina Onvomaha, Jerome A. Singh, C. Shawn Tracy, et al. 2007. "Grand Challenges in Global Health: Community Engagement in Research in Developing Countries." *PLOS Medicine*, 4 (9): e273.
Tronto, Joan C. 1993. *Moral Boundaries: A Political Argument for an Ethic of Care*. Routledge.
Vaduganathan, Muthiah, Jeroen van Meijgaard, Mandeep R. Mehra, Jacob Joseph, Christopher J. O'Donnell, and Haider J. Warraich. 2020. "Prescription Fill Patterns for Commonly Used Drugs During the COVID-19 Pandemic in the United States." *JAMA : The Journal of the American Medical Association*, 323 (24): 2524–6.
Williams, David R., Selina A. Mohammed, Jacinta Leavell, and Chiquita Collins. 2010. "Race, Socioeconomic Status, and Health: Complexities, Ongoing Challenges, and Research Opportunities." *Annals of the New York Academy of Sciences*, 1186 (1): 69–101.
Wolf, Susan M. 1996. "Introduction: Gender and Feminism in Bioethics." In Susan M. Wolf (ed.), *Feminism & Bioethics: Beyond Reproduction*. Oxford University Press.
Yang, Wesley. 2018. *The Souls of Yellow Folk: Essays*. W.W. Norton & Company.
Young, Iris Marion. 1990. *Justice and the Politics of Difference*. Princeton University Press.
Zoltick, Emilie S., Michael D. Linderman, Molly A. McGinniss, et al. for the PeopleSeq Consortium. 2019. "Predispositional Genome Sequencing in Healthy Adults: Design, Participant Characteristics, and Early Outcomes of the PeopleSeq Consortium." *Genome Medicine*, 11: 10.

2

The Wary Relationship between Bioethics and Public Engagement

Gregory E. Kaebnick

In a 2023 essay in the *Hastings Center Report*, the journal I've edited for probably too long, political philosopher Andrew Schroeder issued a stark and surprising challenge to the field of bioethics. He canvassed a range of bioethical and other scholarly opinions on appropriate government policy about whether to impose lockdowns—by which he meant "significant restrictions on people's rights to move about and interact"—during the Covid-19 pandemic. Developing those policy prescriptions required, he noted, identifying which costs and benefits should be weighed and then assigning weights to them. Bioethicists had much to say during the height of the pandemic about the costs and benefits and the appropriate policy conclusions to draw from them. Their arguments were the kind of normative analysis that is the bread and butter of bioethics. But Schroeder waved it all aside: "this sort of reasoning is not suitable to directly guide policy-making in a liberal democracy. In a democracy, policy should be responsive to the public's values and preferences" (Schroeder 2023). The bioethicists' work was "full of insightful and compelling ethical arguments," but useless, insofar as influence on policy is the goal, except as a resource that members of the public could draw on to reach their own opinions (Schroeder 2023).

The problem of how bioethics relates to policy and to the public's values is one I've come up against personally, as probably many in bioethics have. Once, in a debate about using genome editing to modify populations of wild animals, I was challenged by the moderator, the science populist Neil deGrasse Tyson, to say whether I thought a moral philosopher's opinion about science policy should count for more than anybody else's. I denied that I had any special insight into moral truth. I should have pointed out that my concern was exactly the opposite of what he feared: far from trying to squelch public views, I was trying to ensure respectful consideration of them. My anecdotal impression is that many people find the prospect of genome editing of wild animals intrinsically but inchoately morally troubling, and that most scientists and moral philosophers dismiss that concern as irrational mysticism and conservatism. Should we modify malaria-transmitting mosquitoes in ways that drive them into extinction? As many as 500,000 lives could be saved each year (if the technology allowed it, which it does not yet do), and the ecological and public health harms of the modified mosquitoes seem likely to be low, maybe nonexistent. For many bioethicists I've talked to, deliberate extinction via genome editing of Anopheline mosquitoes is nearly a slam dunk. But most nonbioethicists seem to quaver at the prospect, and I tend to think that they should at least be heard.

A large literature now argues that the solution to what is often called the "alignment" problem—the problem of how to ensure that public policy is responsive to the public's values—is a deliberative public engagement exercise in which the public, or a representative slice of it, can learn about a policy problem, think about the values questions at stake in it, and work toward recommendations for the appropriate policy response to it. The result is what the Organisation for Economic Cooperation and Development calls a "deliberative wave" (OECD 2020). Arguments in favor of public engagement have been particularly persuasive on a range of science policy topics that overlap with bioethics: environmental policy-making (National Research Council 2008), nanotechnology (Alexander 2006), and synthetic biology (Presidential Commission for the Study of Bioethical Issues 2010). More recently, public engagement has been endorsed in prominent policy reports on genome engineering (NASEM 2016; NASEM 2017). These reports have brought arguments for public engagement into closer contact with bioethics, but bioethics mostly still treats the idea of public engagement only occasionally and rather skeptically. Political philosophy and science and technology studies have been at the forefront of the movement.

To be sure, bioethics is beginning to think about public engagement. A recent Hastings Center special report, of which I was a coeditor, addressed questions about how public engagement can help guide policy on genome engineering of wild populations of nonhuman organisms (Gusmano et al. 2021). Another used a public engagement process as part of normative analysis of the acceptability of scientific research in behavioral genetics (Martschenko et al. 2023). Another examined the connections between deliberative public engagement processes and the civic virtues and skills necessary for democracy (Kaebnick et al. 2021). In the main body of the *Hastings Center Report*—outside the supplements where appear special reports, which are usually products of Hastings Center research projects—the only discussion of public engagement I can remember is a set of five essays published in 2012 (Blacksher et al. 2012; Solomon et al. 2012; O'Doherty et al. 2012; Goold 2012; Abelson et al. 2012). But my impression is that most people in bioethics share the skeptical assessment expressed by John Conley and others in a 2023 article in the *American Journal of Bioethics*. Conley et al. (2023) charge that some of the expert groups calling for public engagement about human genome editing have failed to live up to their own ideals and have relied on expert-driven processes to generate their recommendations. Moreover, they note, "the evidence for what real-world [public engagement] can accomplish is uncertain" (14).

Conley and colleagues' charge strikes me as unfair. It seems like chastising a doctor for not involving a patient in a decision to seek the patient's consent to try a new intervention that the doctor has developed. It's plain that the patient's consent is needed for the intervention, but does a commitment to patient engagement (let's call it) also mean that the patient's involvement was needed in the decision to propose the intervention and seek the patient's consent? A more reasonable rejoinder would be that the patient could have been involved in the upstream decision of whether to develop the experimental surgery. Maybe so. Certainly, public engagement in upstream decisions about technology development would be desirable. But the need for public engagement and the best strategies for obtaining it have only recently been recognized and are still being debated, and we must start somewhere.

Probably more importantly, as I shall argue, Conley et al. also assume a particular and limited account of why public engagement is needed and what it can accomplish. Nonetheless, they raise important questions about the use of public engagement, the relationship of bioethics to public engagement, and the role of bioethics in policy-making. I will suggest here—though only tentatively—that, given a sophisticated account of public engagement, bioethics can be understood both as part of public engagement and as a corrective to public engagement.

Public Policy and the Public's Values

The argument for deliberative public engagement rests on a suite of claims. One component is an instrumental claim that deliberative public engagement will lead to better policy decisions (Grogan and Gusmano 2007). Experts may end up better informed about the issues at stake in a decision, and informing the public about an issue and asking for input can lead to better public understanding of the issue and better public acceptance of the decision. Additionally, deliberative public engagement cultivates trust between the public and the scientific community (Dietz 2013) and between the public and political leaders (Boulianne 2019). It might foster a sense of political solidarity (Jennings et al. 2021). Simply having an opportunity to learn about an issue, formulate one's thoughts about it, listen respectfully to others, engage in thoughtful discussion, and perhaps refine one's position in light of that discussion can help develop one of the fundamental skills of a democracy, namely, a capacity to live together with people with whom we strenuously disagree (O'Doherty and Burgess 2013). At bottom, however, is the argument invoked by Schroeder that deliberative public engagement is frequently necessary for democratic legitimacy. It's a basic premise of democratic government that people should have a say in the policies that govern their lives. The National Research Council echoed this view in 2008: "public participation is intrinsic to democratic governance" (National Research Council 2008). Mechanisms such as aggregative voting do not always suffice to ensure adequate public participation; deliberative public engagement helps address its problems by creating a mode for participation that is more focused and thoughtful. The 2018 referendum in Ireland to expand abortion rights is a case study: the referendum built on legislative initiatives that themselves were informed by a deliberative public engagement process that created a space in which a difficult political issue could be hashed out thoughtfully, in a way that both reflected and guided the overall public's views (McKay 2019).

Given this suite of considerations, at least one element of Conley and colleagues' critique of public engagement seems to miss the point. Conley et al. (2023) note that the public engagement events that have occurred on human genome editing have issued results that are "strikingly similar" (13) to those of expert bodies, seemingly with the implication that they are adding nothing. But this misunderstands the argument for public engagement. If the argument is based on the claim that public engagement provides democratic legitimacy, then the lack of a difference between the findings of an expert group and a public engagement event is not a strike against it. And beyond legitimacy, engagement might help the public learn about an issue, become engaged with policy-making, and learn to deliberate about them better, all of which might be a good thing for a country that wants to remain a democracy (Kaebnick et al. 2021). After the public has learned about the issue, we might expect the public's views to align with experts' views much of the time, but the alignment doesn't undermine the case for giving the public a say.

To these general considerations might be added that some policy issues are less likely than others to be addressed through normal democratic processes, so that public engagement brings democratic processes and legitimacy that might otherwise be missing. Some policy issues, such as genome editing, aspects of neuroscience, and many other science policy issues, seem especially in need of the learning, listening, and discussing that are the hallmarks of deliberative public engagement. These policy issues are characterized by novelty, uncertainty about outcomes, conceptual vagueness and misunderstanding, moral ambiguity, disagreement, and (in the minds of at least some people) high moral stakes. (Among the questions that need pondering: What is "nature"? What does it mean to talk about human intervention as "preserving" nature? How do genetic interventions compare to other kinds of interventions?)

Without deliberative public engagement, such issues may not receive adequate attention from political leaders, and they also may not receive adequate attention from the public. Many such topics receive comparatively little attention in the media or in conventional political debates. Only a small and quite unrepresentative slice of the wider public is reasonably well informed about genome editing, and perhaps no one is likely to make voting decisions on the basis of their views about it. As a result, the issue is swamped by other political topics and inevitably, and probably quite appropriately, receives almost no political attention. To the extent that the relevant policy decisions do receive attention, they are likely to be influenced by a small group that may well have vested interests in them or may be ideologically dead set against them. Both groups seem likely to be privileged classes and not representative of the overall public (Gusmano 2021). Deliberative public engagement is meant to ensure better representation of the public and better public thinking, as compared to public comment periods or referenda; in theory, it offers the chance to find out what the public thinks *when the public is really thinking*, as the political philosopher and deliberative democracy theorist James Fishkin (2020) puts it.

What mechanisms there are for public participation in policy decisions about many issues seem inadequate as well. For genome modification, by and large, the relevant policy decisions end up getting made mostly at the federal level, and within federal agencies rather than on the political stage. They take the form of regulatory actions that, under the Administrative Procedures Act, must in certain cases be published in the *Federal Register* and remain unsettled while the public has a chance to offer comments on them. But this form of public engagement is very limited. For example, not all instances of creating and releasing genetically modified organisms into the shared environment would even trigger this process, given technical details of the proposals (Kuzma 2021). Nor, for those that do, does a public comment period offer a chance for deliberative public engagement. There is no chance for true deliberation, very few people will ever participate in it, and the views they express may not even count for the agency making the decision. As Jennifer Kuzma has pointed out, organisms that have been genetically modified in ways that might help limit the spread of disease would be regulated by the Food and Drug Administration, but the criteria that the FDA would bring to its decision pertain only to safety for the animal and the efficacy of the drug. "If public comments during rulemaking pertain to general public health or the ecological safety of [the organism], technically, the agency need not consider these comments. It also does not have to consider any ethical concerns or socioeconomic or cultural impacts" (Kuzma 2021, S29).

Yet "ethical concerns or socioeconomic or cultural impacts" might be exactly what most people are most exercised about in the kinds of examples Kuzma is discussing. In the prospect of extirpating a species via genetic modifications (by spreading a trait through a population that forces a severe imbalance in the sex ratio, for example), the core issues at stake may turn on ideals people hold about the human relationship to nature. Perhaps, too, they have unexpressed and admittedly perplexing views about the moral significance within nature of species—a sense that a species is more important than the individuals that make it up, notwithstanding the fact that the species is only a set of some sort and is incapable of having the sensations, thoughts, and feelings that individuals may have. Or perhaps they feel that some kinds of species count for more than others, for reasons that need examining. Or perhaps they believe that eliminating a species would involve risks and uncertainties, and they feel (contrary to standard thinking in behavioral economics) that risk is inherently worse than predictability and uncertainty inherently worse than mere risk, so that one policy option may seem worse to them than another even if a mathematical comparison of the outcomes would favor a different policy choice (Oliver 2018). Part of what's attractive to some people about public engagement is that it might bring these kinds of moral beliefs, which are frequently excluded from policy-making, back into it. Through deliberative public engagement, these beliefs could be expressed and debated and, if they win enough adherents, help guide policy decisions.

Problems for Public Engagement in Bioethics

Nonetheless, there are many problems to be worked through to decide how to use deliberative public engagement on bioethical policy issues. Some of these are logistical problems that turn on the feasibility of deliberative public engagement, but they lead into abstract questions about the desirability of deliberative public engagement. Here, I'll sort these problems into two broad categories. The first is a set of problems that have to do with the broader issue of deciding when deliberative public engagement is warranted. The second is a set of problems that have to do with how deliberative public engagement should be done.

When is deliberative public engagement needed? First, and most prosaically, there's a problem of administrative efficiency. In 2016, a National Academies report on gene drives (a kind of genetic modification that can be passed from generation to generation in a way that could lead to modification of an entire population of wild organisms as a result of releasing just a few modified individuals) argued that gene drives warrant engagement with publics at three levels: in the community where a drive would initially be released, among larger groups of stakeholders who have immediate interests in the release, and, finally, more widely (National Academies, 2016). (I was a member of the committee that issued this report.) As a matter of justice, it seems that local publics should have a special opportunity to shape, and maybe reject, an experimental genetic modification of the shared environment. Stakeholders outside the community might have well-formed perspectives that should be aired. And since gene drives may be capable of spreading widely, people well removed from the site of release, otherwise uninformed about the intervention, seem to have a right to be involved as well. Moreover, even people who have no tangible stake in a proposal to edit a species—who may not be personally harmed or benefited by it—may nonetheless have a deep interest in it. (People in temperate places seem to care about polar bears, for example.) Yet engagement with these different publics might require multiple processes: imagine something like town hall meetings for the community, workshops for stakeholders, and other events for wider publics. Possibly, these events should be iterative (to allow different opinions to come forth, for example), and very likely, different events would be needed at different points in the development of the proposal (from upstream decisions about what to work on through downstream decisions about implementation and risk management). Events like these, crafted to engage a "minipublic"—a small sample of a larger public—take many forms: stakeholder workshops, citizen juries, citizen assemblies, and deliberative polls are a few of these forms. Given their variety, there are no standard protocols for running them, and each must be set up and funded de novo. Doing so takes tons of money and time. Calling for public engagement can begin to look like a way of simply stopping it in its tracks rather than bringing thoughtful public attention to it.

It might be helpful, then, to try to sort out questions that especially need public deliberation from those for which the case for public deliberation seems to be weaker. For example, if the argument in favor of public deliberation depends partly on the novelty, uncertainty, moral ambiguity, and disagreement surrounding a topic, then the argument for deliberation seems to be weaker as proposals become familiar, better understood, and less controversial. Perhaps it's only the first releases of gene drives, for example, that really require public engagement. Similarly, if conventional governance mechanisms are created to allow the public to learn about, discuss, and influence policy proposals, then the need for minipublic events seems less. There are no clear lines, however, about what is warranted when. Gene drive proposals could come in many different forms, involving different organisms, different technical specifications, different ecosystems, different publics, and different goals; arguably, each proposal will involve a high level of novelty for a long time. A proposal to alter mosquitoes in Africa in pursuit of a very important public health goal is not the same as a decision to suppress invasive rats on a Pacific Ocean island in order to save seabirds, and a proposal to eradicate screwworm in order to prevent the economic loss and animal suffering that screwworm infestation causes in livestock is yet another thing. And that's just gene drive proposals. There are many other kinds of proposals for genetically modifying nonhuman organisms, as well as many kinds of proposals for genetically modifying human beings.

This leads to a slightly different question about how questions are framed. The problem isn't just identifying which are novel; it's also sorting them in ways that organize the public engagement appropriately. For genetically modified nonhuman organisms, most commentary holds that the need for public engagement is generated by a specific case: public engagement should focus on the local public or the immediate stakeholders affected by that release, should address the facts of the given case, and occur if and as proposals are put forward by scientists and funders. But these characteristics also mean that public engagement will tend to prioritize local interests in a way that makes wider public policy deferential to local decisions, maybe inappropriately so. In fact, wider policy-making could get stuck: generalization from a few particular cases may not lead to wider policy. And control over wider policy could be de facto conceded to scientists, if it's scientists who decide which technologies to develop and which cases to attempt. The effect will be, as Ben Hurlbut puts it in a different context, that science proposes and society merely reacts (Hurlbut 2015).

This question about framing could arise in somewhat different ways for different policy topics. For deciding about lockdowns in a pandemic, for example, very similar questions arise about whether policy should be decided first at the local level or first at the broader level, and whether a decision is tied to the particular fact picture that is deliberated upon. For many other health policy topics—what should health insurance cover, what health needs warrant research, or how should an affected public be able to shape medical research—the questions will take yet different forms.

Connected to these questions about the implications for wider policy is a final problem about the reach of public engagement's influence over policy. Some policy issues turn on moral issues that are not supposed to be up for debate at all in a liberal democracy. Schroeder holds that a blatantly racist or sexist policy proposal should be off the table from the start and therefore not be put to deliberative public engagement. Lockdowns, he notes, also "implicate other values foundational to democracy, such as the rights to assemble, to vote, and to protest the government." Conversations I've had with scientists about public engagement and the need to align their work with public values suggest that many scientists are very wary about their liberty; they don't want the public weighing in too closely on their research. This is a flip side to one of the things that's attractive about public engagement: by allowing for a richer set of values to come into play in policy-making, it also opens up the possibility that policy could end up based on moral values often thought to be inappropriate for policy-making in a liberal democracy.

How should deliberative public engagement be done? The questions above emerge from work in bioethics. The core question is simply how a given issue that bioethicists have been working on could be appropriately taken to the public. Another trenchant set of questions emerges from work in political theory and in science and technology studies and examines the design of deliberative public engagement events. Some of these questions may call for no more than design changes. Others amount to a serious critique of the current understanding of public engagement. The literature is enormous and complex, and I will merely highlight a few considerations.

First, to allow for meaningful deliberation, discussion must be structured in a way that gives all participants a chance to listen and to be heard. That can be hard to do not just because some people will tend to dominate, some speakers will be boring, and so on, but also because the structure of discourse could be at odds with the goal of equal participation. A discussion hosted in an academic setting may be intimidating, even oppressive, to some participants (Taitingfong and Ullah 2021). An even more fundamental question is whether discussion should forefront academic modes of discourse—unbiased presentation of evidence followed by logical argument. That mode looks to some like the sine qua non of good deliberation (Gutmann and Thompson 1996), but others have argued that it tends to exclude some groups (Young 2001; Davies 2014). It's also worth asking whether, at least on some topics, it would tend to exclude some perspectives. Ideals about the human relationship to nature, for example, can be hard to express and are sometimes seen as emotional or mystical compared to the good, hard logic of utilitarianism.

A related structural design problem has to do with how the public is represented. Some perspectives may dominate deliberation because they belong to dominant demographic groups, and there is a divide among theorists of deliberative public engagement about how to respond to that fact. Some think that a minipublic should strive to be representative of the demographics of the larger public (Fishkin 2018), and others that a minipublic should be weighted toward marginalized groups (Burgess and Tansey 2009).

Finally, many theorists of deliberative democracy now question whether minipublic processes are inherently undemocratic, however they are run. Minipublics may be too small in scale, episodic, cloistered, and controlled to make for genuine deliberative democracy (Curato, Vrudagh, and Bächtiger 2020). The participant pool is just a slice of a larger public, meets briefly, and its discourse is structured in a way that differentiates it from whatever is going on in the larger public (Lafont 2019). As a result, these critics charge, minipublics tend to be conservative in their recommendations, echoing recommendations issued by the experts that tend to control them. (This highlights a sense in which the "striking similarity" that Conley et al. find between the conclusions of public engagement exercises and those of expert groups might be a genuine problem for minipublics—though since it stems from the fact that minipublics are controlled by experts, it's a problem for the expert groups, too. Both, apparently, are conservative.)

Ultimately, these theorists argue, deliberative democracy must be located in the larger society, chaotic and frustrating as that can be. Minipublics may be a tool that contributes to a larger deliberative system—alongside many other social institutions, from legislative bodies to courts to many kinds of nongovernmental bodies; they cannot discharge democratic deliberation by themselves.

None of these issues have been addressed or even much recognized in bioethics, but if bioethics aims at social change, then it must have some relationship to public engagement, and these issues deserve some attention.

A Theory of Bioethics

What does bioethics aim at, and what is its relationship to public engagement? Thinking about the mission of bioethics in terms of its relationship to public engagement gives an opportunity to develop an ideal theory of bioethics in a different way than bioethicists usually do—not a theory about the structure of good moral thinking, but one about its role in public deliberation.

Conley et al. and Schroeder seem to assume that bioethics and public engagement approaches are in competition, each laying claim to be the best way to align policy-making with public values. If so, it would be a strange mistake for an expert group to call for public engagement but fail to do it, as Conley et al. charge. It would be wrongheaded for experts to continue to offer their own recommendations, as Schroeder charges. And there might be cause to ponder the usefulness of public engagement events if the conclusions they reach are "strikingly similar" to those of expert groups, as Conley et al. argue.

But Conley et al. consider only the minipublic approach to public engagement. If public deliberation is understood on the systemic model, there is room for—and need for—many actors on the stage, and both minipublics and bioethics might have multiple roles to play. Theorists of public deliberation who have criticized minipublics have argued that they might yet serve a function if they are understood as part of a deliberative system. Instead of attempting to replace the wider public's deliberation, minipublics might be useful as tools for encouraging wider deliberation: for challenging the public's thinking, for example, or helping to push it in new directions or highlighting issues that the larger public is ignoring (Lafont 2019).

Sometimes, too, perhaps they can still appropriately serve to model or sample the thinking of the public, or of a particular slice of the public, and produce recommendations that lead directly to policy rather than serving merely as input for deliberation by the wider public. That seems to be roughly the purpose of an advisory board in community-engaged research, for example. It might be that some kinds of issues, such as decisions about the direction of public health research undertaken by an academic institution, are not well decided through the wider processes of an overall deliberative system. The focused attention that can be given to them by an advisory group might be more effective and efficient.

In a deliberative system, bioethics—the field collectively and individuals and groups that incorporate bioethicists—is among the many actors on the stage, and perhaps it, too, can serve these two functions. To some extent, bioethics attempts to defend the public's values. That's the point of attempting to develop sets of moral principles and theories that model "common morality" and can guide moral thinking, isn't it? That's surely the point of putting ethicists on National Academies or National Institutes of Health committees that offer advice about the conduct of science. So understood, bioethics tries to help solve the alignment problem directly. As with minipublics, the argument for this use of bioethics would be that some kinds of issues are better decided through these mechanisms or that these mechanisms are useful for bringing issues and ways of framing them to wider public attention.

But bioethics can also take on the task of arguing with the public's values, offering challenges and correctives to them. In thinking about lockdowns or other policy proposals that raise questions of social justice, for example, bioethics might take the role of defending a position that the public widely rejects, in the process attempting to bring the public along. In thinking about science policy, bioethics might challenge widely held assumptions about the implications of a new scientific endeavor.

Bioethics doing work along the first of these lines is often carrying out what Daniel Callahan once called its "regulatory mode," which focuses on finding solutions, looking for compromises and common ground, and generally keeping the railroad running (Callahan 1993). Callahan contrasted regulatory bioethics to what he called its "prophetic mode," in which bioethics is an outsider and critic, raising complaints about business as usual rather than helping it along. The categories are surely not sharp; a bioethics project set up to consider human subjects research might be designed to ensure that research goes forward, which looks like a regulatory goal, yet at the same time calls for significant changes, which looks like prophetic work. Nonetheless, it's plausible to think of bioethics as aiming both to support and to criticize medicine, the medical research establishment, fundamental biological sciences, and so on.

A further question about Callahan's account is about where prophetic bioethics directs its complaints. In Callahan's view, the complaints should be against the medical and scientific establishment, on behalf of the people. We might, however, instead think of prophetic bioethics as complaining wherever complaints seem warranted. Sometimes, medical and scientific authorities certainly are deserving targets, but good prophets must also be ready to challenge the public itself when the need arises. Dan called out medical research for focusing too much on expensive life-saving therapies instead of public health investments that would provide both greater benefits and more equitable benefits. He also thought that the scientific research establishment was wrong to reject some of the public's values, such as the idea that a human life can eventually come to a natural and acceptable end. Such complaints strike me as well worth making. At the same time, the public's views about medical research need not be automatically accepted and defended. The public might, for example, have fears, misapprehensions, biases, and assumptions that need correcting. There is a needed space here for what is called "normative, analytic" bioethics—investigating, say, the implications for research on neural organoids of widely accepted views about the moral status of human beings, or the implications for public health policy of the core liberal commitments to equality and liberty, or the implications for genetic science of the idea of nature.

The result is that bioethics' relationship to public engagement is at least twofold, at least if deliberative public engagement is understood on the systemic model. In some measure, bioethics might contribute directly to public engagement. If public engagement occurs at multiple levels and with many different kinds of publics, then bioethics can be one of the levels—and bioethicists themselves members of the public. And sometimes, too, bioethics will be playing along harmoniously—helping to keep everything running and acting as a kind of arm of other, larger publics. But sometimes, the particular contribution that bioethics makes can take an examining, investigating, even combative role—testing the public's moral beliefs, arguing against them on occasion.

For whom are bioethicists writing if it is participating in public engagement in this complicated way? Schroeder suggests that the only real audience for bioethics is the public, since in his view, it is the public that should control policy on the matters that bioethicists discuss. The measure of success for bioethics is then, for Schroeder, the ability to persuade the public. I wonder if the question of audience isn't more complicated, though. On occasion, surely, it is helpful for bioethics to be directed at other elements of the larger public, which requires that it be comprehensible to those audiences and that it be accompanied by mechanisms to disseminate it to them. Bioethics writing that fits relatively neatly into the regulatory mode—advancing policy suggestions for scientific research or informed consent procedures in the hospital, say—would ideally reach people who are outside bioethics but can use that work. Sometimes, though, when bioethics is examining, investigating, and testing, perhaps it can be thought of as a kind of "test bed" for ideas, and the relevant audience is bioethics itself. Perhaps a piece of scholarship sometimes makes a valuable contribution to the overall development of ideas by carrying out a sidebar discussion that only later, if the ideas survive testing, filters out into the larger deliberative system. An academic conference or journal can be understood as a kind of subsystem that feeds ultimately into the larger system but also whirls along on its own to some extent. Scholars arguing with scholars might foment some creativity that ultimately leads to more productive thinking.

In this vision of how bioethics and minipublic-based public engagement contribute to the overall deliberative democracy, they would stand both in ongoing tension with each other and in mutual support of each other. Since bioethics is based in academe, its claims to provide anything like democratic legitimacy must always be problematic. A field of scholarship that claims to know the public's values better than the public does always needs to be tested by the public. But as scholars dedicated to conceptual clarity, argument form, and consistency, bioethicists can help push public thinking forward. But the details of the relationship between bioethics and public engagement are themselves a topic for bioethics to take up.

Bibliography

Abelson, Julia, Mark E. Warren, and Pierre-Gerlier Forest. 2012. "The Future of Public Deliberation on Health Issues." *Hastings Center Report*, 42 (2): 27–9.

Alexander, Cate. 2006. "Public Participation in Nanotechnology: Report of the National Nanotechnology Initiative Workshop." National Nanotechnology Coordination Office.

Blacksher, Erika, Alice Diebel, Pierre-Gerlier Forest, Susan Dorr Goold, and Julia Abelson. 2012. "What Is Public Deliberation?" *Hastings Center Report* 42(2): 14–17.

Boulianne, Shelley. 2019. "Building Faith in Democracy: Deliberative Events, Trust, and Efficacy." *Political Studies*, 67 (1): 4–30.

Burgess, Michael, and James Tansey. 2009. "Technology, Democracy, and Ethics: Democratic Deficit and the Ethics of Public Engagement." In Edna F. Einsiedel (ed.), *Emerging Technologies: From Hindsight to Foresight*. University of British Columbia Press.

Callahan, Daniel. 1993. "Why America Accepted Bioethics." *The Birth of Bioethics: Hastings Center Report*, 33 (6): supplement: S8–S9.

Conley, John M., Jean Cadigan, Arlene M. Davis, et al. 2023. "The Promise and Reality of Public Engagement in the Governance of Human Genome Editing Research." *American Journal of Bioethics*, 23 (7): 9–23.

Curato, Nicole, Julien Vrudagh, and André Bächtiger, 2020. "Democracy without Shortcuts: Introduction to the Special Issue." *Journal of Deliberative Democracy*, 16 (2): 1–9.

Davies, Sarah R. 2014. "Knowing and Loving: Public Engagement Beyond Discourse." *Science and Technology Studies*, 27 (3): 90–110.

Dietz, Thomas. 2013. "Bringing Values and Deliberation to Science Communication." *Proceedings of the National Academy of Sciences*, 110, suppl. 3: 14081–7.

Fishkin, James. 2018. *Democracy When the People Are Thinking: Revitalizing Our Politics through Public Deliberation*. Oxford University Press.

Goold, Susan Dorr. 2012. "What Is Good Public Deliberation?" *Hastings Center Report*, 42 (2): 24–6.

Grogan, Colleen M., and Michael K. Gusmano. 2007. *Healthy Voices, Unhealthy Silence*. Georgetown University Press.

Gusmano, Michael K. 2021. "Public Deliberation about Gene Editing in the Wild." In Michael K. Gusmano, Gregory E. Kaebnick, Karen J. Maschke, Carolyn P. Neuhaus, and Ben Curran Wills (eds.), *Gene Editing in the Wild: Shaping Decisions through Broad Public Deliberation. Hastings Center Report*, 51 (6) supplement: S2–S10.

Gusmano, Michael K., Gregory E. Kaebnick, Karen J. Maschke, Carolyn P. Neuhaus, and Ben Curran Wills, eds. 2021. *Gene Editing in the Wild: Shaping Decisions through Broad Public Deliberation. Hastings Center Report*, 51 (6) supplement.

Gutmann, Amy, and Dennis Thompson. 1996. *Democracy and Disagreement*. Belknap Press.

Hurlbut, J. Benjamin. 2015. "Reimagining Responsibility in Synthetic Biology." *Journal of Responsible Innovation*, 2 (1): 113–16.

Jennings, Bruce, Michael K. Gusmano, Gregory E. Kaebnick, Carolyn P. Neuhaus, and Mildred Z. Solomon. 2021. "Recommendations for Better Civic Learning: Building and Rebuilding Democracy." In Gregory E. Kaebnick, Michael K. Gusmano, Bruce Jennings, Carolyn P. Neuhaus, and Mildred Z. Solomon (eds.), *Democracy in Crisis: Civic Learning and the Reconstruction of Common Purpose. Hastings Center Report*, 51 (1) supplement: S64–S75.

Kaebnick Gregory E., Michael K. Gusmano, Bruce Jennings, Carolyn P. Neuhaus, and Mildred Z. Solomon, eds. 2021. *Democracy in Crisis: Civic Learning and the Reconstruction of Common Purpose*, in *Hastings Center Report*, 51 (1) supplement.

Kuzma, Jennifer. 2021. "Deficits of Public Deliberation in U.S. Oversight for Gene Edited Organisms." In Michael K. Gusmano, Gregory E. Kaebnick, Karen J. Maschke, Carolyn P. Neuhaus, and Ben Curran Wills (eds.), *Gene Editing in the Wild: Shaping Decisions through Broad Public Deliberation. Hastings Center Report*, 51 (6) supplement: S25–S33.

Lafont, Cristina. 2019. *Democracy without Shortcuts: A Participatory Conception of Deliberative Democracy*. Oxford University Press.

Martschenko, Daphne Olusaseun, Shawneequa L. Callier, Nanibaa' A. Garrison, et al. 2023. "Wrestling with Public Input on an Ethical Analysis of Scientific Research." In Erik Parens and Michelle N. Meyers (eds.), *The Ethical Implications of Social and Behavioral Genomics. Hastings Center Report*, 53 (2) supplement: S50–S65.

McKay, Eva. 2019. "A Jury of Peers." *Foreign Policy*. https://foreignpolicy.com/2019/01/05/a-jury-of-peers/.

National Academies of Sciences, Engineering, and Medicine. 2016. *Gene Drives on the Horizon: Advancing Science, Navigating Uncertainty, and Aligning Research with Public Values*. National Academies Press.

National Academies of Sciences, Engineering, and Medicine. 2017. *Human Genome Editing: Science, Ethics, and Governance*. National Academies Press.

National Research Council. 2008. *Public Participation in Environmental Assessment and Decision Making*. National Academies Press.

O'Doherty, Kieran C., and Michael M. Burgess. 2013. "Public Deliberation to Develop Ethical Norms and Inform Policy for Biobanks: Lessons Learnt and Challenges Remaining." *Research Ethics*, 9 (2): 55–77.

O'Doherty, Kieran, Francois-Pierre Gauvin, Colleen Grogan, and Will Friedman. 2012. "Implementing a Public Deliberative Forum." *Hastings Center Report*, 42 (2): 20–3.

Oliver, Adam. 2018. "Behavioral Economics and the Public Acceptance of Synthetic Biology." In Gregory E. Kaebnick and Michael K. Gusmano (eds.), *Governance of Emerging Technologies: Aligning Policy Analysis with the Public's Values. Hastings Center Report*, 48 (1) supplement: S50–5.

Organisation for Economic Co-operation and Development (OECD). 2020. *Innovative Citizen Participation and New Democratic Institutions: Catching the Deliberative Wave*. OECD Publishing.

Presidential Commission for the Study of Bioethical Issues. 2010. *New Directions: The Ethics of Synthetic Biology and Emerging Technologies*. Presidential Commission for the Study of Bioethical Issues.

Schroeder, S. Andrew. 2023. "Lockdowns, Bioethics, and the Public: Policy-Making in a Liberal Democracy." *Hastings Center Report*, 53 (6): 11–17.

Solomon, Stephanie, and Julia Abelson. 2012. "Why and When Should We Use Public Deliberation?" *Hastings Center Report*, 42 (2): 17–20.

Taitingfong, Riley, and Anika Ullah. 2021. "Empowering Indigenous Knowledge in Deliberations on Gene Editing in the Wild." In Michael K. Gusmano, Gregory E. Kaebnick, Karen J. Maschke, Carolyn P. Neuhaus, and Ben Curran Wills (eds.), *Gene Editing in the Wild: Shaping Decisions through Broad Public Deliberation. Hastings Center Report*, 51 (6) supplement: S74–S84.

Young, Iris Marion. 2001. "Activist Challenges to Deliberative Democracy." *Political Theory*, 29 (5): 670–90.

3

Dialogue as the Medium and Goal of Bioethics

Arthur W. Frank

In June 2022, when Covid-related violence against healthcare workers was often in the news, the *New York Times* advice column *The Ethicist*, written by the philosopher Kwame Anthony Appiah, discussed a problem of medical care. Appiah (2022) responded to a question from a physician whose hospitalized patient made racist and homophobic statements about staff she came into contact with. The physician organized several staff meetings that reached a decision: if the patient did not stop speaking this way, she would be discharged.

To the physician's relief, when the patient was told what the consequences would be if she continued to speak that way, she stopped. But the physician, anticipating such a situation might happen again and that patient might not acquiesce, asks a question: Would it be ethical to discharge such a patient if there is "a very real possibility that she could have died" from the cessation of hospital care? The physician also wonders whether the patient's disease—including "substance-abuse disorder"—"might have interfered with her ability to fully appreciate the consequences of her actions."

Appiah agrees that telling the patient to stop using insulting language was "entirely proper." But he argues that clinicians have a duty of care that takes precedence over the need for a respectful workplace. He draws an analogy to wartime: "a medic can have a responsibility of saving the life of a wounded enemy soldier, even if the soldier has just killed one of the medic's friends." Discharge is not justified if withdrawal of care poses a substantial risk to the patient. Appiah then addresses the issue of power in such a situation:

> [The patient] had no power over the clinicians who attended to her and to whose decisions she was subject. One indication of her lack of status is that your hospital's risk managers evidently decided that the institution could safely eject her without being accountable for the consequences. Though they didn't intend to mete out a punishment that might have amounted to a death sentence, the risk managers effectively put the hospital ahead of the patient.

The case raises multiple issues. One of these is the problem, and ethics, of providing care at a time when more people feel empowered to express publicly feelings that, in the past, they would have realized were inappropriate and kept to themselves. Maybe the patient's speech was a result of her impaired physical condition, but quite possibly not. She may have been instigated by a sense that it's a viable life strategy to push limits—basically, she lives by seeing how much she can get away with. How does an institution like a hospital deal with people who act that way?

A different perspective is to ask whether the patient's racist and homophobic speech was the only idiom she had available to express her anger at the powerlessness that Appiah notes in her situation. The staff might well ask how the patient can speak this way about people who are working hard to treat and hopefully to cure her. She may see things differently. The patient may experience the staff organizing her care in ways that put their needs, and the institutional needs, ahead of what the patient imagines would be optimal care. Appiah suggests this interpretive possibility when he writes that the hospital's risk managers "effectively put the hospital ahead of the patient." The patient may be reacting to a perceived pattern of having her needs subordinated, and lacking an appropriate vocabulary of resistance, she resorts to hateful speech directed toward individuals.

My interest is in what neither the physician nor the philosopher suggests as a possibility. Both seem to frame possible responses as binary alternatives: for the physician, either the patient stops being insulting, or she will be discharged; for the philosopher, either the clinicians decide the patient poses a viable threat of physical violence, or else their duty of care requires continuing to treat her while tolerating her behavior. Neither considers engaging in continuing dialogue with the patient, asking how she understands her situation and what choices she feels she has. Appiah's analogy to wartime hospitals seems unfortunately accurate: in contemporary hospitals, patients are too often regarded as wounded enemies, for whom there remains a duty of care. But what if someone, rather than presenting the patient with an either/or ultimatum, invited her, through nonjudgmental questions, to express what troubles her as the source of her anger? Is such a dialogue—which may not go well at first and will take time—the role of a hospital ethics consultant?[1]

The absence of dialogue in hospitals causes suffering not only on the side of disempowered patients; it also affects clinicians. The physician Brent Carr (2024) describes his experience of requesting and receiving an ethics consultation on a dilemma of whether to treat. Most briefly stated, Carr's patient suffers from prolonged debilitating depression for which ECT (electroconvulsive therapy) has been the only effective treatment. But the patient has a heart condition that gives ECT a substantial risk of being fatal to her. Carr's description of the outcome of the ethics consult that he requested is a testimonial to the lack of dialogue:

> Forty-eight hours [after the consult request], I was asked to proceed with ECT. The resident reported the Ethics Consult was on the chart. It was a succinct summary that stated all the necessary legal obligations had been met, the established lack of capacity had been appropriately documented, attempts to "avoid harm" were present, and affirmed husband was legally able to consent. The Ethics team signed

> off but stated they were available again should the need arise. According to the resident, the Ethics Consultation team had met with the husband but not the team. Brief, simple. Oddly, all team members and students now verbalized how comfortable they were with proceeding with ECT. All hesitation or concern had fully and immediately dissolved after this perfunctory consultation. I attempted to process with the residents and students why there was such an immediate resolution to their concerns. But I was met with silence. (Carr 2024, 15)

But Carr's story does not end in silence. The consultation leaves an aftermath of discontent that is audible but never given public voice: "The nursing staff had voiced their frustration. . . . Medical students confidentially articulated their confusion and concern to only the resident but were apprehensive about expressing their thoughts at a team level" (2024,15).

Carr's conclusion should cause bioethicists to be troubled over what actually counts as "ethics" in not all but too many hospitals: "The ethics consult seemed deprecated somehow—relegated as though it were a solitary lab order that had returned a simple, concrete value. And that was the end of the discussion and concerns" (2024,15). But from Carr's description of how the ethics consultation proceeded—who the ethicist talked to or didn't—and its format as ticking off a series of required boxes, the clinical staff were justified in treating it like "a solitary lab order" with a single conclusion. The consultation affirmed their sense that hospitals value bureaucratic processes and leave little time or space for dialogue.

This chapter is about the tension between clinical situations that cry out for dialogue and institutional structures that systematically shut down dialogue. Carr takes responsibility on himself and his colleagues, writing that consults are "only as good as our willingness to engage in them" (Carr 2024, 16). That may be true, but it is equally true that people's willingness to engage depends on whether the consult clears a space in which that engagement seems not only possible but positively welcome. Again, the consultation that Carr's team received *taught them the limits* of what they could expect from their work environment, just as the ultimatum given to the patient in the Appiah case taught her what to expect as her "care."

To explore the tension in health care between imposed silence and open dialogue, I will first consider, briefly, what seems a relevant distinction between *ethics* as institutionalized practice and ethics as individual moral agency. These two forms of ethics co-exist in a tension that is also mutual dependence; the issue cannot be one or the other, but how to sustain an unstable balance. Then, to better grasp the imbalance between ethics and moral agency in hospitals, I develop a distinction drawn by the philosopher Jürgen Habermas in the 1980s between what he called the lifeworld and systems.

This distinction raises a fundamental question for bioethics: Can hospitals, as systems, be ethical? That question complicates not only the work of hospital-based consulting bioethicists but also the work of being a patient, family member, or clinical staff in a contemporary hospital.

Institutional Ethics, Moral Agency, and Dialogue

In some usages, the terms "ethical life" and "moral life" might be interchangeable, with differences depending on context. Who uses which word in which way varies, but in professional usage, a distinction is generally observed. I find it useful to think instead of *ethics* and *moral agency* as being mutually entangled in everyday life, yet separable for analytic purposes.[2] Their entanglement matters in the two cases this chapter begins with. My argument is that institutions push to insulate ethics from moral agency, and one necessary work of bioethicists is to protect and enable that agency.

The institutional form of ethics is exemplified by the chart entry that Carr reports in his story. Ethics consultation means addressing a number of criteria, and once those boxes are checked off, an action is certified as ethical. Ethics in this sense is procedural and impersonal: the ethicist in Carr's story feels no need to talk to everyone involved; only the competence of the surrogate decision-maker needs to be assured. Such an ethics service accepts that its role is to keep the wheels of the institutional process rolling when some dilemma slows things down. Ethics also provides institutions with accountability, documenting that required precautions were taken. Ethical concern thus turns into institutional liability control; with that priority, the rumbling undercurrent of discontent that Carr describes is inaudible.

In contrast with such ethics, moral agency is pensive; it broods, never sure of itself. Moral concern is what leads the physician to send his question to Appiah's *Ethicist* column. Some time after the patient's discharge, the physician continues to worry whether the right thing was done. Carr writes from a similar ongoing discontent. If ethics outsources decision-making to a template, protocol, or code, what is moral begins with individuals feeling responsible in the sense advocated by the philosopher Emmanuel Levinas (2001): response-ability is one person's ability-to-respond to another. That response reflects obligation both to one's own humanity and the humanity of the other. In moral life, each person is directly responsible to an embodied other, who is somehow a reflection of oneself. By contrast, ethical responsibility is limited: consultants enact what institutions prescribe.

But to define ethics as institutional and moral agency as personal draws another false dichotomy, both because anything personal has its origins already entangled in institutions, and because the persons who act on behalf of institutions do not give up all agency. Institutional designations including patient, healthcare worker, attending physician, or nurse are more than job descriptions. Each is an identity position that individual people are put into, whether by recruitment, conscription, or individual need, and then variously embrace as who they know themselves to be and how they expect others to know them. Any separation between the institutional and the personal is always an idealization; in the messiness of people's actual lives, each is the possibility of the other.

Yet a tension remains, and bioethics, in my account, takes place in the space of that tension. In the Appiah case, it's easy to imagine hospital functionaries not wanting a dialogue in which an ethics consultant explores the patient's racism, including whether it might be somehow connected to her substance abuse issues. Functionaries want to keep treatment focused and responsibility limited; that requires excluding contextualizing issues. In Carr's story, smooth institutional functioning—productivity—is served by an ethics report that does not open up the kind of staff dialogue that Carr regrets did not happen. Most bluntly put, such a dialogue would not be reimbursable; there's no income generation in it, quite the contrary.

If institutional ethics is resistant to dialogue, moral agency is both formed in and enacted through dialogue. Dialogue, as I use the term (Frank 2004), has at least three qualities. First, each person encourages the other's fullest expression of their perspective, recognizing that the other can articulate their perspective only through a process of talk in which each person's responses to the other encourage further reflection. Second, each is willing to have their own perspective changed through the encounter with the perspective of others; each anticipates such changes. And third, there is no final point to the process, although a moment may come when sufficient agreement enables action. Dialogue is time consuming, and it is unsettling in its unpredictability. If participants are committed to a particular outcome, then it's not a dialogue.

Much more could be said about dialogue and how it is a necessary condition of moral relationships, the point being that *moral* always involves being-in-*open*-relation. But what has been said is sufficient to move on to the bioethical problem, which is why the nature of institutions, of which hospitals are a prime example, is to favor procedural ethics over dialogical moral relations.

Institutional Ethics as Colonization

To understand how the tension between institutional ethics and individual moral agency results from what institutions are, and how modernity is based on institutional forms of which hospitals, for all their uniqueness, are a typical example, I turn to Habermas's great work *The Theory of Communicative Action* (1987; Frank 1989). I consider Habermas to have been prophetic: his argument has become more relevant today than when it was written.

Habermas imagines society comprising two aspects that are mutually dependent but can be considered separate for analysis. He calls these *lifeworlds* and *systems*. The lifeworld is where we humans live our daily lives: where people are born, grow up, work, raise children, grow old, and throughout all this, care for each other as individuals. Lifeworlds are intangible yet compelling; their taken-for-grantedness makes them resistant to reflective specification, yet they are the basis of appeals to act or refrain from acting.

A crucial part of growing up in the lifeworld is the acquisition of a sense of what should be done or not done; humans' sense—which can feel like an intuitive certainty—of right and wrong, culpable or justified, sinful or saintly derives from the lifeworld. Attempts are made to codify this sense or disposition in the form of specified values and ethical injunctions, but the force of any articulated values or injunctions depends on a history of individual experiences of watching others act and respond to different actions, modeling behavior and learning whom to take as a model for what, and unfortunately but maybe necessarily, experiences of hurting others and being hurt.

An example is useful both to show the force of the lifeworld and to dispel any idealization of lifeworlds. The sociologist and legal scholar Susan Shapiro (2019) in her ethnography of surrogate decision-making in end-of-life medical care quotes a clinical conference taking place in Chicago. The surrogate decision-maker has power of attorney, but she speaks of her need to respect what the rest of the family, who are in Italy, believe is the right thing to do. They are people she has grown up among and feels responsible to, but her lifeworld is removed from theirs; they, at a distance, cannot see the scene as she does, there in the hospital. A nurse attempts to break the impasse: "But we have a POA saying [the patient] didn't want this," meaning continuing life support in intensive care. The surrogate decision-maker replies, "Yes, but they're going to say I killed him. They're going to blame it all on me" (Shapiro 2019, 203).

The decision-maker is caught in a conflict between lifeworlds. Her family in Italy has its compelling sense of what is right and wrong, but in a Chicago intensive care unit, that sense of rightness does not fit. As I read the case and reflect on what I would do, I recognize the force of the stories I grew up with, in which my parents and grandparents not only accepted but praised older family members' decisions to forego recommended medical treatments because those treatments would have prevented living out their lives as they desired. Those stories shape my sense of what should or should not be done. How, then, can different lifeworlds mediate their differences?

For the project that Habermas calls *communicative action*, what matters is whether any disagreement, such as the one just sketched, can be the topic of dialogue: can differences be talked about with the goal of each eventually understanding the other's stance as *plausible*. "One determines which values are to be rationally accepted and pursued only . . . by making what everyone could want in this situation plausible" (Habermas 1978, 136–7). Over the decades since I first read that, and across conflicts that I have seen during those decades, Habermas's plausibility criterion has become increasingly important because initiating dialogue between polarized parties has become more difficult. Plausibility does not mean agreement with others; it's not even about empathy. Plausibility is about recognizing that the other's perspective makes sense if understood as coming from their lifeworld; their goals and desires make sense in that context. Such plausibility by itself guarantees nothing—one party can find the other's interests and intents plausible yet still trample them. But plausibility is necessary for dialogue.

What Habermas calls communicative action involves the goodwill, and perhaps historical awareness, to recognize the inhumanity and eventual futility of discounting others' perspectives and resorting to domination. Thus, the surrogate decision-maker described by Shapiro refuses the suggestion to cut off deliberation by invoking the power of attorney. To do that would end her communicative relationship with her Italian family. The nurse who proposes invoking the POA is acting not on the basis of a lifeworld awareness with its commitment to communicative action, but on the demands of a system that she represents. We can observe, with regret, that she is doing her job in a way that her administrative superiors would commend.

The difference between lifeworlds and systems hinges on not all communication being *communicative*, as Habermas uses that term. Communicative action is predisposed to seek mutual understanding. Habermas refers to the early twentieth-century social psychologist George Herbert Mead (1970 [1934]), who understood social life becoming possible because people are capable of taking the role or attitude of other persons, imagining themselves in the other's situation. Mead locates the development of this capacity in children's play, in which each child plays at being multiple others and acts toward their playmates as if they were multiple others. As play develops, children learn to organize their assumed roles in relation to what others are playing at being. Learning to play is how children develop a shared commitment to mutual lines of action.

Habermas opposes communicative action to what he calls *strategic action*, which seeks not mutual understanding but self-advantage. Systems are based on strategic action. Strategic action can involve taking the role of the other, but here role-taking enables manipulation, as in salesmanship. A further difference is that communicative action measures gain or success in qualitative terms; in the lifeworld, the value of relationships, of community membership, of acting rightly cannot be measured: value is inherent. Systems act upon quantitative measures: for something to count, it must be countable. Systems run on algorithms that require numbers. In hospitals, care is measured in units of time that have a measured cost, and that cost is weighed against reimbursement. Systems displace ideas of inherent value with measures of comparative productivity, again quantified.

Habermas's distinction between lifeworld and systems enables me to better conceptualize two attitudes toward vulnerability, including nonhuman vulnerabilities of animals, plants, rivers, and landscapes. The difference between these attitudes seems crucial to what we imagine bioethics is for: what its task is. Lifeworld vulnerability begins and ends with self-awareness of living in a fragile body that never outgrows its initial dependency. This body has limited strength and is easily broken. Embodied vulnerability extends to feeling its interdependence: both each individual's dependence on other similarly vulnerable bodies and others' dependence on them. Interdependence is both a liability and also the source of what is good in life, which I gloss as relationships.

Systems, lacking bodies except in a metaphorical sense, utilize vulnerability as a principle of control. Bodies' vulnerability makes them susceptible to being *ordered* in both senses of being commanded and being set in order, like soldiers in formation, office workers in cubicles, or hospitalized patients ordered according to diagnostic categories, treatment schedules, units, and rooms. That ordering alternatively promises and threatens; its benefits can be as real as its penalties.

Vulnerability in the lifeworld is *felt* by each individual in their body and in relation to the bodies of others. Systems *measure* vulnerability in quantitative forms including not only costs but also constant calculations of the balance between individual need and aggregate demand for services. Medical systems are not distinct in valuing quantitative metrics: political systems count votes, and corporations report in monetary gains and losses. Again, what counts for systems is what is countable, and the rest is noise, vaguely heard but not worth attending to.

Habermas then reaches what I consider to be the crux of his argument. Systems depend upon the persons who populate them—whether as staff or clients—having acquired values in the lifeworld and regulating their behavior according to those values. The Appiah case is a good example. A hospital system is disrupted when a patient lacks what the institution expects as a proper sense of deportment: her lifeworld has not prepared her to be disposed to act as the hospital requires; that is, being respectful to staff. Maybe, at worst, her lifeworld makes her feel compelled to use racist and homophobic expressions because these insults count as essential tokens of membership in that lifeworld, expressing an identity she cannot readily let go of.

But here Habermas observes a fundamental contradiction: systems systematically erode the value-generating capacity of lifeworlds, even as they depend on that capacity. Habermas's metaphor is that systems *colonize* lifeworlds. Since he wrote that in the 1980s, the literal and metaphorical usage of colonization has expanded, and perhaps today the metaphor is overloaded. Habermas's argument is that systems first insinuate themselves within lifeworlds and then erode what integrates those lifeworlds. Actions in families and communities become more strategic than communicative; inherent value is displaced by measurables, primarily money.

The systems logic of action that runs governments and corporations gradually comes to pervade the value-generating institutions of families, schools, and communities. In their colonized form, lifeworld institutions no longer produce persons with value orientations that systems require, as the Appiah case illustrates. Systems most often respond by becoming harsher versions of what they inherently are, which in the Appiah case means delivering an ultimatum to the patient: a threat of force to compel compliance. Here we see a fundamental contradiction. Hospitals may be the first institutions to show the corrosive effects of systems colonizing lifeworlds because hospitals, more than other corporate forms, explicitly claim to *care* for individual patients and families. Hospitals make lifeworld claims, yet they run as systems and treat patients, families, and staff according to a system logic of strategic communication and quantitatively measurable value.

Another case example is useful at this point. Several decades ago, our friends' daughter needed surgery for persistent ear infections. Her mother was on the staff of the children's hospital where the surgery occurred and has told this story in grand rounds. Like most children's hospitals, this one expressed its commitment to individualized care and to supporting families. There was a careful presurgical orientation, assuring the child that her mother could remain with her, holding her hand until she went to sleep.

But when the mother was about to enter the operating room with her daughter, the surgeon forbade entry. He told her that if he allowed every parent to stay with their child, the aggregate slowing down would mean a specific number of fewer surgeries each day. Thus, he reneged on the earlier agreement made on his behalf. Hospitals depend on patients and families trusting staff, including "team" members who speak for other team members. I imagine that as a person, the surgeon would readily affirm the principle that lying to anyone, and especially to children, is wrong. But in his systems role as surgeon, he claims exemption from this principle; the need to maximize operating-room capacity makes the situation exceptional. The surgeon is working hard, hospital resources are limited, and that gives him a get-out-of-normal-decency pass. Predictably, his appeal is quantitative: the more operations that can be performed, the more compelling the justification for doing what has to be done to achieve that end.

What has to be done—from a systems perspective—is first getting the family to agree to surgery by making certain promises, then preventing emotional upset on the way to surgery because that would slow things down, and finally reneging at the moment when the parent has the least scope to resist or refuse. Again, the surgeon can justify his action as what the system requires. Recall Appiah writing that risk managers "effectively put the hospital ahead of the patient." The logic of systems always prioritizes institutional needs, with those needs expressed in quantitative forms: it is what systems *are*. Yet such systems logic is ultimately self-defeating.

The surgeon in the story accomplishes an immediate goal without thought to future problems that his action creates, which are problems arising from the loss of trust—trust that the operation of the system depends on.[3] Here we see the full cycle of how systems colonize lifeworlds, and in that process, undermine themselves—they cut off the branch they sit on. The surgical system depends on layers of trust about what will happen and limits on what will happen; that trust centers on the surgeon and extends to his representatives. Withdrawal of that trust—as when a patient refuses to sign a consent form—is a significant disruption to the system. But as trust erodes, such disruptions predictably will increase.

Habermas understands the crisis of modernity to be the inability of lifeworlds to generate ethical predispositions as quickly as systems undermine lifeworld values. That crisis is bioethics' point of entry. Bioethics' task is to repair relationships that systems systematically impair, and it sometimes can do just that.

The physician Laura Hoeksema (2024) describes a hospital ethics consultation called when two care teams were in conflict. "Members of the two care teams advocated passionately for what they thought was best for her. At times, team members were advocating strongly for conflicting interventions. Every member of both teams experienced moral distress related to some aspect of her care" (Hoeksema 2024, 21). Hoeksema offers few specifics of what was said in the consultation, but her description of the outcome exemplifies Habermas's ideal of communicative action: "We came to understand that because of the values we held so dearly and prioritize differently, we had divergent perspectives on her care. This experience helped us clarify our individual values as we reflected on which of our values we felt were being disregarded or infringed upon" (2024, 22). In Habermas's terms, each team came to understand the other's values as plausible, and going a bit further, each person no longer saw their own values as being threatened by others holding different values.

Hoeksema concludes with a description that I believe is a truly profound reflection on how working in hospitals affects people: "As we cared for the patient over several months, team members sometimes became hypo- or hyper-engaged in the face of helplessness" (2024, 22). Habermas would understand that split—disengagement alternating with commitment that admits no compromises—as being a predictable condition of people who live in an increasing divergence between lifeworld values and system imperatives. Again, this split may be worst in institutions like hospitals that most explicitly commit to lifeworld values of care while operating on a logic of systems. That literally drives people crazy.[4]

The Contradictions and Potential of Bioethics

The frequently recognized contradiction that has to be confronted when we ask how bioethics might respond to the crisis of systems colonizing lifeworlds is that bioethics is itself an institutionalized enterprise in which careers depend on employment that is mostly in systems. Doing bioethics depends on getting some form of airtime, which might mean convening a clinical conference, authoring a scholarly publication or commissioned report, or attracting mass media attention. That airtime is controlled by systems. What we call *bioethics* is a loose affiliation of actors who depend in different ways on multiple institutions, including medical centers, universities, and funding bodies operated by governments, nonprofit foundations, and corporations. Bioethics is a diffuse system embedded in other systems.

Yet—bioethics is called into existence by a lifeworld awareness of embodied vulnerability. That awareness makes imperative the need to protect humans, whether they are patients, research subjects, or healthcare workers. That need to protect extends to nonhuman actors with which human life is interdependent, including what we gloss with words like *ecology* and *climate*. Thus, I understand bioethics as an honorably contradictory enterprise: working within systems to defend lifeworlds against those systems, while recognizing that lifeworlds need systems. Bioethics goes wrong when, as in Carr's consultation story, it is reduced to being an accountability mechanism for the system, never even attempting to enable a scene of communicative action. Beyond advocating the need to avoid that reduction of bioethical work, I offer the following modest proposals of what bioethicists might keep in mind as they do their work.

First, bioethical responsibility includes advocating for what I call *extensive responsibility*, although systems will resist that advocacy, favoring limited liability. When the surgeon reneges on his team's presurgical agreement with mother and child, he limits his responsibility to only the work of that day: how many surgeries he can perform. He takes no responsibility for future encounters in which healthcare workers will confront patients who do not trust them, and how the lack of trust will complicate that future work. These healthcare workers will have to do their work, eliciting patients' trust while knowing that what they tell patients is, in practice, untrustworthy. It's the hospital equivalent of corporate executives thinking only in terms of quarterly profits, disregarding unsustainable actions that produced those profits, because capital can always cash in and go elsewhere. Human health has no elsewhere.

To return to my earlier metaphor, extensive responsibility means remembering that you are sitting on the branch, whatever the short-term benefits seem to be in sawing it off. The word *sustainability* has reached a frequency of usage that makes it almost a cliché. We talk about sustainability so much to cover over multiple failures to respect what the word demands. The sustainability of healthcare systems depends on trust. Issues of extensive responsibility often end with a question of whose trust is being either sustained or undermined by someone else's actions.

Second and complementary to that, it's necessary to connect the macro concerns of bioethics—concerns that include attention to inequalities in healthcare access and outcomes, as well as determinants of health such as climate, personal security, and education—with the micro level of ethics consultation, but how to do this is not evident. Appiah gently suggests that the patient's outbursts have a more extensive basis; understanding racism and homophobia as only this patient's internal dispositions ignores how everyone got where they are. Appiah suggests the patient's hostility reflects her powerlessness not only as a patient in the hospital but in her life generally. Addressing the immediate problem by threatening her with discharge is an exemplary instance of failing to take extensive responsibility. Later, she may tell the story of the hospital's ultimatum in ways that affirm the distrust and ill-will of listeners in her lifeworld.

The question is how hospital ethics consultants, employed to delimit problems to the most immediate circumstances, can be empowered to lead those with whom they consult to perceive and respond to all that created the situation in the first place, especially when that situation involves a conflict. The impossible task that should remain an ideal for hospital ethics consultants is to reintegrate, through the medium of deliberation, all the factors that systems seek to separate or ignore, including how the system's own practices have created the situation; these practices include dividing care between two teams, putting a primary value on quantitative metrics of productivity, and giving assurances that are not always fulfilled.

Third, bioethics consultation has the potential to become a model of how people can encounter a dilemma, which may already have deteriorated into a conflict, without polarization. Hoeksema's description of the two teams each coming to respect the values that led to different treatment priorities shows that this depolarization is possible, although such a consultation will not be accomplished in a couple of hours. Mutual listening, and then reflection on one's own stance, takes time.

Polarization should be an expected part of the decision-making process in health care, because treatment decisions often seem either/or, as in sustaining ICU life-support or withdrawing it, and because systems divide people both into hierarchies and into binaries such as lay/professional, privileging one term in that binary opposition. The need is to understand polarization *as a phase* in a process, rather than accepting it as intractable. The decision to present the patient in the Appiah case with an ultimatum rests on accepting polarization as intractable—dialogue never seems considered as an option, and as the hospital milieu is currently designed, that's understandable.

The dialogical stance is that in any dispute or conflict, each party has a rationale—the basis of which often goes well beyond the parameters of the present situation—that deserves to be heard not only by those who disagree, but also by that person themselves, because they are probably not reflectively aware of what has led them to feel as they do: What has disposed their moral and ethical dispositions?

Communicative action, effected in dialogue, has its limits. Dialogue will not resolve the sort of dilemma Carr faces when the only treatment risks death; that blunt reality cannot be changed by talking about it. But dialogue can mitigate team conflict over the dilemma, and crucially it can change how those involved will be affected by a bad outcome, should that occur. Dialogue can create a milieu of mutual support. My own description of this change is *tragic companionship* (Frank 2022).

I would love to see a hospital publicize itself with a statement like: *We cannot always prevent your family's tragedy, but we can accompany you through it.* That would have a welcome honesty; it sets the bar neither higher nor lower, but in an altogether different dimension. However, systems understand themselves as problem-solving, achieving outcomes, and in a word, *succeeding*, at least according to metrics of success. Systems exhibit what the ancient Greeks understood as the tragic flaw of *hubris*, a wild overestimation of one's own invulnerability, precipitating downfall.

Just as I wrote earlier about how systems understand human vulnerability differently from lifeworld understanding, so *care* is understood differently. Systems measure care in a calculation between costs and forms of return on investment, whatever that means for different national healthcare funding. When systems talk about care, they tacitly or explicitly rationalize limits on their own responsibilities. In lifeworlds, the limits of care are the subject of constant brooding: care has no limits in principle, although in practice, caregivers have to confront their own limits of strength, resources, and capacity for sacrifice. In lifeworlds, giving care means companionship sustained through circumstances that, if not exactly tragic, are very sad.

Bioethics does its work at the intersection of lifeworlds and systems, acknowledging their mutual dependence and seeking to rebalance their usually biased relationship. Systems and lifeworlds each need the other, yet they are in tension with each other. I believe Habermas was prophetic when he wrote, about four decades ago, of the tendency of systems to colonize lifeworlds and how that undermines what systems themselves need to continue functioning. Thus, I understand bioethics as a perpetually two-sided work: reinforcing lifeworlds by being a resource for the expression of claims of moral agency and calling upon systems to recognize the ways they undermine what they depend on, especially trust.

A system that does not prioritize its own needs and does not express these needs in quantitative terms may be a contradiction in terms. But that does not mean systems have to be self-destructive. Systems can include the self-correction mechanism of bioethics, restoring dialogues that are always being excluded.

Notes

1 Here as throughout I understand *bioethicist* and *hospital ethics consultant* as roles that often overlap but also can differ: not all bioethicists are interested in hospital ethics consulting, and not all hospital ethics consultants are bioethicists in training, career

path, or disposition. In my usage, a bioethicist understands specific issues within the broadest context of protection of life itself, the bios, and calls upon traditions of moral and ethical thought. To be a bioethicist is a vocation, in the sense of feeling called to do the work. Many hospital ethics consultants have their primary employment in other areas of healthcare and have been recruited or conscripted to work part-time as ethics consultants. Their orientation is to resolve ad hoc questions and conflicts as quickly as possible, which they often do well. Hospital ethics consultants confer institutional legitimacy, and they worry, perhaps most of all, about institutional liability. Again, these roles often overlap, but too often they do not. In an ideal healthcare world, all ethics consultants would be bioethicists, in scope of concern and disposition.

2 I write about moral agency, not *morality*, a word I avoid. Morality seems on the side of institutional ethics, but with an overtone of unquestioning conviction that is not open to dialogue. Morality prescribes rules and parameters within which individuals are told to live, that life being institutionally certified as just, righteous, honorable, or some such word. Morality involves minimal agency, beyond rule following. Morality has little time for gray areas, where the applicability of rules is uncertain.

3 A complementary conceptualization describes the surgeon as an *artificial person*, that is, someone who acts not only on their own moral agency, but rather as action is required by the system for which that person is merely an agent (Frank 2004, 126–32). The political philosopher David Runciman (2023) understands states and corporate forms of institutions, including hospitals, as artificial persons, considering both the considerable benefits derived from these organizational constructions and the dangers of handing over too much authority to them. For my present argument, what matters most is that *artificial persons are created not to have moral agency*—that is part of their value—although they can be designed to act within prescribed ethical boundaries. Understanding what artificial persons are designed to be and not be seems crucial to what can be expected of bioethics.

4 The literature on mental health problems of healthcare workers proliferates; see, as one example, Olfson, Cosgrove, and Wall (2023).

Bibliography

Appiah, A. K. 2022. "Can I Withhold Medical Care from a Bigot?" *The New York Times Magazine*, August 1, 2022.

Carr, B. 2024. "Side Stepping the Issues." *Narrative Inquiry in Bioethics*, 14 (1): 13–16.

Frank, A. W. 1989. "Habermas's Interactionism: The Micro-Macro Link to Politics." *Symbolic Interaction*, 12 (2): 333–60.

Frank, A. W. 2004. *The Renewal of Generosity: Illness, Medicine, and How to Live*. University of Chicago Press.

Frank, A. W. 2022. *King Lear: Shakespeare's Dark Consolations*. Oxford University Press.

Habermas, J. 1978. "Theory and Politics: A Discussion with Herbert Marcuse." *Telos*, 38: 124–53.

Habermas, J. 1987. *The Theory of Communicative Action, Volume II. Lifeworld and System: A Critique of Functionalist Reason*. Boston: Beacon Press.

Hoeksema, L. 2024. "Healing Power." *Narrative Inquiry in Bioethics*, 14 (1): 21–3.

Levinas, E. 2001. *Is It Righteous to Be? Interviews with Emmanuel Levinas*, ed. J. Robbins. Stanford University Press.
Mead, G. H. 1970 [1934]. *Mind, Self, and Society*. University of Chicago Press.
Olfson, M., C. M. Cosgrove, and M. M. Wall. 2023. "Suicide Risks of Health Care Workers in the US." *JAMA*, 330 (12): 1161–6.
Runciman, D. 2023. *The Handover: How We Gave Control of Our Lives to Corporations, States, and AIs*. Liveright.
Shapiro, S. 2019. *Speaking for the Dying: Life-and-Death Decisions in Intensive Care*. University of Chicago Press.

4

The Future of Bioethics, Reconsidered

Howard A. Brody

In 2009, I published a book which was perhaps misnamed *The Future of Bioethics* (Brody 2009). I did not attempt to guess which issues in bioethics would receive the most attention in the future. Instead, I discussed issues that, in my view, deserved more attention than they were then getting. Briefly, the contents included patient-centered care, evidence-based medicine, pay-for-performance, community dialogue, cross-cultural concerns, race and health disparities, disabilities, environmental and global issues, and new technologies.

A number of these issues have received increased attention in the intervening years. I would include cross-cultural concerns, race, disabilities, and environmental issues. Others remain relatively unexplored.

Here I wish to reconsider three areas. At least one example can be given of reawakened interest in community dialogue. There continues to be a tension between patient-centered care and personalized medicine. And recent changes in the US political climate pose a challenge to activist bioethics. Finally, I want to fill in what was missing in my 2009 book by actually addressing "the future of bioethics."

Community Dialogue

As I summarized in *The Future of Bioethics*, "grass roots bioethics" became a popular movement in the 1980s before fading out in the 1990s. Funded by the Prudential Foundation and the Robert Wood Johnson Foundation, grassroots projects engaged ordinary citizens in extended dialogue over issues such as access to health care (Jennings 1988; Garland and Hasnain 1990). Later work further refined the instructions given to dialogue participants (Fleck 1994) and showed that the methods worked as well among minority communities as with the majority white communities which formed the basis of previous dialogue projects (Bonham et al. 2009).

In 2014–16, our group in Galveston, Texas, conducted a series of community dialogues funded by the Patient-Centered Outcomes Research Institute of the Agency for Healthcare Research and Quality. The grant specified that the initial dialogues be on the topic of Patient-Centered Outcomes Research (PCOR) and Comparative Effectiveness

Research (CER) and that participants be sixty-five years or older; later dialogues could be on any topic chosen (Brody et al. 2013). Dialogues were conducted on PCOR and CER ethical issues in four groups—a predominantly white, upper-middle-class group, two African American lower income groups, and a Hispanic group. Following that, dialogues on the ethics of mental health ethics in elderly populations were held in the white group and one of the African American groups (Crowder and Determeyer 2019).

Dialogues were held in two-hour sessions weekly for six weeks. The research team chose background readings on the ethics topics and illustrative case studies. The team then made a list of apparent ethical conclusions reached by the groups, and these were discussed and debated in the final session. Groups could choose either a single majority report or majority and minority reports (none chose the latter). In the second topic (mental health), the groups chose to invite experts on each weekly topic and to spend an additional hour hearing the expert.

Examples of the findings of the groups include conclusions reached by the first two groups (white and African American) on PCOR/CER:

- PCOR and CER require ethically sound relationships between provider and patient (patient-centered care).
- Commercial interests (e.g., pharmaceutical companies) add unnecessary costs and must be restrained.
- Some restrictions on patient choice must be made toward the goal of cost containment, though this was controversial.
- The African American group was more open to allowing patients to choose scientifically invalid treatments based on the personal testimony of other patients (Brody et al. 2013).

Conclusions reached on mental health and aging include:

- Mental health is as important as physical health, and adequate facilities should be provided to address it.
- Everyone should make plans for their own future, including family discussions and advance directives.
- The cost of medications is a critical issue and must be addressed by Medicare and Medicaid.
- Lobbyists for pharmaceutical and insurance companies have no place in health care and should be disallowed.
- Social Security, Medicare, and Medicaid should be expanded to widen the safety net for mental health care (St. Vincent's House 2016).

Several aspects of the dialogues led to the view that the exercise had been successful. The summary statements of the white and African American groups differed somewhat in terms of both topics chosen and views taken on them. The research team noted several examples where the positions taken by the dialogue groups were not the same as the views of the research team. Meetings held after completion of the project showed a large appreciation among participants.

The falling off of interest and participation in community bioethics dialogue after the first stage of popularity in the 1980s reflects in part the difficulty of engaging in the method. One must select appropriate groups in one's community; engage in discussion over general participation and, later, specific topics to be addressed; develop the background materials in an appropriately neutral way; conduct the dialogue sessions; assemble the final reports and present them to the groups for assent; and appropriately publicize the results in the local community. After one has done all this, one has the findings of a single group and must replicate the process with other groups. One can achieve greater efficiency if the same community group is willing to meet at intervals in the future to discuss a series of topics. This is one of the major findings of the Galveston experiment, that two groups were willing to undertake a second topic and showed evidence of having learned from the experience of the first go-around by inviting expert presentations.

The impact that community dialogue is likely to have on policy formulation will depend on factors largely outside the control of the dialogue participants. The "grassroots" dialogue of the 1980s was largely planned around political efforts to design health care systems. By contrast, the dialogue project on PCOR/CER was restricted by the funding agency to that topic, and the actual impact on health policy was accordingly minimal.

A great deal has been written about the requirements of "expertise" in community dialogue, since the main parties do not have the usual academic credentials. My own reaction has been to cut the Gordian knot and refuse to discuss "expertise" at all. The results of a community dialogue can be readily assessed on their own merits, especially when different community groups have addressed the same issue. It is not clear what one adds to these discussions by attributing, or refusing to attribute, some level of expertise to various parties.

Patient-Centered Care versus Personalized Medicine

In *The Future of Bioethics*, I adopted a definition of "patient-centered care" from a 2004 report on "The Future of Family Medicine" by seven national family medicine organizations:

> [B]ased on a physician-patient relationship that is highly satisfying and humanizing to the patient and the physician (as well as other practice clinicians) . . . the patient, not the physician, occupies center stage. From first contact through the completion of the care episode, the patient must meet with consistent and competent care . . . all patients will receive care that is culturally and linguistically appropriate . . . practices strive to meet patient and community needs for integrated care by giving patients what they want and need—preventive care, acute care, rehabilitative care, chronic illness care, and supportive care—when they want and need it by anticipating patient needs and designing services to meet those needs. (Martin et al. 2004, S14)

Practical applications of patient-centered care included improved access (same-day appointments, expanded hours), offices redesigned as patient health resource centers, and expanded services through multidisciplinary teams. The authors regarded all such changes as core elements of practice, not mere cosmetic frills. In 2009, I found it odd that a major group of primary physicians should contemplate such major changes (I would say improvements) in medical care, with potential impacts on patient autonomy, with so little attention from bioethicists. The answer, I suggested, was that this change pertained to primary care. Bioethics has largely ignored developments in primary care and has focused almost exclusively on specialist practice. This gap is probably explained both by a lack of interest in primary care among bioethicists and lack of specific funding for such inquiries.

In the same chapter, I discussed "personalized medicine":

> Scientists at the National Institutes of Health and in academic medicine generally have recently begun to tout the virtues of "personalized medicine." While such a term might mean many things, its overriding focus appears to be the promise of the new genomic science. The argument is that, once we understand the human genome, we need never give (for example) a drug to a patient that will cause an untoward side effect. Before administering the drug, we will do a study of the patient's genome and discover that this patient carries the gene responsible for that adverse drug reaction, so we will prescribe a different drug that does not have these dangers. By knowing the genome, we can precisely tailor medical interventions, both diagnostic and therapeutic, to the individual patient.
>
> Personalized medicine, in this view, might be a great advance. But it would not escape from the reductionist biomedical model that was the core reason why patient-centered care was seen as a necessary alternative. According to this view, we are our DNA. To treat *as a unique person* is simply to know our gene sequences. Such a formula seems inadequate for a truly patient-centered medicine. (Brody 2009, 57, italics in original)

This criticism of personalized medicine is based on the biopsychosocial model of George Engel (Engel 1977). "Patient-centered care" requires attention to the entire range of the model, from cells and tissues to individual psychology and the social sciences. "Personalized medicine" at first sounds similarly broad, but on inquiry is found to be limited to the biochemical and cellular level.

James Tabery has recently provided a detailed review of personalized medicine (Tabery 2023). To a large extent, his book is a biography of Francis Collins, head of the National Institutes of Health for much of the period. Collins is an engaging personality who often brings his guitar to press conferences. Tabery shows both how Collins followed an essentially reductionist approach to personalized medicine, while at the same time using engaging language (like "personalized medicine" itself) to suggest a much broader scope.

Tabery recounts how the NIH assumed in 2003, with the completion of the mapping of the human genome, that the blueprint for effective personalized medicine was at hand. The reality turned out to be quite different. The number of conditions that were determined by single gene substitutions turned out to be quite limited. Diseases like diabetes were caused by basic gene substitutions in a small minority of cases and in most instances were the product of an interacting array of genes.

Personalized medicine "works" for a small number of diseases, mostly cancers, which can be tied to specific gene sequences. Personalized medicine reduces the number of cases that can be treated—of all the cases of a certain cancer, only a minority will have the specific gene sequence. That means for the pharmaceutical company that produces the medicine that treats the cancer, even if it only slows the cancer growth, it reaches a much smaller potential market. The company must produce not only the treatment medication, but also the chemical test that identifies which patients should receive it. The end result is that the combination of testing and treatment is a very expensive proposition. Many patients eventually go bankrupt if they even have sufficient resources to begin the process. Moreover, studies have shown that sending the patient's blood to different labs, or to the same lab at different times, often produces different results as to the suitability of the medication.

The NIH leadership reacted to the promise and the limitations of the new genomic medicine mainly by designing new studies that involved huge pools of research subjects, upwards of hundreds of thousands, to assure that extremely rare gene sequences would be identified. To encourage support for these efforts, the NIH continued to push the promise of personalized medicine, which soon morphed into "precision medicine." The Precision Medicine Initiative Cohort Program became the All of Us Research Program. The publicity about the NIH research efforts continued to stress "getting the right treatment to the right patient at the right time" and studiously avoided acknowledging the fundamentally reductionistic research framework.

Tabery contrasts these research efforts with the study of SIDS deaths ("crib deaths"). In 1991, SIDS was a leading cause of infant mortality. Research in the 1940s had suggested a linkage between these deaths and prone sleep position, but these findings were largely ignored. By the 1980s, observational studies across the globe again focused attention on infant sleep position, and new studies of multiple environmental factors strongly supported sleep position as a causative factor. That led the child health portion of NIH to launch the Back to Sleep campaign, as a result of which infant deaths from SIDS dropped by almost 60 percent. Genome-based research could not have achieved this result.

Activism and Bioethics

Activism in bioethics is often characterized by the phrase, "speaking truth to power." The activist bioethicist is particularly concerned about vulnerable populations. These populations must be assured of a reasonable place in the capabilities list of Amartya Sen and Martha Nussbaum, including the right to full political participation (Nussbaum 2006, 76–8). The activist bioethicist will therefore be especially concerned about vulnerable populations denied equal or full political participation, and in general, with any dominance of authoritarianism over democracy.

It is generally taken for granted that the United States functions as a democracy and that one must treat the two dominant political parties more or less as equals in this endeavor. Unfortunately, this was once true but is no longer the case. One of the two parties has largely abandoned its role within a democratic system and has become more and more a white-supremacist party. Steven Levitsky and Daniel Ziblatt list three characteristics, besides eschewing white supremacy, that a political party must have to qualify as a "loyal" democratic party. First, the party must respect the outcomes of fair elections, win or lose. Second, the party must avoid violence as a means of achieving political ends. Third, the party must reject antidemocratic forces, especially those that appear democratic on the surface but support violent or authoritarian goals. Levitsky and Ziblatt go into detail about how the Republican Party fails on all these measures (Levitsky and Ziblatt 2023, 40–1)

Discrimination against African Americans has gone through two distinct phases since the Second World War. At first, under affirmative action, Blacks showed some advances in university degrees, for example. Then a reverse movement took hold, and the community at large decided that anti-Black bias had now been corrected, and any affirmative action steps in the future would amount to unfair advantages toward the Black community. Black attendance in higher education either held steady at low levels or declined further.

As summarized by Keith Payne (Payne 2017, 157–8):

> A 2011 survey asked a nationally representative sample of white and black Americans to rate how much they thought both blacks and whites were targets of discrimination in each decade from the 1950s to the 2000s. Both groups of respondents agreed that antiblack discrimination had decreased during the course of those decades, although whites thought that it had fallen much more steeply than blacks did. The two groups differed even more strikingly, though, in their perception of antiwhite discrimination. Black respondents thought antiwhite bias was not a problem in the 1950s and was still not a problem today. White respondents, in contrast, believed that antiwhite bias had steadily risen in the period in question. Whites seemed to view discrimination as a zero-sum game. The less discrimination they perceived against blacks, the more they saw it turned against whites. The trend was so stark in the eyes of white respondents that by the 2000s they judged discrimination against whites to be a bigger problem than discrimination against blacks. (Norton and Sommers 2011)
>
> The data, however, tell a very different story. The income gap between white and black families has remained more or less constant since the 1960s. In 1967 the average black family earned 55 percent of what white families earned. In 2011 that figure was 59 percent. (Kochhal and Fry 2014)

The V-Dem (Varieties of Democracy) Institute gives world political parties an "illiberalism" score, measuring deviation from norms like pluralism and civil rights, tolerance of opposition, and rejection of violence. The US Republican Party had a very low score through the late 1990s, but its score greatly increased in the twenty-first century. By 2020, it was less typical of center-right governing parties and more similar to autocratic or authoritarian parties such as the ruling party of Hungary (Luhrman et al. 2020, 1–2).

Few political groups in the United States are openly white supremacist. Instead, the popular position on the political right has become the fear that powerful elites have taken charge and that ordinary folks are suffering as a result. These elites are seen as favoring diversity, so taking an anti-elite stand means stifling efforts at diversity.

As early as Richard Nixon's southern strategy, white-supremacist thinking was disguised as talk of "law and order" and opposition to busing and desegregation. White supremacy has reached new levels in the era of Donald Trump. Levitsky and Ziblatt (2023, 117) write:

> Whereas his Republican rivals were reluctant to use openly racist, nativistic, or demagogic appeals, Trump readily crossed those lines. His unique willingness to say and do things that other Republicans rejected as bigoted, racist, or cruel allowed him to dominate the market for white grievance votes. As the political scientist Ashley Jardina writes, Trump's campaign signaled to white voters that he intended to "maintain the racial hierarchy." (Jardina 2019, 230–45) Indeed, studies show that white Republicans who perceived their group's status to be threatened were most likely to support Trump in the primaries. As Ezra Klein aptly put it, "Trump didn't hijack the Republican Party. He understood it." (Continetti 2022)

These points go to establishing today's Republican Party as dominated by white supremacy. On what basis can I go on and accuse the party of antidemocratic sentiments? The Republican Accountability Project assigned a "democracy grade" to all Republican members of Congress in 2021, based on six criteria:

- Signed amicus briefs to the US Supreme Court to nullify votes in Michigan, Wisconsin, Pennsylvania, and Georgia
- Objected to the certification of the Electoral College vote on January 6, 2021
- Made public statements casting doubt on the 2020 election results
- Did not vote to impeach Trump for his activities on January 6, 2021
- Voted against creating an independent commission to investigate January 6 activities
- Voted against holding Steve Bannon in contempt of Congress for refusing to comply with the congressional subpoena

Of all Republican members of Congress, 161 of 261 took antidemocratic actions on five of the six measures. Another fifty-four adopted antidemocratic positions on four of the six. Only sixteen Republicans adopted consistently democratic positions across the board, and most of these had either been defeated or had retired by 2022. In the 2022 primary election season, the *New York Times* counted more than 100 television ads in which candidates brandished or fired guns. Levitsky and Ziblatt commented,

"We can think of no other major party in any contemporary Western democracy in which candidates so openly embraced violence" (Levitsky and Ziblatt 2023, 125).

Levitsky and Ziblatt are bold in offering solutions to the present predicament, including:

- Create national standards for automatic voting eligibility at the age of eighteen and issue national ID cards
- Make Election Day a Sunday or a national holiday to eliminate any conflict between work and voting
- Abolish the Electoral College and replace it with a national popular vote
- Abolish the Senate filibuster
- Term-limit Supreme Court justices (Levitsky and Ziblatt 2023, 232–5)

This list of measures seems to go well beyond any agenda for activist bioethics, but it arguably is necessary if we are to avoid becoming an authoritarian, white-supremacist state.

Lisa Parker (2022) notes, "Perhaps the pressing question for bioethics is whether reasoned arguments can still persuade" (681), and adds, "The people . . . remain moral equals and are worthy of respect at least insofar as they participate in the knowledge production process, via reasoned argument, civil discourse, and scientific inquiry. Those who lapse into bullying, manipulation, violence, or deception warrant censure" (Parker 2022, 688). But she also notes,

> Bioethics should also help prepare the public to accept evolving knowledge and to participate in the ongoing process of knowledge production. Doing so may require increased understanding of people's feelings, especially their feeling of belonging to communities that constitute an important part of their identities. This may be especially challenging, but especially important when a constitutive part of such a community is its rejection of the processes of knowledge production. Yet we must try. (Parker 2022, 691)

Many would object to my comments on activist bioethics as moving unacceptably from ethics to politics. In reply, I would propose as an example the hearings of Sen. Max Baucus in 2009 on the Affordable Care Act, in which the senator ordered the arrest of attendees who openly supported a single-payer plan (Nichols 2009). Partly as a result of the senator's actions, many millions of Americans today lack health insurance. I would argue that this is an ethical problem as well as a political issue. Thus, the senator's refusal to consider single-payer as a policy option had both ethical and political implications. To say that an issue is political, and therefore is removed from the domain of health care ethics, is arbitrary.

Richard Wilkinson and Kate Pickett argue for greater equality of personal income in the United States, which would at first appear to be a purely political agenda (Wilkinson and Pickett 2011). They claim that making this change would have a number of significant effects:

- Reduced rates of mental illness
- Reduced rates of obesity
- Lower teenage birth rate
- Significant reductions in crime rate with much lower prison populations
- Longer life expectancy
- Thriving economy allowing for greater overtime and vacation
- Greater trust among the population

They provide a series of graphs. Each graph shows the rate of the phenomenon in question (e.g., mental illness) among the world's richest twenty-three nations, ranged against income inequality. The graphs look more or less identical. Japan and the Scandinavian countries show the lowest rate of the problem and also the lowest rate of income inequality. The other countries are arrayed along a line, with rising rates of the problem associated with greater income inequality. One country deviates markedly from the general line. In each instance, the United States shows both a much higher rate of the problem and a much higher rate of income inequality. Wilkinson and Pickett argue that it is highly unlikely, given the similarity among the graphs, that income inequality just happens to be higher in each case; rather, it is much more likely that there is a causal relationship at work here.

Some of the factors that Wilkinson and Pickett have graphed seem clearly to be in the political realm, such as crime rates and economic well-being. Other factors seem to be issues of health—mental health, pregnancy rates, and life expectancy. Wilkinson and Pickett argue that all factors are equally affected by income inequality. Bioethics therefore needs to address income inequality as one causal factor in a number of health care issues. In particular, US bioethics needs to address the question of why income inequality is omitted from most political discussions about health care and other social problems. This is an illustration of the intersection between bioethics and politics.

The Future of Bioethics

Ironically, to some extent, the future of bioethics may be contained in its origins. Van Rensselaer Potter is credited with the creation of the modern concept of bioethics in his 1971 book, *Bioethics: Bridge to the Future*. He drew especially on the tradition of the "land ethic" of Aldo Leopold, stating, "*Ethical values* cannot be separated from *biological facts*. We are in great need of a land ethic, a wildlife ethic, a population ethic, a consumption ethic, an urban ethic, an international ethic" (Potter 1970, 127). Potter's expansive idea of bioethics, however, was soon pushed aside by the narrow concept of the ethics of biomedicine and the individualistic physician-patient or researcher-investigator relationship.

Stephen Gardiner has laid out a notion of bioethics as part of planetary health, drawing on the report of the Rockefeller Foundation-Lancet Commission (Gardiner 2022; Whitmee et al. 2015). First, a planetary bioethics would call attention to the current inequalities between rich and poor nations, the history of colonialism, and the role of rich nations in creating the structure of today's transnational institutions. Second, a planetary bioethics would pay equal attention to future generations and avoid the current practices of exploiting nature's resources today to the detriment of our children and grandchildren in an "intergenerational arms race." Third (and here going beyond what the Foundation called for), a planetary bioethics would avoid anthropocentrism and show respect for the value of both human and nonhuman life. The result, says Gardiner, is a "fully environmentalized vision of bioethics" (Gardiner 2022, 583).

Donna Orange, a psychoanalyst and philosopher, calls for a "radical ethics" to address the climate crisis (Orange 2017). She notes that the questions of climate change and social justice are inextricably linked: "Climate justice theorists agree that we must adopt no solutions to our current emergency except those that improve the lot of the poorest and most vulnerable people. Keeping intact the way of life for those already living luxuriously cannot be the priority that first world nations and their citizens seem to assume it to be" (Orange 2017, xiv).

> [T]he term "climate justice" . . . involves, I think, two inextricable elements: (1) reducing carbon in the atmosphere to the 350 parts per million needed for a livable planet . . . , and (2) doing this in a way that not only does not further harm the world's most vulnerable people, but also restores some measure of basic dignity to their lives. (Orange 2017, 22)

Orange, who lives in California and teaches in New York City, adds that she recently found out that a single one-way flight from home to New York uses up her personal carbon allowance for one year.

Orange links our unwillingness to address climate change to America's lack of awareness of their "original sin" of slavery and colonial settlement: "*Climate injustice is racism*, unconscious perhaps, but racism all the same, inherited of course, but now our guilt and our responsibility" (Orange 2017, 54, italics in original). She calls on her psychoanalytic background to address much that remains unconscious in our daily lives: "I believe that the very cultural myths that hide envy from our view—that every individual can climb out of poverty and have as much as everyone else, and that my wealth does not disadvantage anyone—are based on an avoidance of shame. The same mentality hides from us the consequences of our carbon-and-methane, oil and beef, lives" (Orange 2017, 76).

To arrive at climate justice, Orange believes that no currently popular system of ethics—Kantian or duty ethics, utilitarianism, or virtue ethics—will do the job. She calls instead for a radical ethics of three elements. One is the dialogical phenomenology of Hans-Georg Gadamer; the second is Asian philosophy such as Jainism. She spends most of her time on the third element, Emmanuel Levinas's argument that the start of moral reasoning lies not with the moral agent, but with the suffering of the other. She finds the basis of Levinas's reasoning in the biblical image of Abraham, whose tent was open on all sides and any stranger was bidden to share a meal:

> To keep the tent open today means not only welcoming refugees into our countries, and at least temporarily into our homes, learning their languages, and learning

> what they need to feel less homeless and bereft. It also means turning a corner on the institutional injustices that bring them, that have turned their homes into deserts and war zones. It means reforming our own lives radically, seeing the links between their suffering and our mindless comforts, learning every day. I believe, actually, that only a radical ethics of the fundamental worth of every human life will make the difference we need in the climate crisis. Until we can see, really see, ethically see, that our carbon-hungry "lifestyle" harms, even destroys, the other whose suffering places an infinite responsibility on me, nothing will change, really. (Orange 2017, 120)

Conclusion

So, what is today's bioethicist to do? Organize more community dialogues on new subjects? Work to abolish the Electoral College? Strive to reduce her own carbon footprint?

First, one should adopt a view of bioethics in which each of these activities is an essential stage or ingredient. Arguing with each other that one of us or another is not doing "real" bioethics is a sure recipe for stagnation. Today's "real" bioethics includes standard approaches such as utilitarian and deontological ethics and the four principles, virtue ethics, narrative ethics, and approaches adapted from feminism, to name only some of the methods incorporated. Anyone adopting a novel approach may be viewed merely as seeking to expand the methodological armamentarium of bioethics.

Second, it is worth noting that each of the four sections of this chapter has alluded to community dialogue in one form or another. To my knowledge, learning the basics of running a community dialogue process is not a part of the training in most graduate programs of bioethics. My generation of (older) bioethicists thought it was our job to write papers by ourselves or along with a few colleagues, and to teach courses in the accepted graduate school manner. The future of bioethics seems to demand a much more robust role for public dialogue.

Bibliography

Bonham, V. L., T. Citrin, S. M. Modell, T. H. Franklin, E. W. B. Bleicher, and L. M. Fleck. 2009. "Community Based Dialogue: Engaging Communities of Color in the United States' Genetics Policy Conversation." *Journal of Health Politics, Policy, and Law*, 34 (3): 325–59.

Brody, H. 2009. *The Future of Bioethics*. Oxford University Press.

Brody, H., S. A. Croisant, J. W. Crowder, and J. P. Banda. 2015. "Ethical Issues in Patient-Centered Outcomes Research and Comparative Effectiveness Research: A Pilot Study of Community Dialogue." *Journal of Empirical Research on Human Research Ethics*, 10(1): 22–30.

Continetti, M. 2022. "Donald Trump Didn't Hijack the G.O.P. He Understood It." *The Ezra Klein Show*, May 6, 2022.

Crowder, J. W., and P. L. Determeyer. 2019. "Optimizing Community Bioethics Dialogues: Reflections on Enhancing Bi-directional Engagement on Health Care Concerns." *Narrative Inquiry in Bioethics*, 9 (3): 259–73.
Engel, G. L. 1977. "The Need for a New Medical Model: A Challenge to Biomedicine." *Science*, 196: 129–36.
Fleck, L. M. 1994. "Just Caring: Oregon, Health Care Rationing, and Informed Democratic Deliberation." *Journal of Medicine and Philosophy*, 19: 367–88.
Gardiner, S. M. 2022. "Environmentalizing Bioethics: Planetary Health in a Perfect Moral Storm." *Perspectives in Biology and Medicine*, 65 (4): 569–85.
Garland, M. J., and R. Hasnain. 1990. "Health Care in Common: Setting Priorities in Oregon." *Hastings Center Report*, 20 (5): 16–18.
Jardina, A. 2019. *White Identity Politics*. Cambridge University Press.
Jennings, B. 1988. "A Grassroots Movement in Bioethics." *Hastings Center Report*, 18 (S3): 1–15.
Kochhal, R., and R. Fry. 2014. "Wealth Inequality Has Widened Along Racial, Ethnic Lines Since End of Great Recession." *Pew Research Center*, December 12, 2014. www.pewresearch.org/fact-tank/2014/12/12/racial-wealth-gaps-great-recession
Levitsky, S., and D. Ziblatt. 2023. *Tyranny of the Minority*. Crown.
Luhrmann, A. et al. 2020. "New Global Data on Political Parties: V-Party." V-Dem Institute Briefing Papers No. 9, Oct. 26, 2020: 1–2.
Martin, J. C., R. F. Avant, M. A. Bowman et al. 2004. "The Future of Family Medicine: A Collaborative Project of the Family Medicine Community." *Annals of Family Medicine*, 2 (S1): S3–S32.
Nichols, John. 2009. "Baucus Healthcare Plan: Arrest Doctors, Nurses." *The Nation*, May 12, 2009. https://www.thenation.com/article/archive/baucus-healthcare-plan-arrest-doctors-nurses/(accessed January 2, 2024).
Norton, M. I., and S. R. Sommers. 2011. "Whites See Racism as a Zero-sum Game That They Are Now Losing." *Perspectives on Psychological Science*, 6: 215–18.
Nussbaum, M. 2006. *Frontiers of Justice: Disability, Nationality, Species Membership*. Belknap Press of Harvard University Press.
Orange, D. M. 2017. *Climate Crisis, Psychoanalysis, and Radical Ethics*. Routledge.
Parker, L. S. 2022. "Bioethics in the Current Climate." *Perspectives in Biology and Medicine*, 65 (4): 680–93.
Payne, K. 2017. *The Broken Ladder: How Inequality Affects the Way We Think, Live, and Die*. Viking.
Potter, V. R. 1970. "Bioethics, the Science of Survival." *Perspectives in Biology and Medicine*, 14: 127–53.
St. Vincent's House and Galveston Island Community Research Advisory Committee. 2016. "Community Bioethics Dialogue: Mental Health and Seniors. Final Report." March 28, 2016. https://hopeandhealingcenter.org/wp-content/uploads/St-Vincents-and-GICRAC-FINAL-Report-Mental-Health-03282016.pdf (accessed October 20, 2023).
Tabery, J. 2023. *Tyranny of the Gene: Personalized Medicine and Its Threat to Public Health*. Alfred A. Knopf.
Whitmee, S. et al. 2015. "Safeguarding Human Health in the Anthropocene Epoch: Report of The Rockefeller Foundation–Lancet Commission on Planetary Health." *Lancet*, 386 (10007): 1973–2028.
Wilkinson, R., and K. Pickett. 2011. *The Spirit Level: Why Greater Equality Makes Societies Stronger*. Bloomsbury Press.

Witnessing Difference and Responding to Vulnerability

5

Othering, Recognition, and Health Justice

Nancy M. P. King

Bioethics needs to take better account of structural injustice. The field's vision has been impeded by a too-easy focus on individual autonomy, which deflects attention from the social and structural barriers that help traditionally privileged communities maintain minoritized groups as inherently inferior "others." Justice requires us to look beyond the walls of hospitals, clinics, and medical academia to address and ameliorate the structural injustices that give rise to health disparities—and to do so long before differential access to health services becomes an issue for underserved patients. This change in focus is no simple matter. It demands engagement in challenging multidisciplinary collaborations, which enable us to understand the sociohistorical complexities of health and illness, appreciate the factors that contribute to shaming and blaming those "others" who are not "us," and work to lessen the discomfort with uncertainty that impedes equity. All of this necessary work takes bioethics well beyond the well-trodden pathways of our usual scholarship and practice. But we simply have to reach higher to do health justice (King, Churchill, and Henderson 2022. See also Powers and Faden 2006).

A Brief History and Theory of Othering

"Othering" is a matter of health justice because it is a human problem of long standing; the habit of dividing ourselves into discrete groups of "us" and "others" is pervasive and has become even more extensive and entrenched in recent times. Just when we imagined that global communication could help break down the barriers dividing groups from one another, those barriers appear to have strengthened.

The many profound divides between "us" and "them" matter for health care in multiple ways, and for health in even more ways. These divides are reflected in health disparities, and thus become matters of health justice. This chapter touches on history, theory, and narrative to examine othering, to connect it with social and structural inequities, and to chart a path forward to do health justice.

Othering begins from an unavoidable reality: each of us is "me" and, starting from birth, everyone else is fundamentally an "other." Many of the scholars who have been important to philosophical bioethics—Levinas, for instance (Bergo 2019)—have addressed the relationship between self and other. Hospitality and solidarity are based on service to and alliance with the other (Jennings and Dawson 2015). Thus, what makes othering problematic is not the reality of the distinction between self and other, but what follows from categorizing a reference "self" group and stigmatizing and blaming the "others" outside it.

In 2008, law professor Charity Scott published an essay in the *Hastings Center Report* on "Belief in a Just World" (Scott 2008). It remains a striking example of the rationale behind othering and blaming. In the essay, Scott describes an effort to inform the public about and strengthen support for PeachCare, Georgia's version of the state children's health insurance plan. The *Atlanta Journal-Constitution* profiled a family whose children were benefiting because PeachCare made it possible for their parents to provide them with adequate health care. But to everyone's surprise, the response from readers was not at all sympathetic to the family. Readers blamed the parents for having too many children and not working at better-paying jobs, thus freeloading on the hardworking taxpayers of Georgia. As Scott explains, the public strongly supported PeachCare when asked about it in the abstract, but their views about "deserving" families did not seem to match that general support. Instead, a belief that the world is just engenders what seems to be a paradoxical response. If the world is just, then people get what they deserve and deserve what they get. The harder they try to succeed, the more blameworthy they are likely to be if they fail (Appelbaum, Lenon, and Aber 2003). Belief in a just world thus neatly enables othering: those who are in need can be blamed and stigmatized for their lack of success, and the prosperous can be distinguished as inherently different from people who fail.

Belief in a just world perpetuates othering through its inability to acknowledge the possibility of structural injustice. Because structural injustices disadvantage individuals by restricting their opportunities regardless of their efforts, it seems that it should be possible to effectively counter belief in a just world by demonstrating the reality of the social structures that perpetuate disparities adversely affecting "deserving others." Instead, belief in a just world simply bypasses consideration of social and structural influences, leaving room for nothing more than individuals' choices and actions.

This focus on individuals is recognizable and arguably familiar in some religious reasoning and may be echoed by health care workers frustrated by patients' failures to adhere to providers' recommendations. Its emphasis on free choice and individual responsibility is easily extended to concluding that failure comes only to those who are lazy, disobedient, or weak-willed. For example, patients with obesity who are unable to lose weight are often blamed and shamed and characterized as lacking in willpower, regarded as plainly other by people with "normal" BMIs. It will be interesting to see whether what is being learned about Wegovy and similar drugs can destigmatize obesity, since America's obvious social and cultural obsession with junk food and fast food hasn't seemed to promote recognition of the structural forces affecting diet and nutrition.

Professor Scott's essay connects belief in a just world with public health ethics. Unfortunately, if we have learned anything from the COVID-19 pandemic, it is that public health ethics is complicated, controversial, and contested. And in order to understand more about why othering is so common, so detrimental, and so antipathetic to considerations of solidarity and structural justice in health and health care, we need to start well before the pandemic.

Consider the beginnings of bioethics. The 1960s and 70s saw enormous growth in attention to civil and political rights for minoritized groups like women and people of color; bioethics' focus on the rights of patients fit perfectly. Patient autonomy fundamentally changed the physician-patient relationship by emphasizing the authority of decisionally capable patients to make health care choices for themselves, using information and recommendations from their physicians without being expected to follow all medical recommendations.

That important change, along with most other key controversies in bioethics, requires continuous contextual consideration in both scholarship and practice. In this instance, ongoing attention to autonomy has helped strengthen bioethics' focus on individuals rather than groups or institutions. Public health focuses explicitly on communities and populations; therefore, public health ethics might be expected to help bioethics broaden its focus beyond the individual.

Paradoxically, however, that might not always work. Fifteen years ago, Jeff Kahn and Anna Mastroianni published a chapter on public health ethics in the *Oxford Handbook of Bioethics* (Kahn and Mastroianni 2009). It is thoughtful and impressively encyclopedic, and it describes public health as always in tension with individual rights. The authors link bioethics' origins to the civil rights movements of the 1970s and argue that the principles of bioethics "arguably operate best when the perspective of decision making is the individual patient or research subject" (Kahn and Mastroianni 2009, 675, referring generally to Beauchamp and Childress). Most importantly, they emphasize that public health can justify "overriding individual rights" (Kahn and Mastroianni 2009, 673). They view the tension between communities and individuals as a conflict; resolving the conflict in favor of the public's health must mean that an individual's rights are overridden. This clash appears to leave no room for nuance or continuum; it is about "me" versus a collective "other."

Whenever the need for public health action arises, it is essential to make a nuanced and contextual assessment of whether and when to override individual rights; that is what public health ethics is all about. When public health and safety are employed to justify collective action, the existence of a potential conflict with individual rights might simply strengthen the conviction that individual autonomy is and should be paramount, as we saw during the COVID-19 pandemic. Resistance to lockdown measures, masking, and vaccination transformed a public health crisis into an us-versus-other conflict with extensive stigmatization of others, reinforcing the perception that the individual "me" versus whoever is or are the others is always a zero-sum fight. That perception arises from a desire to make things simple and clear once and for all: no need to deal with uncertainty or nuance.

Some Stories about Othering

When I was in law school, I took a course on law and psychiatry. The psychiatrist who was a co-instructor told the class that he regarded everyone, including himself, as somewhere on a continuum of mental illness and mental health. It hadn't occurred to me that a continuum view was possible or plausible, yet it made far more sense than viewing people with mental illness as other, belonging to a separate category of people completely distinguishable from, and lesser than, people regarded as "sane" and "normal." Yet mental illness is almost universally othered, perhaps because it is both difficult to understand (see, e.g., Hudson 2023) and frightening to contemplate. The distance of othering provides reassurance, however illusory that bright line might be. It took me a long time to recognize the bravery of the teaching psychiatrist's continuum view.

Fauci, the documentary that premiered in fall 2021 about the career of Dr. Anthony Fauci, provides interesting insights into how othering in American health care and public health has both persisted and transformed in recent times (Hoffman and Tobias 2021). The documentary examines American responses to HIV and Ebola and briefly touches on COVID-19. The story of HIV is familiar: identified after Kaposi's sarcoma became known as the "gay cancer," HIV infection and AIDS resulted in stories of PPE-clad health-care providers sliding food trays into hospital rooms and backing away. The fear of contagion othered gay men, injection drug users, Black and brown people all over the world, and even children with hemophilia (remember Ryan White?). Tony Fauci and Larry Kramer have both eloquently discussed how Fauci came to understand why people with HIV sought faster research progress (Fauci 2024). Since those early years, developments in research and treatment have made HIV infection into a complex chronic disease and even rendered it largely preventable.

Nonetheless, HIV infection is still stigmatized. Its stigmatization in China played a central role in He Jiankui's transgressive "CRISPR babies" project. His goal was to genetically edit zygotes to be resistant to HIV, so that the resulting gene-edited adults would be unlikely to become infected with HIV and thus would not be othered by it. The HIV-discordant couples who enrolled in He's research may have done so in order to conceive and bear children without risking infection of the woman or the fetus. It is well known that sperm washing and IVF, both essential to He's research, are very effective in preventing infection in the woman and offspring of discordant couples, but assisted reproduction is prohibited in China for anyone who is HIV-positive (Rana 2019).

Ebola infection presented a similar story of panic and isolation, at least initially. (Progress has since been made; see, e.g., World Health Organization 2023.) When nurse Kaci Hickox returned from relief work with Ebola patients in West Africa, she was imprisoned in an outdoor tent on the grounds of a New Jersey hospital, despite negative test results (Gatter 2016). Widespread panic ensued in New York City after Dr. Craig Spencer, who also returned from relief work with Ebola patients, traveled on the subway before being diagnosed with Ebola (Spencer 2015). The fear of contagion with a deadly disease othered Black people and an entire continent, even though the route of transmission is physical contact with infected bodily fluids, as with HIV; mere proximity is harmless. The development of successful treatment—with Spencer as an elite white poster boy for the same—has not yet completely eliminated the stigma.

When COVID-19 infection became widespread, the extent and nature of othering in the pandemic became complex, even paradoxical. The scale and severity of the infection, the rapidity with which information was shared about routes of transmission, the lack of information about effective prevention, and the continual development of a wide variety of treatment methods combined to isolate those infected and separate them from loved ones. This was truly tragic, but not initially associated with stigmatization or blame; health-care providers worked exceedingly hard, often at great personal risk, to save the lives of those infected.

Othering came instead from an unexpected direction. Before vaccines were developed, masking, the closing of businesses and schools, and other attempts to slow viral spread had life-disrupting consequences, including loss of income and jobs, business closures, evictions, and supply chain problems. As a result, public health efforts were widely criticized, particularly by those who were reluctant to believe how serious COVID-19 infection could be. The exponential growth of social media, with its echo chamber effect, helped to blame and other those who sought to protect themselves and the public by following public health guidance. In turn, those who sought to protect themselves and their loved ones blamed and othered a growing population of extreme science skeptics. Tolerance for uncertainty almost disappeared as perspectives hardened.

The development of vaccines, the failure of public discussion about the meaning of vaccine effectiveness, and the politicization of views about science have extended and expanded the othering of divergent views. With effective vaccines widely available, health-care providers have continued to struggle to avoid blaming infected unvaccinated patients; yet unvaccinated status is a point of pride for some, and failure to obtain boosters and vaccines for new COVID variants is now common. Vaccination status supports reciprocal othering: the vaccinated and masked are blamed for any requirements that may still at times impede normal daily life, and the unvaccinated and unmasked are blamed for making normal life difficult for anyone seeking to avoid infection. Since the emergence of new variants and infections from new strains have continued, the paradox of reciprocal othering seems destined to continue, even as preventive and protective measures diminish.

Little of this is new, of course. Long before the spread of COVID-19 vaccination conspiracy theories, polio eradication worldwide has periodically been hampered by rumors that the vaccine contains nefarious ingredients (Jegede 2007). In the global North, childhood vaccination remains deeply contested and compromised by Andrew Wakefield's amply discredited research. But the wholesale adoption of pro- and anti-COVID-19 vaccination stigmatization and blame on a population-level scale seems unprecedented (Moreno, Sandor, and Schmidt 2021).

Othering has appeared in many health contexts and has long played a role in responding to patients and those at risk of illness. Pregnant people have been kept out of the workforce, subjected to a range of discriminatory practices, and blamed for their diets, habits, and activities during pregnancy. Nonsmoking women with lung cancer often experience delays in diagnosis and are often considered untruthful after diagnosis because smokers are othered and blamed for that disease.

Race correction in clinical algorithms (Vyas, Eisenstein, and Jones 2020) is just one of many examples of race-based othering. There is an extensive and persistent litany of pernicious misconceptions based on a patient's skin color, including false beliefs about pain sensitivity combined with skepticism about reported pain. In the days of the one-drop rule, being diagnosed with thalassemia—often mistaken for sickle-cell disease—could lead more rapidly to a determination that the patient must be Black than to treatment recommendations. Contemporary research literature is still far too likely to include statements that amount to "We controlled for everything else and there is still a disparity between Black and white patients, so there is probably a genetic explanation." Examples are as pervasive as bioethics' failure to address them (Hoberman 2016).

Racism also displays othering's paradoxical effects. Social scientists have described survey research results showing that "highlighting COVID-19 racial disparities can reduce support for safety precautions among white U.S. residents" (Skinner-Dorkenoo et al. 2022, 1). The authors note:

> Reading about the persistent inequalities that produced COVID-19 racial disparities reduced fear of COVID-19, empathy for those vulnerable to COVID-19, and support for safety precautions. These findings suggest that publicizing racial health disparities has the potential to create a vicious cycle wherein raising awareness reduces support for the very policies that could protect public health and reduce disparities. (Skinner-Dorkenoo et al. 2022)

This result is not surprising if we acknowledge that White Americans might prefer to continue othering Black Americans, and therefore might regard public health protections as less necessary because they are not Black. As the authors conclude:

> Our findings suggest that alerting the public to racial health disparities (such as those observed with COVID-19) has the potential to perpetuate systemic racial inequalities—by reducing White U.S. residents' concerns about public health issues and support for policies aimed at protecting public health. . . . Thus, publicizing COVID-19 racial disparities could reduce support for the very policies that aim to limit the toll of the pandemic, creating a vicious cycle wherein raising awareness of systemic racial health disparities results in public responses that actually exacerbate these disparities. (Skinner-Dorkenoo et al. 2022, 1)

The need to assert a distinction between "us" and "others" thus appears to preclude the possibility that anyone other than "us" might be unfairly treated, even when that unfairness arises from social structures, like public-facing employment during a pandemic, that have little or nothing to do with individual effort or desert. This perspective accords with the persistence of the belief that race has genetic reality—

there could be no easier argument for a perfect, permanent, and unbreachable gulf between white and Black individuals, including patients. That othering actually puts us all at greater risk—physical, political, and moral—is obvious, but difficult to counter.

What Can We Do about Othering?

For nearly all living things, survival depends on the collective resistance of "us" groups to predation by dangerous "other" groups. This means that countering othering is inherently difficult because it requires promoting solidarity with those who are not the same as us or members of our "us" group. Solidarity thus demonstrates the possibility of changing and enlarging who counts as "us"; humans change and expand our group identifications all the time. As we move through life, we develop friendship groups that differ from the family groups in which we grew up. This distinguishes us from most other living things, ironically reinforcing the view that humans are fundamentally different from nonhuman animals and making animals "other." (Our long-standing and long criticized uses of fauna and flora exclusively for human benefit are countered by the One Health concept, which is in part an attempt to acknowledge continuity between humans and animals and to extend solidarity to all living things (Centers for Disease Control and Prevention n.d.).)

Solidarity preserves important differences between "us" and "other" without the adverse consequences of the distinction. According to Jennings and Dawson, solidarity "does not negate diversity at all but, rather, establishes the grounds of its respect, protection, and perpetuation. It amounts to saying that I stand here both as a human person dependent upon the integrity of a complex human community and as a human being with needs and rights common to my kind, my humanity" (Jennings and Dawson 2015, 37).

For Jennings and Dawson, solidarity is essential to overcoming a society that prioritizes othering and corresponds closely with belief in a just world:

> a society in which the interests of each individual (including one's health status) are seen as sui generis and fundamentally distinct from the interests of others. . . . If my interests are fulfilled and yours are not, then I gain and you lose: I am fortunate, you unfortunate; I am skillful and successful, and you are not. . . . If I am healthy and you are sick, your low level of health does not affect in any way my high level of health because we are essentially separate beings. . . . The factors leading to health (or illness) are assessed for each individual separately and serially. And they are normatively assessed serially as well: in the biography of each individual, we find healthy or risky behavior, responsible or irresponsible conduct, compliance with scientific recommendations concerning a healthy lifestyle or foolish and self-indulgent choices. . . . A vision of the individual agent unencumbered, as it were, by solidarity is a vision that stresses the uniqueness of each person and emphasizes difference and separation rather than sameness and commonality. (Jennings and Dawson 2015: 32–3)

The challenge of moving away from this vision and responding to othering is central to health justice and must be made a routine part of bioethics moving forward. Autonomous individuals need relationships, communities, and the support of solidarity in order to promote and protect health and increase health equity. We have to be able to show that the zero-sum game is simply wrong.

There are three actions that bioethics scholars and practitioners should take to support solidarity and counter othering: seeking comfort with uncertainty, identifying and ameliorating social and structural injustice, and promoting meaningful conversation and engagement. Each is difficult; all are complementary, intertwined, and therefore contemporaneous. Most challenging, all three should be undertaken not only within health care and on behalf of patients but also outside healthcare institutions in order to address the social and structural injustices that adversely affect the health of individuals and groups who are not yet patients.

Unequal Treatment, the groundbreaking Institute of Medicine (IOM) report that tried to identify and address race-based inequities in health care, was published over two decades ago (Smedley, Stith, and Nelson 2003). The observations of the IOM are largely unchanged today, despite the report's conclusions and recommendations, which identified structural aspects of the health-care system as causal and recommended systemic reforms (including increases in treatment access and affordability), better data collection, and improved provider education. In 2023, the National Academies of Sciences, Engineering and Medicine was asked to update the IOM report. The update, *Ending Unequal Treatment* (National Academies of Sciences, Engineering and Medicine 2024), reaches very similar conclusions.

Uncertainty

The IOM report described uncertainty in health-care providers as one cause of unequal treatment and identified provider education as one potential means of reducing the uncertainty that results in differential diagnosis and treatment across groups more and less familiar to a given provider. Bioethics can do more to confront uncertainty and the deep desire to make it go away, but this effort should extend beyond health care providers. Uncertainty is unsettling to everyone; most of us try hard to avoid it. Uncertainty accounts for much of the natural human fear of illness; science and medicine promise to conquer it with answers and engender faith for that reason. But science and medicine are increasingly rejected when the answers they provide change or are imperfect or incomplete. Uncertainty is also warded off by belief in a just world, which posits that there are clear ways to distinguish "us" from "others" and thus keep us safe.

Although public and provider education about uncertainty can indeed help, locating the source of othering solely in the individual, directing education toward individuals alone, can inadvertently perpetuate the othering feedback loop. That's why identifying and ameliorating the mechanisms and institutions that support othering by perpetuating inequities is equally essential. Many of those structural sources are found within health care: race-corrected clinical algorithms, differential access to specialty care, and more

(Churchill, King, and Henderson 2020). *Ending Unequal Treatment* details many vital recommendations focused on structural injustices that cause significant health care inequities. But there are even more fundamental sources of structural injustices that affect individuals through their perceived group memberships, including but not limited to rapidly increasing inequalities in opportunity, employment, income and wealth, education, neighborhood quality, and municipal service provision (Churchill, King, and Henderson 2022; see also Powers and Faden 2006).

Social and Structural Justice

Without addressing structural injustice, the pernicious habit of othering cannot be overcome. But understanding and addressing structural injustice takes bioethics beyond its health care comfort zone: the social, structural, legal, and policy supports for othering represent the complex context that surrounds and grounds health and illness. This social context has profound health effects well before health care, or even public health, is at issue at all (Berwick 2020). The social drivers of health influence health and illness throughout lifespans and across generations, yet structural injustice is not usually recognized as part of the territory of bioethics. If we hope to help providers, patients, policymakers, and the public address uncertainty better, stop blaming and shaming others, and expand and strengthen the connections between people and public health, then we have to stretch ourselves as well.

Everyone in bioethics must embrace doing justice as readily as we study, write, and teach about autonomy, beneficence, and nonmaleficence—even though justice is difficult and diffuse. In order to do this, we need to recognize what social epidemiologists, public health scholars and practitioners, and other social scientists have long articulated: that there is a nuanced relationship between scientific and societal causes of health disparities (Matthew 2022; Villarosa 2022). Broad multidisciplinary communication and collaboration across bioethics, the social sciences, medicine, and public health are necessary to integrate genetics, biochemistry, and other relevant scientific perspectives with political and social policies and practices like zoning, infrastructure, funding, and even physiological responses to chronic stress (King, Churchill, and Henderson 2022; Williams, Lawrence, and Davis 2019). Bioethics should both encourage and participate in research seeking to establish causal relationships between structural injustices and health disparities and to identify and test structural reforms to improve health (King 2022). This research should be a central goal of academic learning health systems (National Academies 2024).

Conversation and Engagement

Progress in these essential ways requires effective communication. There have been many unsuccessful efforts to change the conversation about health justice and othering.

Productive conversation has lately become even more difficult, but the need for it is ongoing. As Jennings and Dawson point out, societies tell stories about themselves, and individuals tell stories about their places in society. "One vital function of bioethics is to inform and shape those stories. Bioethics has the potential to offer society a keener insight and perception of what is ethically at stake in controversies concerning health, science, and society" (Jennings and Dawson 2015, 31).

One of the reasons why bioethics has not yet succeeded in changing the conversation is that conversation is necessarily mutual. Opening oneself to conversation with others is difficult, fraught with potential errors, and even threatening. It entails both willingness and ability to talk together. The science fiction novel *The City in the Middle of the Night*, by Charlie Jane Anders (2019), is about othering: othering based on class distinctions in one city-state, othering based on rivalry between two city-states with very different cultures, and othering that makes a sentient native species into a food animal for human colonists on a hostile and alien planet. All these layers of malignant othering are enabled by resistance to communication and failures of the moral imagination whereby we recognize the limits of our own perspectives. Mutual conversation can facilitate that recognition and help expand the limits of our perception. Human characters in the novel are continually forced to confront their limited views and the consequent misinterpretations of others' words and actions, all caused by failing both to share information with others and to be receptive to the information others seek to share (see, e.g., Anders 2019, 179–83, 190–6, 199–201, 206–8). We must be ready to engage in unexpected ways and with unanticipated conversation partners. Ted Chiang's (2016) short story "The Great Silence" offers a profound example; the speaker is a parrot, who notes the eagerness of humans to seek conversation with extraterrestrials while failing to realize the potential partnerships here at home (Chiang 2016; see also Yong 2022).

There are many ways to talk together, and some are more productive than others. In a convocation address at St. John's College nearly thirty years ago, philosopher Michael Dink described four ways of thinking about engaging in discussion, which is the centerpiece of a St. John's College education. One model is based on the story of the blind men and the elephant, in which each person recognizes the partiality of an individual viewpoint, and all perspectives combine to reach a single common and more correct perception. The question to ask about this model is whether talking together is merely a means of achieving a correct viewpoint.

Another model is Darwinian, positing that discussion is a competition in which only the best viewpoints will survive. The question to ask, of course, is what we mean by "best" and whether it has any inherent meaning aside from survival.

A third model looks to deliberative discussion, which is intended to facilitate decision and action. This model often becomes primarily a negotiation; like the Darwinian model, it risks replacing the pursuit of ends having independent value with a view of negotiation as nothing more than a power play.

Recognizing the shortcomings of each of these models of conversation leads to a very different conclusion:

> that there is some sense in which conversation with one another is more fundamental than and prior to any conception of the goal that we hope to achieve through that conversation. Openness to what others have to say, respect for them as sources of intelligibility, a willingness to share our thinking and to risk having it criticized and rejected, a readiness to be moved and changed in response to what others say . . . perhaps . . . conversation with others is an essential condition for having a common and intelligible world about which we can seek to achieve clarity or in which we can pursue our ends.

It may thus be essential to understand conversation as having "a dignity and worth not derived from its goal" (Dink 1999).

Conversation, understood this way, is plainly the beginning of engagement. The obligation of engagement has been masterfully articulated in a brief essay by Tod Chambers. He argues "that bioethics as a field has a vested interest in actively fostering cross-political engagement" because "all academics need to . . . engage with those who have a different worldview and, in doing so, make ourselves conscious of our assumptions. This does not mean that we must abandon our values if challenged, but that we, as academics, have a primary responsibility to justify them" (Chambers 2023, 2).

Because engagement is unlikely to overcome all differences of opinion, bioethics must also help create "public policies that preserve a recognition of moral disagreement so that, even in those situations where one position must win over another, the values of the losing position are still in some fundamental manner respected in the policy" (Chambers 2023,2). This does not extend to taking seriously any argument made in bad faith, nor does it mean engaging with those who refuse to attend to facts. But "bioethics has a basal obligation to actively create forums for those of good faith to engage with each other" (Chambers 2023,2; for a very similar perspective, see also Holm 2009).

Conclusion

When we practice and teach human engagement, we necessarily recognize the inherent dignity and worth of those with whom we seek to talk and engage. And there can be no more powerful antidote to stigmatizing, shaming, and blaming the other than that core recognition. Replacing othering with justice in health care, public health, and human research thus requires profound structural change and continual engagement. This is hard work and an ongoing effort; bioethics has barely begun to make it. Yet we in bioethics have always sought to take seriously the experience, the reality, the humanity of all others. Building a healthy world together can only proceed from that deceptively simple beginning.

Bibliography

Anders, Charlie Jane. 2019. *The City in the Middle of the Night*. Tor Publishing Group.

Appelbaum, Lauren D., Mary Clare Lennon, and John Lawrence Aber. 2003. "How Belief in a Just World Influences Views of Public Policy." National Center for Children in Poverty. Columbia University.

Beauchamp, Tom L., and James Childress. 2019. *Principles of Biomedical Ethics*, 8th ed. Oxford University Press.

Bergo, B. 2019. "Emmanuel Levinas." In E. N. Zalta and Uri Nodelman (eds.), *Stanford Encyclopedia of Philosophy*. https://plato.stanford.edu/archives/fall2019/entries/levinas/.

Berwick, Donald M. 2020. "The Moral Determinants of Health." *Journal of the American Medical Association*, 324 (3): 225–6.

Centers for Disease Control and Prevention (CDC). n.d. *One Health*. https://www.cdc.gov/onehealth/index.html (accessed January 5, 2024).

Chambers, Tod. 2023. "The Obligation of Engagement." *Hastings Center Report*, 53 (1): 2.

Chiang, Ted. 2016. "The Great Silence." In *The Best American Science Fiction and Fantasy* 2016. Houghton Mifflin Harcourt.

Churchill, Larry R., Nancy M. P. King, and Gail E. Henderson. 2020. "The Future of Bioethics: It Shouldn't Take a Pandemic." *Hastings Center Report*, 50 (3): 54–6.

Dink, Michael. 1999. "What Do We Hope to Achieve in Discussion?" *St. John's Reporter* Spring: 6.

Fauci, Anthony. 2024. *On Call: On Call: A Doctor's Journey in Public Service*. Penguin.

Gatter, R. 2016. "Quarantine Controversy: Kaci Hickox versus Governor Chris Christie." *Hastings Center Report*, 46 (3): 7–8.

Hoberman, J. 2016. "Why Bioethics Has a Race Problem." *Hastings Center Report*, 46 (2): 12–18.

Hoffman, T., and J. Tobias. 2021. *Fauci*. National Geographic. https://films.nationalgeographic.com/fauci.

Holm, Soren. 2009. "Policy-Making in Pluralistic Societies." In Bonnie Steinbock (ed.), *Oxford Handbook of Bioethics*, 153–74. Oxford University Press.

Hudson, Annika. 2023. "The Words that Stick Forever." *Mad in America*, December 22, 2023. https://www.madinamerica.com/2023/12/words-that-stick-forever/?mc_cid=11c19dea23&mc_eid=781acec84d.

Jegede, A. S. 2007. "What Led to the Nigerian Boycott of the Polio Vaccination Campaign?" *PLoS Med*, 4 (3): 417–22.

Jennings, B., and A. Dawson. 2015. "Solidarity in the Moral Imagination of Bioethics." *Hastings Center Report*, 45 (5): 31–8.

Kahn, Jeffrey P., and Mastroianni, Anna C. 2009. "The Implications of Public Health for Bioethics." In Bonnie Steinbock (ed.), *Oxford Handbook of Bioethics*. Oxford University Press.

King, Nancy. M. P. 2020. "Justice and Domestic Health Research." *Ethics and Human Research*, 42 (3): 41–2.

King, Nancy M. P., Gail E. Henderson, and Larry R. Churchill. 2021. "Beyond the Medical Model: Retooling Bioethics for the Work Ahead." *American Journal of Bioethics*, 21 (2): 53–5.

King, Nancy M. P, Larry R. Churchill, and Gail E. Henderson. 2022. *Bioethics Reenvisioned: A Path Toward Health Justice*. University of North Carolina Press Press.
Matthew, Dayna Bowen. 2022. *Just Health: Treating Structural Racism to Heal America*. New York University Press.
Moreno, J., J. Sandor, and U. Schmidt. 2021. "The Vaccination Cold War." *Hastings Center Report*, 51 (5): 12–17.
National Academies of Sciences, Engineering and Medicine. 2024. *Ending Unequal Treatment: Strategies to Achieve Equitable Health Care and Optimal Health for All*. National Academies Press.
Powers, Madison, and Ruth Faden. 2006. *Social Justice: The Moral Foundations of Public Health and Health Policy*. Oxford University Press.
Rana, P. 2019. "How a Chinese Scientist Broke the Rules to Create the First Gene-Edited Babies." *Wall Street Journal*, May 10. https://www.wsj.com/articles/how-a-chinese-scientist-broke-the-rules-to-create-the-first-gene-edited-babies-11557506697.
Scott, C. 2008. "Belief in a Just World: A Case Study in Public Health Ethics." *Hastings Center Report*, 38 (1): 16–19.
Skinner-Dorkenoo, A. L., A. Sarmal, Kasheena G. Rogbeer, Chloe J. André, Bhumi Patel, and Leah Cha. 2022. "Highlighting COVID-19 Racial Disparities Can Reduce Support for Safety Precautions Among White U.S. Residents." *Social Science and Medicine*, 301: 1–8.
Smedley, B. D., A. Y. Stith, and A. R. Nelson. 2003. *Unequal Treatment: Confronting Racial and Ethnic Disparities in Health Care*. National Academies Press.
Spencer, C. 2015. "Having and Fighting Ebola: Public Health Lessons from a Clinician Turned Patient." *New England Journal of Medicine*, 372 (12): 1089–91.
Villarosa, Linda. 2022. *Under the Skin: The Hidden Toll of Racism on American Lives and on the Health of Our Nation*. Knopf Doubleday.
Vyas, Darshali A., Leo G. Eisenstein, and David S. Jones. 2020. "Hidden in Plain Sight — Reconsidering the Use of Race Correction in Clinical Algorithms." *New England Journal of Medicine*, 383 (9): 874–82.
Williams, D. R., J. A. Lawrence, and B. A. Davis. 2019. "Racism and Health: Evidence and Needed Research." *Annual Review of Public Health*, 40: 105–25.
World Health Organization. 2023. "Uganda Declares End of Ebola Disease Outbreak," January 11, 2023. https://www.afro.who.int/countries/uganda/news/uganda-declares-end-ebola-disease-outbreak.
Yong, Ed. 2022. *An Immense World*. Random House.

6

Bioethics and Incarceration

Takunda Matose and Elizabeth Lanphier

The field of bioethics is deeply connected with incarceration. Whether it's the military-style incarceration of Nazi concentration camps and the medical experimentation that ensued in them,[1] or the instances of coerced experimentation in carceral facilities like the malaria experiments at Illinois' Stateville Prison, bioethical issues arising from settings of incarceration have been part of bioethical thinking for decades. Although historical medical events don't lend themselves to any singular bioethical analysis (Schicktanz, Michl, and Stoff 2021), legacies related to medical experimentation and incarceration are, arguably, central to the field's inception and founding. They have been a source of certain core bioethical documents that remain part of most genealogies of bioethics (see, for example, the Hastings Center Bioethics Timeline[2] or the chronology of events in Robert Baker's 2024 book *Making Modern Medical Ethics*). These include the Nuremberg Code and the explicit and specific protection of "prisoners" as a vulnerable population within federal research ethics regulations. These events have also yielded theoretical attention in bioethics, including how the concepts of autonomy, exploitation, and coercion are conceptualized with regard to vulnerability.

Incarceration continues to be an important topic for contemporary American bioethics as well. For example, a 2023 *Hastings Center Report* special issue was dedicated to health and incarceration. In that issue, as Sean Valles (2023) notes in the opening of his article commemorating fifty years of mass incarceration in the United States of America, bioethics scholarship on incarceration is certainly deep, if a bit narrow. While this depth of scholarship is commendable, we take this opportunity to not only evaluate its narrowness but also interrogate the relationship between bioethics scholarship and incarceration. Has the field's depth regarding directions and questions related to incarceration diverted attention away from the possibility of other pressing bioethical concerns that incarceration raises? Is the field's inattention[3] to that which falls outside the narrow depth into which it leans occluding important work that bioethics can and should be doing to better address contemporary problems of incarceration? Might widening the lens of bioethical considerations related to incarceration yield productive insights to enrich the field in terms of both its theoretical foundations and its practical impact?

In this chapter, we posit that carceral settings are communal spaces, and that individuals affected by the criminal legal system are themselves members of society more broadly. Consequently, we argue for two main points. First, we argue that bioethicists should engage more expansively with different aspects of incarceration. Second, we argue for a transformation of bioethics itself based on insights gained through that expansive engagement.

Incarceration and Bioethical Inquiry

The intersection between bioethics and carceral health has historically touched three areas: biomedical research, clinical ethics, and normative and conceptual work. On the research front, bioethical deliberation has focused on questions of coercion, exploitation, and vulnerability. As noted above, the core principles for permissible medical experimentation articulated in the Nuremberg Code were developed as a direct response to the research abuses of concentration camp incarceration in Nazi Germany and are central to the self-identity and foundation of bioethics. Bioethical inquiry into research and incarceration continues to be influenced by this seminal document.

In keeping with the core principles articulated in the Nuremberg Code, contemporary questions on research and incarceration focus on improving carceral conditions and addressing issues like certain infectious diseases that disproportionately affect incarcerated persons. In the United States, this focus is seen in documents like the *Belmont Report* and the "Common Rule." As a response to reports of research abuse of incarcerated and unfree individuals, these documents establish the importance of conducting medical research only when there is clear, voluntary, and uncoerced consent. Additionally, these documents identify incarcerated persons as a vulnerable population and provide them with research protections above those available to less vulnerable research populations.

Clinically, bioethical inquiry also aims to address issues that are uniquely produced or exacerbated by incarceration. For example, how can people who are incarcerated receive health care that is equivalent to the care provided to people outside of carceral contexts (e.g., Eichelberger, Wertli, and Nguyen 2023)? Or how should we mitigate and address communicable infections that are more transmissible or prevalent within congregate living settings like carceral facilities (e.g., Lehtmets and Pont 2014)? There are also questions about how to address the mental health problems that disproportionately impact people who are incarcerated (e.g., Lehtmets and Pont 2014).

As some of these examples suggest, recognizing the unjust conditions of historically coerced experiments in carceral contexts has also been essential to how the concepts of vulnerability, coercion, and informed consent more broadly have been articulated in bioethics. Similarly, incarceration raises important questions regarding legal and ethical obligations to access healthcare since the constraints of incarceration press on many assumptions about healthcare, rights, and bioethical principles like autonomy and justice. These questions have been central to several key legal cases like *Estelle v. Gamble* (1976) and *Costello v. Wainwright* (1977) that have in turn influenced how and what we think about what is owed to incarcerated persons. Thus, the questions arising from carceral contexts in bioethics also influence *normative* and *conceptual* considerations in bioethics applied to both research and clinical care.

Incarceration in Bioethics' Present

Given this background, recent efforts at concerted engagement with questions of incarceration in bioethics are an extension of a longer history. As these examples show, bioethics *is* and has been involved in carceral health, and incarceration can be thought of as playing a central role in the development of bioethics, particularly in US bioethics. At the same time, bioethics has been central to the development and maintenance of ethical standards for various dimensions related to carceral health. Primarily, bioethics has been influential in righting prior wrongs regarding how research and clinical care occur in carceral contexts, but not in interrogating the bioethics of incarceration itself. This means that in research, bioethics has helped respond to prior injustices and unethical research with guiding norms and standards for ethical research in carceral contexts as with the National Commission for the Protection of Human Subjects of Biomedical and Behavioral Research and the creation of the *Belmont Report*. Regarding clinical care, clinical ethicists are sometimes consulted by hospital systems treating patients who are part of the criminal legal system. Such involvement in criminal legal systems can at times be incidental to ethical dilemmas in patient care or can be a key contributor to them.

Yet, we believe traditional bioethical principles and frameworks—some of which have developed explicitly in response to injustices that occurred in carceral settings—have proved inadequate for addressing bigger picture ethical problems arising in carceral healthcare. The existing frameworks are at times insufficient to address research and clinical needs in carceral contexts. Sometimes they may in fact be harmful in how they work against the health interests and health justice for incarcerated folks.

For example, respect for autonomy is often cited as a central principle in biomedical ethics. Yet, as is also often the case in situations outside of carceral contexts, merely *naming* the concept of autonomy without explaining what autonomy is and how to support or achieve it doesn't do much to clarify what it ought to mean for the specific research or clinical case in which it is being invoked (i.e., Dive and Newson 2018). What autonomy ought to mean regarding research and clinical engagement for incarcerated individuals, for whom incarceration is a means of constraining their autonomy in certain domains, is even more complicated. And a concept like autonomy may prove harmful if unreflectively applied in carceral contexts, as we discuss in relation to our examples below.

The impact of the Covid-19 pandemic on incarcerated populations and the communities in which they are incarcerated illustrated that health is not only something that needs to be managed within carceral facilities (Lanphier and Behne 2023), but that carceral facilities impact community health (Gifford 2019). The Covid-19 pandemic thus draws new attention to thinking about incarceration as a problem for public health and public health ethics that may not be resolved through existing bioethical approaches. It also provided examples of the unique ways that questions like fair access to healthcare, surrogate decision-making for incapacitated persons, and participation in research studies in carceral contexts are not easily resolved with traditional bioethical approaches, as we illustrate in more detail below.

Theories of Incarceration

A full review of the literature theorizing the purpose and justification of incarceration is outside the scope of this chapter; however, we need to briefly acknolwedge the literature debating both the purpose of incarceration and the logic justifying the state's authority to incarcerate. These debates impact normative bioethical arguments regarding health and incarceration broadly, and considerations regarding research or clinical care in carceral contexts. Moreover, there are practical aspects of how incarceration functions in the United States, separate from its intended or theoretical purpose, that impact the scope of healthcare rights and duties related to incarcerated populations.

There are four main theories of punishment: retribution, deterrence, incapacitation, and rehabilitation (Patch 2013). A retributivist account uses incarceration to impose a punishment on an individual that is meant to be proportional to the seriousness of the crime for which they are found guilty, while deterrence is meant to impose a cost for committing a crime that deters an individual from committing it. Both models presume that individuals are making decisions to engage in criminal activities with a good deal of free will. Using the language of bioethics, we might say these models presume individuals are making highly autonomous choices, are aware of the risks of engaging in criminal activity, and choose to do so in the context of having reasonable alternatives. Such presumptions may or may not be correct.

Two other models of incarceration, incapacitation and rehabilitation, take what might be considered health or public health-related approaches. Incapacitation as a theory of punishment presumes that people who commit criminal offenses may do so again, and incarceration incapacitates them from doing so, for the public good. Gregg Caruso (2021) has a version of an incapacitation theory that he considers a public health "quarantine" model. One challenge with incapacitation theories is that it is not possible to know which offenders will commit future offenses, unlike quarantining individuals with known infectious disease or exposure. Rehabilitative theories take the function of incarceration to be rehabilitating the incarcerated individual to reenter society as an effective citizen. However, unlike in the case of a medical patient requiring physical or occupational therapy after illness or injury, there is no clear prescription for rehabilitation for criminal offenses, if meaningfully rehabilitative services are available at all.

Regardless of the theory of punishment operative in incarceration, practically incarceration always serves a punitive function. The state assumes the ability to circumscribe the rights and privileges ordinarily granted to its citizenry when incarceration constrains the rights to freedom of movement that non-incarcerated individuals ought to enjoy. At the same time, as we discuss later, the state's decision to confine an individual to a specific location for punitive purposes also entails a custodial relationship to those it incarcerates. The incarcerated person becomes almost entirely dependent on the state, and their well-being becomes the state's responsibility. This custodial role toward incarcerated persons requires the state to provide for the incarcerated individual's basic needs.

Carceral Settings, Healthcare, and Bioethics

Healthcare is among those basic needs, though the scope of the state's obligation to fulfill it is variable. US Supreme Court decisions have established a constitutionally protected right to healthcare for incarcerated individuals (including the already mentioned *Estelle v. Gamble* 1976, and *Deshaney v. Winnebago County* 1989). Yet this putative right does not entail a guarantee of healthcare access, either in terms of availability or affordability of care. Many incarcerated individuals in the United States pay hefty co-pays to access basic medical care and high prices via prison commissaries for routine over-the-counter medications, let alone specialized prescriptions or medical care (Avila 2022). But to the extent that Supreme Court decisions set precedents requiring healthcare provision for prisoners, it's still telling that such healthcare often must be secured through further legal action on the part of incarcerated persons and is not simply the default. Importantly, we want to highlight how prisoners' healthcare options were restricted enough for them to require legal intervention to achieve whatever protections they have received, and that legal action continues to be necessary to assert rights to access treatment.

Returning to unreflective applications of a concept like autonomy in carceral contexts, harm can occur in at least two ways. One way in which harm occurs is when it's assumed that all competent adults are free to exercise autonomous healthcare choices without accounting for the significant constraints on such choices faced by competent incarcerated adults. Another way in which harm occurs is when it is assumed that the punitive function of incarceration constrains the autonomy of incarcerated individuals to such an extent that they are presumed unable to make *any* autonomous decisions, including regarding their own medical care. The first type of harm ignores the limitations to expressions of autonomy faced by the incarcerated. The second harm removes the medical decision-making agency of the incarcerated and overextends the custodial role of incarceration to act as the individual's medical custodian.

In failing to register the alternative expressions of autonomy that are necessitated and possible within carceral contexts, both these harms ultimately render incarcerated individuals *more* vulnerable, even by a kind of analysis initially intended to underscore the vulnerability of incarcerated individuals and protect them as patients or research subjects from exploitation or coercion. At the same time, the combination of an incarcerated individual's lack of free movement (to seek out healthcare) and the state's minimal fulfillment of its custodial role (to maintain incarcerated persons' well-being) effectively constrains one's medical autonomy regarding the range of available medical options for their healthcare needs. Yet this valence of medical autonomy in carceral contexts often goes underappreciated in the clinical and research ethics literature.

Building on this general tension regarding the application of a bioethical principle of autonomy in carceral contexts, we'll briefly sketch three kinds of cases related to carceral health that are typified in the bioethics literature but that we argue remain inadequately addressed. These cases include research participation, surrogate decision-making, and access to medical care. Each could be the topic of its own essay, and our aim here is to merely illustrate where traditional bioethical approaches fall short when applying these topics in carceral contexts. In response to what we see as current bioethical inadequacies of thought, and action, the rest of this chapter turns to an account of how incarceration should have a bigger impact on bioethics and how in turn bioethics should impact incarceration.

Research Participation

Even bioethicists who interface little if at all with incarcerated individuals are likely aware that US federal regulations on research identify "prisoners" among the vulnerable groups warranting special protections. The Common Rule states that the purpose of this additional guidance is to provide direction "Inasmuch as prisoners may be under constraints because of their incarceration which could affect their ability to make a truly voluntary and uncoerced decision whether or not to participate as subjects in research" (45 CFR §46.302). Biomedical and behavioral research with "prisoners" permitted by the regulations is largely limited to that which is about the direct study *of* incarceration and carceral facilities or conditions recognized as disproportionately impacting incarcerated persons (45 CFR §46.306).

There are at least three things to note about such research protections, which originate from an unjust history of experimentation on incarcerated populations but remain inadequate to address the scope of vulnerabilities entailed by incarceration. One is that designating prisoners as a vulnerable population in research does not protect them from potential quasi-research abuses conducted outside of clinical trials, to which carceral conditions may render them acutely vulnerable. For example, during the Covid-19 pandemic, one carceral facility administered ivermectin to incarcerated individuals without their knowledge or consent, and outside of any official treatment or research protocol (Hernandez 2022).

Second, the Common Rule's attention to *possible* coercion or the compromising of voluntariness of consent is important but should not be confused with implying that, by definition, the conditions of incarceration negate voluntary consent or are necessarily coercive such that incarcerated individuals are unable to make sufficiently autonomous decisions.

The third thing to note is that requiring research conducted with incarcerated individuals to be narrowly about incarceration or carceral populations is yet another constraint on autonomous decision-making to self-determine one's own priorities for research participation. It might also exclude individuals from research from which they may directly or indirectly benefit. Taken together, these points raise questions about whether the very regulations put in place to protect a vulnerable group do not, at times, render the population more vulnerable.

Surrogate Decision-Making

Another source of vulnerability for incarcerated individuals, but in the clinical context, is through the presumption that their carceral status makes them unable to provide consent to medical treatment. As mentioned above, this presumption may occur if clinicians or ethicists assume that the state has the authority to control medical decisions as part of its punitive control. In such cases, healthcare teams may inadvertently further undermine autonomy by deferring to the carceral facility's decisions for incarcerated patients who retain medical decision-making capacity (as a clinical determination) and competency (as a legal determination).

That said, an incarcerated patient can lack medical decision-making capacity due to their clinical status and require a surrogate decision-maker. In these cases, identifying the appropriate surrogate for incarcerated patients may be a matter of following and applying state laws (Scarlet, DeMartino, and Siegler 2019). However, state laws, such as those that indicate a department of corrections official should act as the surrogate, may not reflect standard ethical approaches to surrogate decision-making. In some cases, healthcare facilities seek guidance from carceral facilities for patient decision-making, even when there are patient-chosen surrogates involved, due to deference or uncertainty about authority (Batbold et al. 2024). Although involvement in patient decision-making might align with the state's custodial function toward incarcerated persons, the state's concurrent punitive function undermines the possibility that it could make fair medical decisions on the individual's behalf without significant conflicts of interest.

Moreover, a corrections official is unlikely to know the patient's values and preferences to apply the optimal standard of adult surrogate decision-making, substituted judgment. Ideally, incarcerated patients would have someone who knows their values and preferences make medical decisions on their behalf as any other patient would. The designation of the appropriate surrogate would follow a state's hierarchy for appointing decision-makers in the absence of a pre-appointed proxy or power of attorney, which often involves identifying appropriate family or friend decision-makers. However, this also introduces challenges. For example, the state likely applies its punitive powers to control when and if an incarcerated person can have contact with their family and friends (i.e., phone and visitation restrictions) and extends this control to when an incarcerated individual is hospitalized or otherwise obtaining medical treatment. In some cases, individuals may be incarcerated for criminal offenses against family members who would appear on a typical hierarchy of surrogate decision-makers. In other cases, these relationships have been disrupted for so long that it's not clear whether family and friends are best positioned to know the incarcerated person's values or preferences. In cases like these, the state could play a relevant role in delineating who should not be approached as a decision-maker but may also overreach in this role.

Identifying appropriate surrogate decision-makers can be fraught in many situations in which incapacitated patients do not have pre-appointed surrogates (and even in some cases in which they do, and they are not fulfilling their duties as surrogates) regardless of carceral status. These situations often raise questions of who has authority to make decisions, who may have conflicts of interest, and how they are making decisions. While it may on the surface appear that these questions are simplified for incapacitated incarcerated patients, we contend that standard ethics of surrogate decision-making interact with the roles and realities of incarceration in ways that only complicate matters further.

Access to Medical Care

Guidance imported from research regulations into clinical care recognizes the ways in which incarcerated individuals may be vulnerable to coercion in their medical decision-making or may understandably worry about medical abuses in ways that compromise relationships with medical providers and treatment planning. Even in cases where incarcerated individuals are recognized as their own medical decision-makers, questions may arise regarding whether their consent to treatment is sufficiently voluntary if they may, for example, perceive potential nonmedical benefits from pursuing a particular treatment (i.e., being able to recover in the hospital rather than having to return to the carceral facility) or may not perceive the significance of potential harms (i.e., if a harmful outcome seems less risky given their baseline living conditions). Other questions may arise regarding whether consent is sufficiently informed if, for example, an incarcerated patient is counseled on the risks, benefits, and alternatives of treatment but does not have access to those alternatives.

That is to say that the very treatment options to which one does, or does not, have access create other potential, and often overlooked, constraints on medical decision-making in carceral contexts. The state has a custodial function to protect incarcerated persons' basic needs, and medical treatment is a constitutionally protected right and need for incarcerated populations in the United States. However, protecting health and well-being as a *basic* need does not articulate the specific level of healthcare provision the state must fulfill (short of through lawsuits when incarcerated individuals claim the state has failed to fulfill its duties, which, when successful, result in specific obligations on the part of the state). And although the state as custodian effectively becomes the payor for healthcare for those it incarcerates, it can, like many payors, implement co-pays that deter or in some cases prohibit accessing timely, needed medical care.

Moreover, the punitive function of incarceration to limit incarcerated individuals' freedom of movement practically delimits their access to medical care, which must either be brought into the facility or coordinated at an outside facility. Accessing care becomes at the discretion of the carceral institution rather than initiated by the care-seeking individual and can impact obtaining medical diagnoses and treatments as well as treatment options if they are constrained by practical access to resources, caregivers, transportation, or specialized care.

While both the potential cost of medical care and its logistics are barriers for many individuals regardless of carceral status, they exacerbate barriers for those in carceral settings. Although incarceration may not negate one's general moral or cognitive capacity to make autonomous decisions, the lack of access to meaningful choices constrains medical autonomy in ways that standard deployments of autonomy and debates about it in the literature don't easily address, let alone resolve.

Moreover, the constellation of these issues—research participation, surrogate decision-making, and access to care—challenges the assumption that the vulnerability of incarcerated persons means they are best protected when their care is entrusted to the state. This model renders incarcerated persons susceptible to the whims of the same state that is also placing them in the vulnerable position of being incarcerated. The very nature of this vulnerability might occasionally warrant *expanding* access to research and developing different approaches to health care access and delivery for incarcerated populations. Additionally, the nature of vulnerability in carceral contexts (e.g., Victor 2019) might warrant reconceptualizing how bioethics applies and understands these issues.

Relationality in Carceral Contexts and Bioethics

In our view, then, incarceration introduces considerations and challenges into these bioethical areas of inquiry that bring into question some standard bioethical responses. At the same time, we want to suggest that some of these considerations might be relevant to non-carceral issues in bioethics, particularly for patients and research subjects at the margins (of society, of kinship structures, of healthcare access, of capacity, etc.). Yet these cases remain inadequately addressed by standard bioethical responses. One reason for this inadequacy is that despite bioethicists expressing a variety of views on each of these topics, they generally operate through a relatively limited set of frameworks that don't fully account for how different conditional factors can affect people with the same bioethical issues. Our objective in the rest of this chapter is to explore a few considerations that help explain why incarceration troubles standard bioethical frameworks before suggesting how bioethics might better meet these challenges.

One reason why incarceration poses a significant challenge for many bioethical frameworks is the unique way it disrupts, distorts, and produces relationality. Incarceration often begins with disrupted relationality. This disrupted relationality is apparent in two competing models of criminality. The interactionist model accounts for social causes and characterizes criminalized behavior in terms of structural and relational failures. In contrast, the positivist model characterizes criminalized behavior in terms of psychological, cognitive, or biological causes.

As we have previously argued (Lanphier, Matose, and Abdur'Rahman 2020), we are partial to the interactionist model given the way it captures how many incarcerated individuals are not afforded the kind of economic, social, and moral scaffolding necessary to avoid the criminal legal system. Nonetheless, even on the positivist model, criminalized behavior is often characterized in terms of a disrupted relationship between victims and presumed perpetrators. On either model, however, incarceration also clearly disrupts the families and communities of the incarcerated person.

In the same way that incarceration disrupts relationality, it also distorts it. As we've previously suggested, and as others have argued, both incarcerated persons and corrections staff often come from similar socioeconomic circumstances (e.g., Hallinan 2001). In other words, shared circumstances often drive both groups to carceral contexts. Yet, these shared backgrounds are obscured by the power dynamics and carceral logics that turn incarcerated persons and corrections staff into antagonistic groups. Consequently, members of both groups have a distorted view of those with whom they might otherwise be in solidarity.

Yet incarceration also produces new forms of relationality and relational connections. For instance, within carceral contexts, new forms of relationality are created in carceral communities constituted by individuals who might not otherwise be in community together. Incarceration creates a single carceral population out of people who would have very different relationships outside carceral contexts. While incarceration thus creates new possibilities for solidarity, it nonetheless can reproduce broader social inequalities in a way that can create tensions between various carceral populations. This possibility shows that while all incarcerated persons can experience vulnerability by virtue of their social status as incarcerated persons, some will inevitably experience further intersecting forces of oppression by virtue of their economic status, racialization, or gender status. Thus, intersectionality remains a factor in considering the communal dynamics of incarceration. All this means that people in carceral contexts encounter all the hallmarks of community. They form both positive and negative relationships with one another and must figure out how to navigate those relationships, including through social cooperation and problem-solving or face emergent dysfunction and harm above and beyond even what is mandated under various carceral logics.

Incarceration produces another distinct form of relationality that arises between the state and the incarcerated person. We've discussed the punitive and custodial functions of incarceration, which occur concurrently. These two dimensions of incarceration are another form of relationship, one that creates a complex web that requires deciphering which elements of incarceration are features of its custodial function of incarceration and which features are part of its punitive function. Importantly, delineating these various elements and determining whether and how they must be carried out becomes an ethical concern, particularly in ostensibly liberal democratic societies where the actions of the state are carried out on behalf of the citizenry.

If some version of what we're suggesting here is correct, then carceral institutions, and the criminal legal system more broadly, are all communal contexts where health-relevant ethical concerns should be expected to arise in the same way they might arise in society more broadly. Carceral institutions could be thought of as health care settings in direct and indirect ways. Directly, they affect and determine the health of incarcerated persons through their function as spaces of complete custodial control over incarcerated persons' lives, including the healthcare resources to which they do or do not have access. Indirectly, they are settings that could potentially enhance health by affording opportunities for mental and physical health improvement, but that perhaps more often undermine health by creating poor conditions for mental health (i.e., violent, untrustworthy, or isolating environments) and physical health (i.e., poor nutrition options, sometimes limited opportunity for physical activity, crowded conditions prone to communicable disease, etc.). Similarly, carceral institutions and the criminal legal system often have significant environmental and socioeconomic impacts on surrounding communities, further suggesting links to health reaching well beyond the confines of the carceral facility.

In many respects, these features of incarceration and the criminal legal system make them appropriate sites for bioethical engagement. However, as the inadequacies highlighted earlier suggest, bioethical engagement has been limited to a discrete set of issues in which merely applying existing bioethical frameworks generally falls short. But, even if these frameworks adequately addressed that discrete set of issues, we contend that those issues are not reflective of the full complement of bioethical concerns arising in both incarceration and the criminal legal system. The predominant bioethical engagement seems to presuppose that bioethical concerns arising in incarceration are like concerns that arise in non-carceral healthcare settings. If this is the case, then bioethical tools and frameworks developed for non-carceral settings should easily and appropriately translate to the criminal legal system. But if we're right and incarceration produces unique ethical issues, then bioethical engagement has not been adequately expansive, and its tools and frameworks might not be best for tackling the kinds of bioethical issues created by incarceration.

Incarceration and Bioethical Futures

There are at least three approaches the field of bioethics could take to the bioethical issues *within* carceral contexts and the bioethical issues raised *by* incarceration: continuation, revision, and abolition. In what follows, we attempt to provide an articulation of each of these approaches along with an assessment of their merits and disadvantages.

One approach to the issues we've raised would be to continue applying prevalent bioethical frameworks to ethical issues arising within carceral contexts, but to understand the range of relevant bioethical issues and questions applicable to these settings much more broadly. This approach would certainly improve upon the current situation since there are more issues to consider than the ones that tend to be engaged by bioethicists. Yet, as we've suggested, the impact of this approach might be limited. While a broader set of carceral questions would be brought within the purview of bioethics, the tools bioethics uses to address them may remain inadequate. This approach would deploy standard bioethics tools like respect for autonomy to the ethical issues of incarceration. Yet, as we've suggested, a principle like respect for autonomy likely needs reconceptualization to be applicable for incarceration given how the criminal legal system impacts the paradigmatic features of autonomy.

Another approach that might be more responsive to this latter concern is to revise bioethical engagement such that existing frameworks better reflect issues that are idiosyncratic to incarceration. A related approach might be a more radical revision, not of bioethical frameworks, but rather of the very modes of theorizing that bioethics engages. This would entail the development of new frameworks that rely on conceptual tools that capture carceral realities. The advantage of either of these revisionist strategies is that engagement with carceral questions can build on existing efforts in bioethics to think expansively about its very role and scope.

Revising bioethical theories and methods by being intentionally sensitive to how they could be better equipped to respond to existing issues in incarceration aligns with similar projects, some reflected in this collection, to rethink bioethical methods and concepts relevant to a wider notion of "bios." It is part of a project of reimagining bioethics for issues as wide-ranging as climate change and the Anthropocene to deliberative democracy. This approach might allow for the most immediate positive impact on the health and well-being of incarcerated persons and the communities in which they live and to which they return. Nonetheless, this approach has the drawback of accepting a kind of conservatism that, while potentially revolutionizing bioethics, might nevertheless be inadequate for challenging broader structural, political, and ethical issues with incarceration itself.

The approach that might best respond to this final worry would be to advocate for the abolition of the carceral system, as bioethicists like Jennifer James (2023) have argued. There is a compelling argument to be made for abolition, particularly in places like the United States where the criminal legal system not only results in disproportionately high rates of incarceration relative to its population but also replicates and exacerbates broader social inequities along racial and economic lines. The argument for abolition should be even stronger for bioethicists given the totalizing impact on health and well-being that incarceration has. Incarceration raises concerns regarding justice (a traditional bioethical principle, though one for which the shape and meaning of the term need to continually be articulated and refined when invoked) and also for key contributors to health as a social or structural determinant of health. That said, prison abolition often presents an ideal form of justice. As a result, abolitionists should address what we should do in the unjust meantime, to use Alison Jaggar's phrase (2019) about the period during which ideal conditions of justice are pursued but not achieved. The call to address the unjust meantime requires us to recognize that incarceration is an imperfect form of justice that still requires attention as more ideal justice is progressively realized.

Our view is that these approaches need not be mutually exclusive. Bioethics should be descriptive, normative, aspirational, and transformative. This means that bioethicists should meet bioethical concerns where they are, and in the world as it is, even as they think about and point to the world as it should be. If our view is right, then some of the discourse on both sides of the prison abolition debate might be misguided to the extent that it inadequately fails to engage and address extant issues in incarceration. For instance, as suggested above, some prison abolitionists fail to adequately address what we should do in the unjust meantime between current carceral injustice and abolition. On the other hand, defenders of incarceration (reformists) like Tommie Shelby (2022) and Thomas Douglas (2014) quickly premise their arguments on idealized societies and circumstances they conjure up. Both approaches are misguided and obscure what we take to be a central truth about any world in which incarceration exists; it is a necessarily nonideal and flawed world that requires immediate and concerted intervention in the pursuit of justice. Importantly, this is true about both the world in which incarceration can be defended as a necessity and one in which it is so indefensible that it needs to be abolished. In either case, the question of how to address extant injustice and harm remains.

It's also worth noting that the debate between reformists and abolitionists likely stems from competing conceptions of the type of justice that should be pursued when harms or wrongs occur. In general, incarceration—and the criminal legal system more broadly—aims at a particular kind of justice that frames the incarcerated as wrongdoers who need to be removed temporarily or permanently from society. The type of justice pursued by abolitionists, on the other hand, reframes those involved with the criminal legal system as members of society. While bioethical approaches focusing on access to healthcare for incarcerated populations need not (and perhaps typically do not) adopt abolitionist perspectives on *criminal* justice, they often share the abolitionist view of the incarcerated person as a member of society in matters of *healthcare* justice. In practice, those interacting with incarcerated patients in healthcare settings, including healthcare workers and ethicists, may hold commitments to a traditional or reformist view of criminal justice that regards incarcerated patients as outside of society. These traditional or reformist commitments are likely in tension with commitments to treat these patients as members of society who are nonetheless due healthcare justice.

The difference in how the incarcerated are framed between traditional, reformist, and abolitionist conceptions of justice might also foreground distinctions in moral philosophy between moral subjects and moral objects. Incarceration tends to frame the incarcerated as moral subjects or persons who ought to be held accountable in particular ways. Whereas abolitionist conceptions of justice, as well as bioethical ones, might consider incarcerated persons as moral objects, or persons to whom something is owed. As moral philosophers have argued, these two conceptions of individuals are often not mutually exclusive, and our objective is not to suggest that one or the other ought to take precedence. We only highlight that this difference might play a role not only in disagreements between views of justice for the purposes of criminal justice but also in tensions between criminal and bioethical justice that occur in the theory and the practice of administering medical care to incarcerated persons or including them in clinical research. This disagreement doesn't obviate the need to address the ethical issues that arise in the current system by suggesting it is merely a matter of conceptual difference. Instead, it shows how these challenging conceptual differences complicate resolutions to the ethical issues in practice.

Revolutionizing Bioethics; Revolutionizing Incarceration

So, what does a bigger impact for bioethics look like and how should the present injustice and harm of incarceration be addressed? Our aim in this chapter has been to highlight existing tensions while calling for more expansive bioethics engagement on the kinds of ethical issues that arise due to incarceration to produce specific recommendations. In that spirit, we conclude by pointing back to where we started this chapter. As we noted, incarceration has been an integral part of the origins and development of bioethics. However, for bioethics to have a bigger impact on incarceration, this engagement cannot and should not remain a historical artifact. Incarceration continues to generate ethical issues that are relevant to and interact with various approaches to bioethics.

Conceptual Work

We call on bioethicists doing conceptual work to pursue a few lines of inquiry. For example, what lessons can be gleaned from examining incarceration, and how can they inform existing frameworks and concepts? Similarly, given the inherently interdisciplinary nature of bioethics, what are the theories and perspectives that can be brought into the scope of bioethics to aid in this project of expanding the reach and impact of bioethics further into incarceration? There are also important conceptual questions about the role, function, powers, and responsibility of the state when it outsources management of carceral systems to the proliferating private and for-profit prison sector in the United States. Bioethics may be poised to analyze these questions considering parallels to for-profit healthcare systems in the United States and the contrast with socialized health systems in other nations. Finally, what concepts can be dispensed with, and where is there a conceptual lacuna that needs to be filled with further work?

Empirical and Applied Bioethics

We also call on bioethicists to reflect on their methodological approaches to build on the trend toward centering patient experience and diverse experiences. We believe that building on these approaches will allow more inclusive engagement with incarcerated populations and those impacted by the criminal legal system. These populations have been largely left out of being methodological informants and partners in clinical research, but also in bioethical research more broadly. As our own experience collaborating with incarcerated and formerly incarcerated colleagues shows

(Lanphier, Matose, and Abdur'Rahman 2020, Lanphier and Behne 2023), individuals with relevant direct experience are willing and capable partners in the process of reimagining strategies for addressing questions at the intersection of bioethics and incarceration. Growing interest in participatory bioethics research with incarcerated people also shows promise in this area (e.g., Abma, Voskes, and Widdershoven 2017). But even without direct partnership, there are ample opportunities for revolutionizing bioethical methodology through the incorporation of perspectives offered by those whose lives have been impacted by incarceration and the criminal legal system.

Activism and Advocacy

Finally, we call on bioethicists who see their role as involving activism and advocacy to agitate when we see misalignment between our political and social systems and health and well-being. Just as we might advocate for all sorts of other policies that impact health—even indirectly—we should understand incarceration and the criminal legal system to be a site of advocacy and activism. At the same time, we encourage epistemic humility, recognizing that others—often outside of academia, and deeply embedded in carceral systems and the lives of those impacted by them—are already actively working in these areas. As bioethicists, our engagement ought to be measured, additive, and respectful.

Bioethics and incarceration already intersect in each of these areas we've named. Consequently, we see this chapter as an invitation for all bioethicists whose work touches these areas to recognize and acknowledge how their work might be relevant to and could be influenced by incarceration. In other words, this chapter is an invitation to expand on existing efforts to account for how incarceration provides insights into both the possibility and limitations of ethical life. This is part of the bioethical project of addressing ethical failings in the bios. Scholars like Jennifer James and Andrea Pitts are already cognizant of this intersection and have been doing important work in each of these areas. We invite the field to recognize and build on their contributions and participate in their efforts. At the same time, we are calling for the bioethical engagement with incarceration to be reciprocal. That is, bioethicists should revise and expand their frameworks as they intervene on the ethical issues of incarceration. Doing so can only improve what we do while producing a bigger impact for our efforts.

Notes

1 Carl Elliot, in discussing his 2024 book *The Occasional Human Sacrifice* on research abuses with the Noncompliant Podcast, described how one of the whistleblowers about abuses at Willowbrook, a residence that housed and conducted research on intellectually disabled children, referred to it as "an American concentration camp." Attention to carceral logics in bioethics is not only relevant to those involved in the criminal legal system. https://noncompliantpodcast.com/2024/04/11/willowbrook

-whistleblowers-human-rights-carl-elliott-on-his-new-book-the-occasional-human-sacrifice/

2 The timeline is an online resource that can be found at https://www.thehastingscenter.org/bioethics-timeline/

3 The body of work that does reside at the intersection of bioethics and incarceration largely comes from more continental traditions and Foucauldian analysis. Yet these conceptual approaches are often outside the core methodologies for what is primarily an analytic, case-based style of American or English-speaking bioethics. Our own thinking is influenced by contemporary continental and pluralist thinkers on incarceration, including Andrea Pitts, Sarah Tyson, and Lisa Guenther, and by feminist philosophy and bioethics, another literature on the sidelines of mainstream bioethics.

Bibliography

Abma, Tineke A., Yolande Voskes, and Guy Widdershoven. 2017. "Participatory Bioethics Research and its Social Impact: The Case of Coercion Reduction in Psychiatry." *Bioethics*, 144–52.

Avila, Cecille Joan. 2022 "Prison Health Care is Only Available if You Can Afford It." *Prism*, October 31, 2022. https://prismreports.org/2022/10/31/prison-health-care-hidden-costs/.

Baker, Robert. 2024. *Making Modern Medical Ethics: How African Americans, Anti-Nazis, Bureaucrats, Feminists, Veterans, and Whistleblowing Moralists Created Bioethics*. MIT Press.

Batbold, Sarah, Jennifer D. Duke, Kirsten A. Riggan, and Erin S. DeMartino. 2024. "Decision-making for Hospitalized Incarcerated Patients Lacking Decisional Capacity." *JAMA Internal Medicine*, 184 (1): 28–35.

Caruso, Gregg D. 2021. *Rejecting Retributivism*. Cambridge University Press.

Costello v. Wainwright. 1977. 430 U.S. 325 (U.S. Supreme Court, 21 March).

DeShaney v. Winnebago Cty. DSS. 1989. 489 U.S. 189 (U.S. Supreme Court, 22 February).

Dive, Lisa, and Ainsley J. Newson. 2018. "Reconceptualizing Autonomy for Bioethics." *Kennedy Institute of Ethics Journal*, 28 (2): 171–203.

Douglas, Thomas. 2014. "Criminal Rehabilitation Through Medical Intervention: Moral Liability and the Right to Bodily Integrity." *The Journal of Ethics* 18 (2): 101–22.

Eichelberger, Markus, Maria M. Wertli, and Toan T Nguyen. 2023. "Equivalence of Care, Confidentiality, and Professional Independence Must Underpin the Hospital Care of Individuals Experiencing Incarceration." *BMC Medical Ethics* 24 (13).

Estelle v. Gamble. 1976. 429 U.S. 97 (U.S. Supreme Court, 30 November).

Gifford, Elizabeth J. 2019. "How Incarceration Affects the Health of Communities and Families." *North Carolina Medical Journal*, 80 (6): 372–5.

Hallinan, Joseph T. 2001. *Going Up the River: Travels in a Prison Nation*. Random House Publishing Group.

Hernandez, Joe. 2022. "Arkansas Inmates are Suing After Being Given Ivermectin to Treat COVID-19." *NPR*, January 18, 2022. https://www.npr.org/2022/01/18/1073846967/arkansas-inmates-ivermectin-lawsuit-covid-19.

Jaggar, Alison M. 2019. "Thinking About Justice in the Unjust Meantime." *Feminist Philosophy Quarterly*, 5 (2): 9.

James, Jennifer E. 2023. "The Problem Is Not (Merely) Mass Incarceration: Incarceration as a Bioethical Crisis and Abolition as a Moral Obligation." *Hastings Center Report*, 53 (6): 35–7.
Lanphier, Elizabeth, and M. Forrest Behne. 2023. "Prisons, Pandemics, and Personal Responsibility." In Katherine Sorrels, Lora Arduser, Danielle Bessett, Vanessa Carbonell, Michelle McGowan, and Edward Wallace (eds.), *Ohio under COVID*. University of Michigan Press.
Lanphier, Elizabeth, Takunda Matose, and Abu Ali Abdur'Rahman. 2020. "(Re)Imagining (Re)habilitation: An Argument from Death Row." *Public Philosophy Journal*, 2 (2).
Lehtmets, Andres, and Jörg Pont. 2014. *Prison Health Care and Medical Ethics*. Council of Europe.
National Commission on COVID-19 and Criminal Justice. 2020. "Impact Report: COVID-19 and Prisons." December 6, 2020. https://covid19.counciloncj.org/2020/12/06/impact-report-covid-19-and-prisons/.
Patch, Kimberly L. 2013. "Sentencing Reform Act: Reconsidering Rehabilitation as a Critical Consideration in Sentencing." *New England Journal of Criminal and Civil Confinement*, 39: 165–91.
Scarlet, Sara, Erin S. DeMartino, and Mark Siegler. 2019. "Surrogate Decision Making for Incarcerated Patients." *JAMA Internal Medicine*, 179 (7): 861–2.
Schicktanz, S., S. Michl, and H. Stoff. 2021. "Bioethics and the Argumentative Legacy of Atrocities in Medical History: Reflections on a Complex Relationship." *Bioethics*, 35 (6): 499–507.
Shelby, Tommie. 2022. *The Idea of Prison Abolition*. Princeton University Press.
Valles, Sean A. 2023. "Fifty Years of U.S. Mass Incarceration and What It Means for Bioethics." *Hastings Center Report*, 53 (6): 25–35.
Victor, Eilzabeth. 2019. *Vulnerability and Incarceration*. Lexington Books.

7

Toward a Phenomenology of Aging

Implications for Bioethics

Larry R. Churchill and David Schenck

Both medicine and the dominant US culture continue to misunderstand aging. In so doing, they not only mischaracterize and stereotype the elderly; they also tend to cut us off from the deeper wells of meaning that can emerge from becoming older. Bioethics, which is too often just a reflection of both contemporary social worries and a medicalized understanding of human problems, has been largely complicit in this until recently. In building upon existing bioethics work and highlighting the spiritual possibilities for growth, our aim is to contribute to the more complete and realistic view of aging that is needed to shape the work of bioethics, medical practitioners, and the larger culture.

Getting beyond Stereotypes

Four popular images of aging, created and fed by our consumerist culture and prevalent in advertising, have had an oversized influence. These images need careful reexamination and critique and should finally to be discarded.

What we claim in naming these stereotypes is not entirely new for bioethics. Several scholars working in and around bioethics have had aging on their agendas for some time. The Hastings Center published an excellent set of essays in 2018 entitled *What Makes a Good Life in Late Life? Citizenship and Justice in Aging Societies*, with a wide-raging collection by bioethicists, gerontologists, public health experts, and others (Berlinger, de Medeiros, and Solomon 2018). Kate de Medeiros, a gerontologist and coeditor of this volume, has stated well the tendency to label older persons that we want to develop and examine here. She claims:

> To think like a gerontologist is to consider the cultural and societal values—past and present—that shape the experience of aging to recognize people as complex beings whose individual lives do not follow predictable patterns or easily identified trajectories, and *to recognize our own habits of regarding older persons as "other"*

> *and the consequences of "othering" for older persons and social systems.* (de Medeiros 2018, S10, emphasis added)

This emphasis dovetails nicely with Nancy King's essay on "othering" in this volume.

One image we have identified portrays the elderly as *docile, harmless, kindly creatures*, delighted to spend more time in leisure with their grandchildren. They (we!) are often pictured as happy in their retirement homes, playing cards, watching daytime dramas, and playing golf or shuffleboard in a sunny venue. It is a picture of passivity toward political concerns except for taxes, property values, and the government programs that sustain their economic advantage. In this image what best characterizes the elderly is a benign tranquility.

Another image also sees the elderly as beyond their productive years, but not passively "out to pasture." Rather, the image is one of *overly entitled seniors*, taking up far more than their share of social and political space, better off financially than their children yet demanding the best amenities wherever they go. This view may be a backlash to the recognition that more than twice as much public money is spent on the elderly through Medicare and Social Security than on other age groups and most notably, children. This image is reinforced by policy changes such as Medicare Advantage, and its embrace of wellness services and through changes in medical practice, such as the rise of concierge medicine.

Medicine and popular culture collude in a third stereotype, thinking of *aging as an illness and the aged primarily as patients*. This image is fed by the seemingly endless analyses of the costs of caring for the aging, the looming bankruptcy of Medicare, the prohibitive costs of long-term care, and the inevitable warehousing of the frail elderly in custodial institutions.

Finally, there is the aspirational image presented by antiaging medical research, which dovetails with antiaging commercial products to suggest that the good life is all about *retaining or restoring youthfulness*. The goal of "forever young" is fed by moon shot efforts to reverse-engineer our basic molecular structures, espoused especially by the scions of Silicon Valley and their funders. In this image, as with others, consumerism skews the sense of who the aging are and what is possible as one nears the end of one's life.

That these images and many like them are deeply flawed is well recognized. As Bruce Jennings has observed, quoting James Meek, just under the surface is "a rhetoric of immigrant fear, of the neurosis that a stable, long-established society is on the verge of being swamped by outsiders from far away, except that these 'outsiders' were born far away in time, rather than space" (Jennings 2018, S19). The demographics of aging in modern Western societies only increases this fear and feeds and exacerbates the "othering" embedded in the "outsider" label. We might all recognize these stereotypes as "ageist." In a perceptive analysis, Joel Micheal Reynolds notes that "ableism is at the core of ageism," underscoring how the powerful social and cultural determinants of our current ableism assumptions in policy thinking also contaminate thinking about aging (Reynolds 2018, S33).

Neglected in each stereotype is the arduous daily work of many elders in simply living tolerable lives and helping others to do so. These efforts rarely figure into social or governmental economic assessments of what the elderly contribute to the social fabric. Moreover, many of the elderly live on Social Security income alone, or with very modest pensions or savings, making do with incomes just above the poverty level.[1] We rarely hear about these elders, but they are a far larger number than the affluent elderly of the second stereotype. Also, many elders remain politically active and champion issues that affect future generations, with a concern that extends well beyond worries about their own families to include generations of people that will follow them. Like most stereotypes, the popular images sketched above fail to account for the great diversity in elders, emphasized by de Medeiros, in how they live and what they value. Most important, the elderly are portrayed not only as one-dimensional but also static, as no longer growing and changing and especially, we will argue, growing in spiritual domains not previously open to them when they were younger.

Yet despite these helpful analyses, we claim that too little attention has been given to the felt experiences of aging as a successive series of losses, sometimes coming slowly, at other times cascading into disability. A crucial component of the elderly world is the fact of our existence in time and the inevitability of aging bodies and altered selves. It is this to which too little attention—attention without a therapeutic or social agenda—has been given. This can be a frightening image to consider, which is one reason the popular stereotypes don't include it. But alarming as they can sometimes be, these losses—and the adjustments and adaptations we make to accept and accommodate them—present unique opportunities for growth. This is the area to which too little attention has been paid. Despite recent advances, the customary dominant feature in bioethics work is usually the plight of the aging *patient*, where growing older is already pathologized, typically accompanied by a range of health policy remedies reasserting the dignity of the elderly in spite of the burdens of caring for them. There are, to be sure, some excellent analyses of how social and health policy can better accommodate the aged.[2] Yet seldom has aging been considered in bioethics with anything like the careful, thick descriptions of experiences that portray illness, or the work of health care professionals. It is time to correct this lacuna in the field and refocus on aging and its place in bioethical discourse.

The description that follows focuses on mundane problems of mobility, dexterity, and mental acuity. In the last section, we discuss the implications for bioethics as a field of work.

Phenomenology and Aging

Over its roughly fifty-year history, bioethics has benefited from several works that could count as phenomenologies of illness, the workings of physicians, and nursing and its challenges.[3] There are also highly descriptive accounts of patients as they move through various phases of particular illnesses such as cancer, along with treatments and their sequelae.[4] Similar studies of aging are hard to find.[5]

By "phenomenology" we mean the effort to give attention and describe something without an explanatory framework in order to see things as they are, rather than how we want them to be, or think they ought to be. We take our working definition primarily from Maurice Merleau-Ponty and his preface to *The Phenomenology of Perception*, where he states that phenomenology must be "practiced and identified as a manner or style of thinking" that existed before it was formalized into a school of thought by philosophers such as Husserl or Heidegger (Merleau-Ponty, 1962).

By such a practice, Merleau-Ponty intends to point to the "facticity" of a world already there before reflection, a world in which we are inseparably intertwined. A large component of that world is the fact of our aging bodies and aging selves. It is this to which little attention—attention without a therapeutic or social agenda—has been given. Phenomenology requires close attention and description. We aim for only a modest beginning. A more comprehensive phenomenology of aging is a book unto itself, perhaps a full shelf of volumes. We seek here simply to make a start in hopes that others will see the value of this task and contribute.

Losses of Mobility, Dexterity, and Memory

The examples taken up below are drawn from our own experiences as septuagenarians and those of our friends and colleagues. We are also relying on our work over decades with patients in hospitals, hospices, and clinics, as well as our reading, study, and engagement with the arts. This is, however, an admittedly highly selective and skewed sampling. We intend not exhaustive accounts, but illustrative ones. If the reader feels an inclination to explore these issues and help produce a more adequate set of examples, our efforts here will have succeeded.

Mobility

Balance is the new imperative for the aged. Merely walking can be a problem. Walking aids, such as canes and forearm crutches, often become necessary. After a fall, there's an increasing fear of more falls and their consequences (concussions, subdural hematomas, fractures). The precariousness increases when one is out of one's familiar living space. Walking across a parking lot, on wet grass, on gravel or cobblestones can all present challenges. Yet even in familiar settings couch surfing (moving through one's living areas within touching distance of a piece of furniture or a wall) may be needed to provide additional proprioceptive input for the balance.

Stairs can be especially challenging. Loss of confidence in leg strength and coordination means stairs always present a falling risk, especially if there are four steps or more. Stairs without rails are forbidden unless the arm or shoulder of a large person is available for support and safety. When using stairs, one goes more slowly, with a hand always free to grip the rail or banister. Any task requiring both hands to be occupied while descending the stairs is now too risky, and ascending with both hands occupied means being ready to drop something if needed. In stairways where no rail is present, no attempt is made. No banister means no entry.

Getting dressed, once unproblematic, can also prevent hazards. Getting pants on, especially early in the day, can be a risky undertaking. Simply standing on one leg while slipping one leg in and pulling up is no longer a trustworthy maneuver. It is best to sit on the bed or lean back against a wall, with a hand free to balance on a chest, table, or chair. Putting shoes on requires sitting on the bed or in a chair and involves bending over and twisting in unusual and often painful ways. A long-handled shoehorn is sometimes necessary.

When getting out of bed, it becomes important to feel the calves against the bedside and reach out to put fingers on a nearby wall to be sure one is properly balanced before taking one's first two or three steps.

Low car seats now require forethought and calculation. A butt-first entry is often the only way in, mindfully guided by hands on the door jam, then swinging the legs around is required, often assisted by the roof strap. One must also have enough hand and arm strength to situate oneself and buckle the seatbelt. And then there's the reversal of all this when exiting the vehicle.

For bathrooms, grab bars in showers become indispensable, as do "guard rails" and grab bars for toilets. Using the toilet involves sitting down and getting back up, bending and twisting. Is the seat too low? Where are the grab bars? Is the floor slick? Getting into and out of a tub is an especially hazardous maneuver, requiring forethought and strategy. A hot bath becomes a rare luxury.

Dexterity

Careful use of the hands is of paramount importance as arms weaken and tremors develop. Avoiding accidents becomes a constant concern, especially in the kitchen. Deliberate and calculated movements are essential for cooking—for handling pots of boiling water, placing casseroles in the oven, and moving hot dishes. Using the stove, oven, and toaster oven becomes hazardous. One often begins to knock things over while preparing meals, leading to working next to the sink for ease of cleanup, and having tops and covers on everything possible.

Eating and drinking involve using both hands. The shift to using metal and plastic cups and mugs to avoid breaking glass, plates, and even ceramics is necessary. Carrying food on a tray—fast food, cafeteria, buffet—is no longer an option. More coffee stains now adorn the carpet.

Weaker hands and arms are a constant reminder of aging. Opening a new jar—of mayonnaise, pickles, or peanut butter—is now often impossible without grips. Turning a screw or driving a nail becomes much more difficult. Lifting boxes, heavy books, or a stack of plates is potentially dangerous. Carrying anything now requires calculation: Does the object weigh too much? Is it balanced? Can it be gripped securely? How far does it need to be carried?

Writing and using the computer now require careful attention. Handwriting can become difficult to impossible due to tremors or arthritis. Using a computer is becoming more and more inefficient when hands are cramped in pain or shifting about uncontrollably.

Getting dressed presents mobility and flexibility issues, but also issues of dexterity. Buttons can be especially troublesome, as well as clothes fasteners of all kinds. Buttons on sleeves or collars mostly impossible. At some point, ties, zippers, and belts present problems, as does getting one's arms into tight coats or sweaters and getting gloves on properly.

Memory Loss

Managing the household brings many pitfalls. There is a standard list of challenges that is useful—the *Seven Instrumental Activities of Daily Living*: using the telephone and computer; shopping (especially for groceries); preparing meals; housekeeping; using transportation; taking medication; managing finances. What groceries were bought last week? There's the recipe heard yesterday and now forgotten, which could explain why there are strange items on shelves and in the refrigerator. Where is that new casserole dish bought last week? Has the stove or the oven been left on?

Relating to one's family becomes more complicated. What was the last thing you did with your grandchild? What is her favorite book? There's the puzzle of the name of your son-in-law—and eventually of your daughter. And when is that birthday?

One loses language skills. Nouns seem to be the first things to go. The names of people known for thirty years, and those of other people one knows can't be recalled. Names of objects, ideas, concepts, as well as book titles, authors, actors, and the names of comedies and tragedies are also forgotten. Some items are readily accessible to memory, some are periodically inaccessible, while others are lost in the black hole of the mind. Spoonerisms become more frequent. These gaffes are named for the Reverend William A. Spooner, a late nineteenth-century English cleric famous for saying things such as "It is kisstomary to cuss the bride." These can be sheer nonsense, sometimes humorous, and sometimes embarrassing.

Handling the medical system gets more frustrating, and errors in following directives become more frequent. What the doctor said in this morning's appointment can't be recalled when the time comes to give an account of the visit to one's partner.

Amanda Grenier and Christopher Phillipson have argued that "precarity" is a very useful concept to describe the amplified risks that elders encounter, and they claim that ethical considerations are needed to frame adequate social responses to increased precarity (Grenier and Philipson 2018). Our experiences and those of others described above underline a need for greater use of this concept, and that moral notions of justice, equity, dignity, and obligations of care cannot be absent in any effort to move forward. Yet beyond that, we want to illustrate a power the elderly possess that is often ignored in the aging literature that presents under the heading of "Openings" below.

Reactive Responses: Denial, Anger, Frustration, Anxiety

That slow war of attrition that we will inevitably lose has begun. Some months one loses much ground, other months less. Sometimes this is because of one's efforts, or lack thereof—exercise, physical therapy, nutrition. But often enough it seems random, leaving one feeling even more vulnerable, more at the mercy of capricious and hardly benevolent gods. Here are a few representative quotes.

- "Damn, I've spilled the coffee. And of course, I knock something over now every time I go into the kitchen. When will I be able to go outside again without crutches? Ever? Ah, I've thrown boxes across the room and ripped the recycling to shreds, out of frustration, again—feeling any better now? And there's that doorframe I run into so often—if I keep kicking it, I'm going to break my foot, as if I needed that, too. I snapped at the nurse at the clinic this morning and sulked like an angry teenager all through my appointment with the doctor. Are these medical people worthless? Am I?"
- "Not to mention that I hate having to be so careful. There's so much fear. Fear of accidents, injuries, broken bones (especially a hip!); of 'tomahawk' or 'face-plant' falls, concussions, brain bleeds; of deep cuts, severe burns. The kitchen, the bathroom, and all steps are particularly dangerous."
- "How could I forget to pay the rent this month? I didn't recognize my ex-wife, the mother of my children, in the supermarket last week. And I had to stop my presentation today—a long, long pause—uncomfortable for everyone—because I lost my place in the slides and had no idea how to go on."
- "And then the worries. Short-term: Who can help if I fall? Is there a hospital or clinic close by? How much time before EMTs can get here? And then there's the long-term. I haven't even gotten to the hard stuff yet—major illness, major accident, crippling dementia. Who will take care of me as I continue to decline? When will the money run out?"
- "The new range and intensity of anxieties. It's spread to more and more activities (driving at night, facing steep steps, meeting new people, giving a lecture) and places (heights, MRIs, elevators) that never caused anxiety in the past. And anything that caused anxiety in past now generates almost unbearable sensations."

Is there something beyond these reactive responses? What are the ways of being-in-the-world that are possible as the active phase of life is passing? And this is especially important in a society such as ours in which ageism and ableism are still so prominent. Can losses be seen as a transition to relief, and perhaps even an opening to something more? Is there a path into a new phase that doesn't feel like deprivation and failure, that doesn't involve fighting or denying aging? Our claim is that the very things thought of as deprivations of aging and diminishment of the body can be precisely the locations of existential openings.

Openings

Opportunities can be found in small pieces of life as well as large ones. Notice, for example, how the physical limitations of being bound more closely to a chair or a stool, a table or a counter encourage paying attention to things previously unseen: time to notice, for example, the way the spider weaves her web, the way layered and textured light changes as it breaks through the trees and finds its way to the window, the sheer beauty of a bare tree, its limbs configured in ways that delight and stir curiosity about its life, its health, and its placement, or the textures of fabrics, the boldness of colors, the hues of wood in the room around me.

Notice, as well, changes in one's social world. People now come to us when we are seated and not mobile. They offer themselves in new ways—sometimes helpful, sometimes brusque. What can now be seen about relatives—children, grandchildren, cousins, in-laws—from this perspective? How different is it to have a small child climb into one's lap instead of having to bend down to pick the child up? We are dependent in new ways and have to find novel ways to ask for help, to express gratitude, to overcome embarrassment. Limitations imposed by biology force us to find creative ways of living in the world our new restrictions have made. How can I inhabit gratefully the life my now-altered body offers me?

For example, with mobility challenges one can move one's attention "inside the knees" to investigate balance. For the aged, the floor can move, like the deck of a ship or the stern of a small boat. It's hard to stand. When walking through the house, watch how postures have to shift, how one has to place one's feet to avoid running into walls or furniture. And no falling! How does the body feel as a possible fall begins? Notice how your arms and trunk react to that danger. Mobility issues change the way one indwells one's body, which in turn alters space and time. And while this is a negative compared to one's previous functioning, it can also be the occasion for wonder, and surprisingly, deep gratitude for the years of mobility one had, and for the mobility one still has.

Limitations can provide opportunities for imaginative exercises, as well as greater precision in observation. To investigate dexterity challenges of weakness and tremor, try acting as if it isn't the hand that's shaking, but the objects one is reaching for. Looking out from the fingers, see exactly how hard things are to grasp. Notice the sensations in the fingers while trying to open the new jar of peanut butter. One's access to every piece of one's world has been altered, and most importantly, not just diminished but in some ways enhanced.

Memory losses change time. They alter the way one holds the past. They determine the way one moves into the future. What is it like to turn to the past in story, in daydream, in fantasy? Apply the same questions to the future. Watch to see if this means one is losing the past and the future. How does that process feel in the body? The redeeming quality in this loss is the power to reinterpret. Less attention to clock time and the sequential rhythms it demands can mean a release from the tyranny of chronological time. Attention to the contours of bodily time, as opposed to chronological time, can lead to experiences of being "out-of-time," traditionally recognized as a hallmark of deepening relationships with the cosmic order. This degree of life scrutiny is awareness practice and can be accompanied by a new sense of awe not available to me when I was younger and took effortless functioning for granted.

One can now take up the process of undoing emotional burdens that mar one's daily life, rather than being at their mercy. One needs to address emotional states and reactive behaviors, knowing them to be powerful drivers of the active, ego-dominated life that needs to be left behind to open the way to a new world.

How can one check one's impatience? There is, first, the awareness of where it arises in the body. Do you feel it in your throat, in your chest, in your arms? And then attending to that place and allowing the impatience to be there without acting on it. Let it pass. Retrain your reaction. This same exercise can be done with anger or with sadness.

Think carefully about what it takes to be balanced in behavior. Study texts that project lives of equanimity and take them as teachers. Be aware of behaviors you want to change: speaking sharply when frustrated, slapping the wall when angry, going on buying sprees when depressed. Look for emotional reactions that spoil your life and that of others you care about.

Find the ways you make yourself suffer; find ways to release the grip of pain-causing habits. Commit yourself to this work as the path to greater equanimity. Suffering and loss, and how these twin inevitabilities are understood, is one of the perennial themes of most religious and spiritual traditions. This essay is about suffering the disorder of diminishment of body and mind, how we respond to it, and the openings available to us to reorder our lives.

In summary, accepting limitations in mobility, dexterity, and memory loss presents openings for growth. Such acceptance can make possible the achievement of whole new levels and complexities of meaning in one's life. It can nurture new stories for mobility, dexterity, and memory loss while helping one to escape stories of life as steady and ongoing diminishment.

All three of the challenges described—mobility, dexterity, and memory loss—serve to confirm what we know intellectually, but likely have not absorbed in our bodies. This is the knowledge that we, as individuals and as a species, are no different from any other existent beings. We face the certain prospect of decline and dissolution. We face inevitable aging and death. Aging, our bodies begin releasing their grip on pieces of the world we have borrowed. This prospect generates a certain fear, if not terror, in us, as well as many textures of grief, loss, and longing. Sometimes sharp and aching; sometimes, if we are fortunate, gentle and fond. Coming to terms with aging means owning our embodiment, both the diminishment of our bodily functioning, and the possibilities for being grounded differently and more creatively in and through the openings now available to us precisely through that diminishment.

We hasten to add that we claim no special standing for ourselves here. We see glimpses of growth in ourselves and in others. In some, we see far more than glimpses. But we are here seeking to describe a horizon—a perceived destination never to be reached. We are pointing to possibilities, aspirations experienced but not completely grasped.

Implications for Bioethics

Earlier in this chapter, we sketched popular portraits of the elderly and suggested that they are marked by several shortcomings. These images are too homogeneous, failing to account for the great diversity in elders, too influenced by commercial estimates of worth, and overly medicalized, seeing the elderly predominantly through the lens of illness and pathology. Each of these portraits is also an exercise in "othering," the alienation of the aged from the rest of society. We argued that like all stereotypes, these portraits are naïve in their assumptions of what aging is like and detrimental to our understanding of this late phase of life. The main agenda of this chapter has been to describe with detail and accuracy some of the mundane experiences of growing old. We have argued that what appear to be completely negative stories of loss and disablement actually present new opportunities for growth.

In order to do its work properly, bioethics must rely on accurate accounts of what human beings experience and the meaning structures, stories, and values that permeate these experiences. Yet the predominant story of the elderly in bioethics relies heavily on a medical understanding of the aging patient, so that the losses of mobility, dexterity, and memory we described are seen as occasions for professional intervention. This is clearly sometimes needed and fine as far as it goes, but it is hardly the full story. In short, bioethics focused on the elderly draws largely from a tradition of medical ethics that sees the fundamental issues as about whether and to what extent to ameliorate bodily losses with drugs or surgeries. Reverberating through this approach is the notion that aging is an altogether negative experience, without inherent positive meaning, so that all efforts to diminish the impact of aging are viewed as welcome. Drug and surgical advertising to make us younger are the more blatant and candid expressions of this devaluing.

Our task here has been to illustrate mundane experiences of elders as credible sources of a larger picture and a deeper truth. This has several implications for bioethics.

First, bioethics needs to pay more attention to elders' stories and accredit them as genuine sources of truth. Without knowing and accrediting these larger stories, bioethics will continue to fall prey to the thin and largely negative portraits of our youth-obsessed culture and to exclusively medical solutions to the problems of aging. Accrediting stories of loss and diminishment opens the realm of meaning-making to what are best described as spiritual aspects of life. This does not mean making a larger place for organized religion or theology in bioethics. It does mean broadening our interpretive grids beyond the standard values of bioethics—autonomy, beneficence, and justice. Humans are not just beings who seek autonomous activities, beneficent relations, and just actions and institutions. They are also creatures who continually strive to make sense of their experiences.

This kind of sense-making is readily apparent to those bioethicists who do clinical work, for the severely ill and their families often make use of these and other resources. Meaning-making work should also be seen as characterizing the elderly, and especially elders who are struggling to understand the losses that accompany aging. Resources for understanding are also evident in the accounts of significantly handicapped and disabled persons we have encountered, both in clinical and ordinary life settings. Rather than seeing their lives as ones of diminishment and loss, many less able individuals consider themselves to be much more than their diagnoses and limitations, as fully human, with no diminishment of value, and sometimes better than "normal." They often see themselves as better than normal because they have adapted in surprising and creative ways, and also because sometimes their losses have taught them things about life that were inaccessible before their disability. There is a lesson here for how the losses of aging should be viewed, and how bioethics can appreciate aging persons.

Second, careful descriptions of the mundane life of elders can show us where social and health care priorities need to be placed. We currently have a set of social policies emphasizing medical interventions and life-extending technologies. When these technologies fail, as they all eventually do, we often resort to warehousing the elderly, effectively segregating them from the younger and healthier population. Over thirty years ago, Daniel Callahan offered a different vision of caring for the elderly, one that emphasized social support for independent living, assistance with the tasks of daily living, and de-emphasizing the use of expensive and scarce medical technologies (Callahan 1987). His suggestions were greeted as realistic and salutary by some and as blatant ageism by others. Callahan reiterated and affirmed his convictions more recently (Callahan 2018) and his position is complemented by bioethicist and public health scholar Lauren Taylor, who says that policies that seek flourishing in the aged are unlikely to achieve their aims through health care, at least in part because the health care sector is prone to underestimate and mismeasure the true value of social support services (Taylor 2018). We argue that Callahan's and Taylor's policy priorities are a better fit than the current, medico-centric politics for the life and world of elders we describe in this chapter. Careful attention to such policy priorities should be high on the list for future work in bioethics.

Tom Cole, the acclaimed historian of aging, observes that the current economic commitments of Western societies to unlimited growth through scientific management exact a large cultural and moral price, portraying the elderly as peripheral and of inferior status (Cole 1992). Bioethics, insofar as it is a humanistic discipline, has as its role the promotion and lifting up of all people thought to be of inferior status. Over the past fifty years bioethics has famously done this for the sick and hospitalized, imbuing them with the status of persons who must he consulted, listened to, and whose values matter. A similar effort has been made by bioethics, with arguably lesser effect, to those who are less able, to women, to minorities, and to the dying. In this chapter we are seeking to make the case for the elderly as a cohort of humanity who likewise have tended to occupy an "inferior status." In part this is a function of the stereotypes we have examined and discarded; in part it is a product of the fear in our culture of growing older with its inevitably diminishments. If bioethics can embrace loss and diminishment as opportunities for growth, and the elderly as capable of an enlightenment not easily accessible to younger cohorts, it will have moved toward doing for the elderly what it has done for patients more generally. Such an embrace and affirmation would mark a much-needed maturity for the field.

Notes

1 Of note, the average income of persons sixty-five and older in 2023 was $75,274, yet the median income for this group was $47,620, while average expenses for the elderly were $48,872, according to https://www.fool.com/research/average-retirement-income/ accessed January 11, 2024.
2 See Joanna Lynn. 2016. *Medicaring Communities: Getting What We Want and Need in Frail Old Age at an Affordable Cost*. Altarum Institute.
3 Many accounts of illnesses, doctoring, and nursing do not describe themselves as "phenomenological" but are presented in the spirit of accuracy to facts, rich and careful description, and awareness of bias in presentation. Among these, on the works of clinicians, we would note Eric Cassell on interviewing and caring for patients, Andrew Jameton on nursing and its moral ambivalences, Kathryn Montgomery on the thinking of doctors, Larry Churchill and David Schenck on the phenomenon of healing from both clinician and patient perspectives, David Loxterkamp on family medicine, John Berger on the life of a country practitioner, Abraham Verghese on medicine as a calling, and many others.
4 We have in mind both the stories of illness from scholars like Martha Montello, Rita Charon, Suzanne Poirer, Anne Hudson Jones, as well as the many first-person narratives from patients, such as those of Harold Brodkey, Arthur Frank, Kay Jamison, Reynolds Price, Raymond Carver, Jill Bolte Taylor, and Anatole Broyard, and many others.
5 One notable exception is the stories of older men recorded and edited by Thomas R. Cole in *Old Man Country: My Search for Meaning Among the Elders* (Oxford University Press, 2020).

Bibliography

Berlinger, Nancy, Kate de Medeiros, and Mildred Solomon, "What Makes for a Good Life in Late Life? Citizenship and Justice in Aging Societies. *Hastings Center Report* 48 (5), 2018.

Callahan, Daniel. 1987. *Setting Limits: Medical Goals in an Aging Society*. Simon and Schuster.

Callahan, Daniel. 2018. "Aging: Drawing a Map for the Future." In *What Makes A Good Life in Late Life? Citizenship and Justice in Aging Societies, Hastings Center Report* 48 (5) supplement: S80–4.

Cole, Thomas R. 1992. *The Journey of Life: A Cultural History of Aging in America*. Cambridge University Press.

De Medeiros, Kate. 2018. "What Can Thinking Like a Gerontologist Bring to Bioethics?" In *What Makes for a Good Life in Late Life? Hastings Center Report* 48 (5): S10–S14.
Dunn, Michael. 2018. "Realizing and Maintaining Capabilities: Late Life as a Social Project." In *What Makes for a Good Life in Late Life? Hastings Center Report* 48 (5): S25–S30.
Grenier, Amanda, and Christopher Philipson. 2018. "Precarious Aging: Insecurity and Risk in Late Life." In *What Makes for a Good Life in Late Life? Hastings Center Report* 48 (5): S15–S18.
Jennings, Bruce. 2018. "Solidarity and Care Coming of Age: New Reasons in the Politics of Social Welfare Policy." In *What Makes for a Good Life in Late Life? Hastings Center Report* 48 (5): S19–S24.
Merleau-Ponty, Maurice. 1962. *Phenomenology of Perception*, translated by Colin Smith. Routledge and Kegan Paul.
Reynolds, Joel Michael. 2018. "The Extended Body: On Aging, Disability and Well-Being." In *What Makes for a Good Life in Late Life? Hastings Center Report* 48 (5): S31–6.
Taylor, Lauren A. 2018. "How Do We Fund Flourishing: Maybe Not through Health Care." In *What Makes for a Good Life in Late Life? Hastings Center Report* 48 (5): S62–6.

8

What Is Past Is Prologue

Searching for Social Justice Advocacy in Bioethics

Virginia A. Brown

This chapter seeks to offer insight into how returning to the past to retrieve an overlooked element of the Belmont Report could offer the necessary guidance and justification needed to unify how we, in the field of bioethics, can engage in social justice advocacy by understanding and addressing how race, class, gender, ability, and other historically marginalized identities intersect to differently advantage and disadvantage not only individuals, but communities as well, in receiving equitable treatment in health and health care.

Locating Social Justice via Intersectionality

In the 2022 article "On the Shoulders of Giants: A Reckoning with Social Justice," Bogdan-Lovis et al. asked four bioethics "luminaries" to assign a grade for the field's performance in addressing racial injustice. D+ responded the pioneering bioethics scholars Patricia A. King, Claretta Y. Dupree, Anita L. Allen, and Lawrence J. Prograis, Jr. (Bogdan-Lovis, Kelly-Blake, and Jiang 2022).[1] Such poor performance demands remediation. Yet where does addressing bioethics negligence to racial injustice, and social justice more broadly, begin? Answer: it begins by recognizing and responding to the historic and contemporary intersections that race, class, and gender create in delivering unequal treatment in medical practice and research and the resulting inequitable outcomes in health and health care experienced by Black and other historically marginalized peoples.

Our individual and collective racial, economic, and gender identities (past and present) merge and emerge as part of an intra/interpersonal dialogue and experience—creating our "lived experience." As bioethicists, especially for those at the bedside or bioethicists engaged with medical humanities and narrative practices, the story being heard and interpreted, too often, does little to interrogate and report an unabridged telling of how intersectionality, in all its forms, is at play. To better understand the relationship of intersectionality to the field of bioethics begins with a brief account of its origin and application in the field of law.

The phrase intersectionality, penned by legal scholar Kimberlé Crenshaw, served as a metaphor to describe the unique position that Black women found themselves in when seeking redress for workplace discrimination (Crenshaw 1989). Crenshaw revealed how antidiscrimination laws regarding race or sex were inadequate in addressing the unique discrimination Black women experienced when their race and sex created a compounded and thus more complex form of oppression. A decade after Crenshaw, Patricia Hill-Collins (2000) furthered the metaphor of intersectionality as a "form of critical analysis . . . essential to resistant knowledge projects" (Hill Collins et al. 2021, 693). Intersectionality, having left its metaphorical descriptor behind, began its transformation into social science praxis.

When applied to bioethics, I argue that intersectionality functions as a form of investigation, a methodological approach of inquiry that attends "to the integration between what is structured--the historical and enduring institutions that constitute and naturalize social power--and what is dynamic--the ways that power is continuously reproduced and contested in real time" (Bello and Mancini 2016, 15). Moreover, applying intersectionality in bioethics "can challenge an uncritical use of race" (Byeon, Sellers, and Bonham 2019, 20). Intersectionality can function as a "framework [that] might enrich patient-clinician encounters, increase patient centeredness, and help navigate better clinical experiences" (Wilson et al. 2019, 11) resulting in, not only "the potential to create solidarity and cohesion" (Roberts and Jesudason 2013, 313), but also an approach that "offer[s] bioethics a precious opportunity to understand more deeply and work towards addressing barriers to human flourishing and justice" (Ray et al. 2023, 259). So, how ought we bioethicists—who come from a range of disciplines to this field—recognize that which we have failed to realize: the role that power and privilege impart when it comes to the production and reproduction of the benefits and burdens associated with health and health care?

The Belmont Report and Intersectionality

Intersectionality offers a method of praxis, understood as a form of inquiry and action that works to confront and disrupt heretofore implicit and therefore unexamined (because they are unrecognized) forms of power that shape the health experiences of historically marginalized people. Yet, one might ask, what does this have to do with bioethics? In a word, plenty!

A brief review of The Belmont Report (National Commission for the Protection of Human Subjects of Biomedical and Behavioral Research 1979, referred to from here forward as The Belmont Report 1979) reveals that the National Research Act of 1974 authorized the creation of the National Commission for the Protection of Human Subjects of Biomedical and Behavioral Research. The commission's formation arose out of the backdrop of the social and technological forces of the 1960s and early 1970s (e.g., access to dialysis, Karen Ann Quinlan and end of life, and *Roe v. Wade*) (Jonsen 2007; Shelstad 1999). The catalyst for the commission culminated with the revelation of the United States Public Health Service Study of Untreated Syphilis at Tuskegee in 1972 (Brandt 1978; Jones 1981; Gamble 1997). The commission was convened and tasked to identify

> the boundaries between biomedical and behavioral research and the accepted and routine practice of medicine, (ii) the role of assessment of risk-benefit criteria in the determination of the appropriateness of research involving human subjects, (iii) appropriate guidelines for the selection of human subjects for participation in such research and (iv) the nature and definition of informed consent in various research settings. (The Belmont Report 1979)

The commission members realized

> that they were being asked to explore the ethical foundations for human research more deeply than had any extant statements. They decided that a closed retreat should be held . . . so that a freewheeling discussion could explore the nature and role of ethical principles for human research. (Jonsen 2005, 3)

The retreat was held in February 1976 at the Belmont House, a conference center in Elkridge, Maryland, owned at that time by the Smithsonian Institution. It was there that the eponymous Belmont Report would establish the ethical principles of respect for persons, beneficence, and justice as the guidelines for the protection of human subjects in research.

In a rereading of The Report, Commissioner Jonsen wrote that the text "for the next generation should retain almost unchanged the current text." However, "it should be surrounded by an appreciation of these broader, wider perspectives," including "how should we describe the frontier, for example, between personal autonomy and social justice?" (Jonsen 2005, 10). This frontier, I argue, requires the realization that power and privilege, as stated previously, are not only replicated but should be challenged as they function at the intersection of individual and community. This intersection makes space for a bioethics praxis that emphasizes the centering of personal stories in a society that unjustly distributes social benefits and burdens when seeking to understand and respond to social justice as advocacy.

A close read of The Report indicates that "[s]ocial justice [in research] requires that distinctions be drawn between classes of subjects that ought, and ought not, to participate in any particular kind of research based on the ability of members of that class to bear burdens and on the appropriateness of placing further burdens on already burdened persons" (The Belmont Report 1979). While no definitions are offered about who comprises these "classes of subjects," it should not be construed, for example, as socioeconomic status or as a typology, but rather it can be argued "classes of subjects" refers to an underdeveloped reference to the role of intersectionality as it functions in distributing burdens and benefits not only to individuals but also to communities as well.

The Belmont Report's second reference to social justice calls for an "order of preference in the selection of classes of subjects." However, it does not call out a specific theoretical position or methodological approach for addressing this "order of preference." More importantly, though, it explicitly states that "*injustice arises from social, racial, sexual and cultural biases institutionalized in society*" (emphasis added). Additionally, The Belmont Report notes that despite the best efforts of Institutional Review Boards to ensure the fair and equitable treatment of participants by the institution and researchers alike, "unjust social patterns may nevertheless appear in the overall distribution of the burdens and benefits of research." The Belmont Report foreshadows intersectionality and the injustices that can (and do) arise based on such intersections of identities. How this realization has failed to be operationalized in bioethics inquiry is beyond the scope of this chapter, nonetheless the need to recover and examine its importance is imperative.[2]

The Future Is Now

Carbado et al. (2013) capture well the collective "failure to attend to intersectionality's movement [which] has limited too many scholars' ability to see the theory in places in which it is already doing work and to imagine other places to which the theory might be taken" (303). And this other place, to which the praxis of intersectionality should be taken, is bioethics. Intersectionality offers the field of bioethics guidance and the necessary methodological approach to investigate and respond to the demands of social justice.

The justification for this praxis of intersectionality is grounded in the reality that structural inequality, fueled by prejudice and the corresponding practices, policies, and laws that reinforce such bigoted beliefs, interact to produce and reproduce policy and practice which have perpetuated and continue to exacerbate disparate outcomes in health and health care for historically marginalized peoples. In a country where one's zip code can predict one's life expectancy (Baciu et al. 2017), it is imperative to expand bioethics' responsibility to clearly advocate for social justice, by examining ethical issues through an intersectional lens.

Bioethicists, writ large, have neither recognized, understood, nor operationalized the reference to intersectionality in The Belmont Report. The Report suggests an additive approach to competing identities. Simply put, adding and subtracting categories of burdens until an acceptable balance is achieved has been and continues to be the approach. Understanding how intersectionality merges and shapes the experiences of historically marginalized individuals and the communities they represent helps us to make the implicit (i.e., intersectionality) explicit, thereby allowing for the development of intersectional frameworks to arise to redress these wrongs.

Bioethics' failure to attend to the field's lack of diversity and the corresponding challenges (Ravitsky et al. 2024) that this has created is well documented (Parsi 2016; Myser 2003, Toolkit: Black Bioethics), yet for this writer the recognition is not revelatory. Regrettably, missing from the discussion is a centering of the contributions of bioethics scholars, many of whom are Black, whose voices and work have been overlooked. The challenges confronting today's bioethicists who are Black are not new. Such scholars as James E. Bowman, Vence Bonham, LaVera Crawley, Annette Dula, Troy Duster, Robert F. Murray, Jr., Marian Gray Secundy, Vanessa Northington Gamble, Verle E. Headings, Patricia King, Benjamin Roy, and September Williams[3] represent a few of the forebearers in bioethics scholarship that have contributed to the literature since the nascent days of the field. Rediscovering their contributions fosters greater epistemic humility by encouraging intergenerational dialogue. Rooting out systemic oppression is not new; however, finding it in places where we did not expect it, like bioethics, is.

Simply put, the past is prologue and how we come to know the world is fragile and dependent on multiple ways of knowing and understanding. As Kamala Harris[4] reminds us "You think you just fell out of a coconut tree? You exist in the context of all in which you live and what came before you" (Hessee 2024). And like the Sankofa,[5] we must return to the past to retrieve that which has been forgotten in order to "frame a better, bolder, and braver bioethics [one] that prioritizes social justice" (Fletcher et al. 2022, S6) because we do stand on the shoulders of giants.

Notes

1 Each of the scholars, respectively, offered individual grades, C, D, C-, and D, which determined this averaged grade.

2 Central to the issue of injustice "institutionalized in society" is the question of trust and trustworthiness. When seeking to address issues of injustice, I offer LaVera Crawley's foundational article: Crawley, L.M., 2001. "African-American Participation in Clinical Trials: Situating Trust and Trustworthiness." *Journal of the National Medical Association 93* (12 Supplement). In this article, she reminds us "to reframe the discourse on mistrust as the breech of trust" as we cannot reestablish trust where it has never been established (15S).

3 This list is by no means exhaustive and only represents this author's firsthand acquaintance with each.

4 As of this writing, she is the current United States Vice President and presumptive Democratic nominee for President.

5 See Appiah Kubi Kwarteng (2016). *The Sankofa Bird and Reflection*. Sankofa is the symbol of the mythical bird that stands with its feet firmly planted. It is this wisdom in learning from the past that ensures a strong future. Often translated as "go back and get it," the adage is said as follows: "Always remember the past for therein lies the future, if forgotten we are destined to repeat it." This is the foundation upon which intergenerational dialogues are built.

Bibliography

Baciu, A., Y. Negussie, A. Geller, et al., eds. 2017. "The State of Health Disparities in the United States - Communities in Action - NCBI Bookshelf." In *Communities in Action: Pathways to Health Equity*. National Academies Press.

Bello, Barbara Giovanna, and Letizia Mancini. 2016. "Talking about Intersectionality. Interview with Kimberlé W. Crenshaw." *SOCIOLOGIA DEL DIRITTO*, no. 2.

Bogdan-Lovis, Elizabeth, Karen Kelly-Blake, and Wendy Jiang. 2022. "On the Shoulders of Giants: A Reckoning with Social Justice." *Hastings Center Report*, 52: S72–8.

Brandt, Allan M. 1978. "The Experiment and Hew's Ethical Review Racism and Research: The Case of the Tuskegee Syphilis Study." *Hastings Center Report*, 8 (6): 21–9.

Byeon, Yen Ji Julia, Sherrill L. Sellers, and Vence L. Bonham. 2019. "Intersectionality and Clinical Decision Making: The Role of Race." *American Journal of Bioethics*, 19 (2): 20–2.

Carbado, Devon W., Kimberlé Williams Crenshaw, Vickie M. Mays, and Barbara Tomlinson. 2013. "Intersectionality: Mapping the Movements of a Theory." *Du Bois Review: Social Science Research on Race*, 10 (2): 303–12.

Crawley, LaVera M. 2001. "African-American Participation in Clinical Trials: Situating Trust and Trustworthiness." *Journal of the National Medical Association*, 93 (12 Supplement): 14S–17S.

Crenshaw, Kimberlé. 1989. "Demarginalizing the Intersection of Race and Sex: A Black Feminist Critique of Antidiscrimination Doctrine, Feminist Theory and Antiracist Politics." *University of Chicago Legal Forum*, 140: 139–67.

Fletcher, Faith E., Keisha S. Ray, Virginia A. Brown, and Patrick T. Smith. 2022. "Addressing Anti-Black Racism in Bioethics: Responding to the Call." *Hastings Center*, 52 (2): S3–S11.

Gamble, Vanessa Northington. 1997. "Under the Shadow of Tuskegee: African Americans and Health Care." *American Journal of Public Health*, 87 (11): 1773–8.

Hessee, Monica. 2024. "Kamala Harris and the Coconut Tree of Hope." *The Washington Post*, July 3, 2024. https://www.washingtonpost.com/style/power/2024/07/03/kamala-harris-as-joe-biden-replacement/.

Hill Collins, Patricia. 2000. *Black Feminist Thought*. Routledge.

Hill Collins, Patricia, Elaini Cristina Gonzaga da Silva, Emek Ergun, Inger Furseth, Kanisha D Bond, and Jone Martínez-Palacios. 2021. "Intersectionality as Critical Social Theory: Intersectionality as Critical Social Theory, Patricia Hill Collins, Duke University Press, 2019." *Contemporary Political Theory*, 20 (3): 690–725.

Jones, James H. 1981. *Bad Blood: The Tuskegee Syphilis Experiment*. Collier Macmillan.

Jonsen, A. 2005. "On the Origins and Future of the Belmont Report." In James F Childress, Eric M. Meslin, and Harold T. Shapiro (eds.), *Belmont Revisited: Ethical Principles for Research with Human Subjects*. Georgetown University Press.

Jonsen, Albert R. 2007. "The God Squad and the Origins of Transplantation Ethics and Policy." *Journal of Law, Medicine & Ethics*, 35 (2): 238–40.

Myser, Catherine. 2003. "Differences from Somewhere: The Normativity of Whiteness in Bioethics in the United States." *The American Journal of Bioethics*, 3 (2): 1–11.

National Commission for the Protection of Human Subjects of Biomedical and Behavioral Research. 1979. *The Belmont report: Ethical Principles and Guidelines for the Protection of Human Subjects of Research*. U.S. Department of Health and Human Services.

https://www.hhs.gov/ohrp/regulations-and-policy/belmont-report/read-the-belmont-report/index.html

Parsi, Kayhan. 2016. "The Unbearable Whiteness of Bioethics: Exhorting Bioethicists to Address Racism." *The American Journal of Bioethics*, 16 (4): 1–2.

Ravitsky, Vardit, Nancy Berlinger, Virginia A. Brown, Faith E. Fletcher, and Danielle M. Pacia. 2024. "Diversifying Bioethics: Taking Action, Making Progress, Sustaining Success." *The American Journal of Bioethics*, 24(9): 25–7.

Ray, Keisha, Faith E. Fletcher, Daphne O. Martschenko, and Jennifer E. James. 2023. "Black Bioethics in the Age of Black Lives Matter." *Journal of Medical Humanities*, 44 (2): 251–67.

Roberts, Dorothy, and Sujatha Jesudason. 2013. "Movement Intersectionality: The Case of Race, Gender, Disability, and Genetic Technologies." *Du Bois Review: Social Science Research on Race*, 10 (2): 313–28.

Shelstad, Kirsten. 1999. "Landmark United States Biomedical Ethics Cases: A Selected Bibliography." *Medical Reference Services Quarterly*, 18 (2): 27–53.

Toolkit: Bioethics and Black People. 2020. "#BlackBioethics." *Bioethics Today*. https://bioethicstoday.org/blog/toolkit-bioethics-and-race-blackbioethics/# (accessed July 31, 2024).

Wilson, Yolonda, Amina White, Akilah Jefferson, and Marion Danis. 2019. "Intersectionality in Clinical Medicine: The Need for a Conceptual Framework." *American Journal of Bioethics*, 19 (2): 8–19.

Bioethics Response to Global Warming

9

Bioethics for a World on Fire

Travis N. Rieder

Bioethics is intended to be action-guiding. Indeed, bioethics may be the paradigm case of an action-guiding field of ethics. The core case studies in much of classical bioethics involve urgent problems to which an answer must be provided, because not acting constitutes an action. Doctors (and families) must decide how aggressively to treat a comatose patient when the patient's wishes weren't made clear ahead of time. Research studies must either be allowed or not, perhaps depending on whether subjects could provide genuinely autonomous consent. When ventilators, medicines, or any other healthcare resources are scarce, they must be distributed somehow. Insofar as bioethicists have traditionally tackled questions like these, they are working in a field where providing concrete recommendations and evaluating actions and policies are crucial *desiderata*.

One of the core claims of this chapter is that all of us are now facing an enormous class of ethical decisions that are properly classified as bioethical, but about which the field of bioethics has largely been silent. It is not offering action guidance, nor is it really even recognizing the issues as presenting problems for the field. And this, I will hypothesize, is because the structure of the modern world has changed in such a way that these cases fall through the cracks of classical bioethical reasoning. The tools we have used in the past no longer work, and so the problems are not readily identified as bioethical problems (though the moral distress we feel is part of the evidence that they are).

The structural feature of the world that I'm referring to is that the global human society has gotten so large so quickly, and our technology has connected us in so many ways that are so complicated, that our tiny, individual actions implicate us in many structures and systems that we don't intentionally choose, and which are morally problematic. Climate change is the paradigm case here, as the uncoordinated actions of 8 billion people are warming the planet in a way that causes massive harm, and so each of us knows we are contributing to the problem, though the power we have to affect it is infinitesimally small. The reason this raises an ethical puzzle is that our bioethical reasoning is good at dealing with individual cases in which our actions impact others (think clinical and research ethics); and it's good at dealing with cases of policy in order to address structural or systemic problems (think public health ethics and health policy); but it's not good at dealing with *individual moral responsibility for structural or systemic problems.*

The result is that many of us feel like we have a moral responsibility to change our actions in the face of structural problems that we contribute to, but our moral tools aren't well-equipped for explaining that responsibility (let alone telling us what to do). Given this reality, I will argue that we need a new set of moral tools for helping us to navigate the new world in which we find ourselves—we need to do what I have elsewhere called "catastrophe ethics" (Rieder 2024). These tools must be aimed not only at specialists in particular fields such as medicine, science, or public health, but at *everyone*, since we are all playing a tiny role in producing disaster.

The Puzzle of Individual Ethics in the Modern World

What I call "the Puzzle" of individual ethics is the felt sense that many modern problems morally implicate individuals, combined with two claims: (1) that our individual actions are meaningless in terms of their impact on the problems; and (2) as a result, we not only don't have any duties to do one thing or the other in such cases, but it's ethically problematic to focus on the ethics of individual action at all. In this section, I'll first describe how climate change presents a paradigmatic version of this Puzzle before showing that it arises elsewhere as well.

Many of us feel the moral pull of being good environmental citizens. We recycle or compost (or feel that we should). Some of us buy energy-efficient vehicles and appliances. Some of us even bike or walk more to limit driving. We might feel like we shouldn't fly too often. Or perhaps we should go vegetarian or vegan, since animal-sourced foods have a relatively high carbon footprint.

Dangerous climate change occurs when *trillions* of tons of greenhouse gases (GHGs) like CO_2 accumulate in the atmosphere. Precisely how many tons of GHGs we're talking about depends on what level you set as "dangerous"—holding warming to no more than 2 degrees Celsius global average requires limiting the all-time anthropogenic budget to less than 3.7 trillion tons of CO_2 equivalent (Allen et al. 2009); keeping warming to the more ambitious limit of 1.5 degrees Celsius would reduce that budget by some—perhaps by as much as a trillion tons (Lamboll et al. 2023)—but in either case, the scale is absolutely massive. Dangerous climate change is the result of billions of people emitting GHGs over the course of many decades.

Compare that, then, with the emissions that a typical individual can generate from any particular action. Even a gratuitous action like taking a joyride in a fuel-inefficient vehicle, or "joyguzzling," has been estimated to result in 14 kilograms of CO_2 (Sinnott-Armstrong 2005). A transatlantic flight might result in a full ton of CO_2. Even the combined emissions of a full year of activity for the average American—some of the wealthiest people in the world—are only about 14 tons of CO_2 (CO_2 Emissions 2020). Smaller choices, then, like eating meat for a single meal, make one responsible for a truly negligible amount of GHG emissions.

The scale of the problem thus absolutely dwarfs any of our individual contributions to it. Even our most environmentally significant actions, like flying, typically add less than one-trillionth of the amount of GHGs that compose the problem. The scale of climate change is so large that it is generally insensitive to individual choice.

Although some philosophers have tried gallantly to rescue the idea that we are still obligated to reduce our carbon footprint, I have argued elsewhere that these arguments are largely unconvincing (Rieder and Bernstein 2020). When our individual actions do not meaningfully contribute to the problem, it seems strikingly difficult to justify the claim that we are obligated to refrain from doing so anyway.

But the case against individual ethics actually gets worse. According to some, it's not only not wrong to emit GHGs. It's ethically problematic to focus on individual responsibility in the first place. This is because the actual power to make things better lies with systems and institutions (like governments and large corporations), so focusing on individuals places the responsibility for change—and potentially the blame for failing to change—on the wrong parties.

The climate scientist Michael Mann makes a version of this argument, claiming that energy companies push narratives of individual responsibility because they know that doing so is an effective way to *deflect* responsibility from them (where it should be) onto individuals. He cites the example of the company BP developing the world's first carbon footprint calculator as an example. It's not that they wanted people thinking about carbon emissions; it's that, so long as people are thinking about emissions, they want us pointing our fingers at one another, rather than at them (Mann 2021). This strategy of deflection suggests an empirical prediction: that if we focus on individual responsibility for climate change, we are less likely to be effective at creating large-scale change.

But there is also a moral component to the worry: it's *wrong* to hold the wrong parties accountable. Especially when individuals are harmed by the choices of more powerful players, to then blame those individuals for not changing the structures in which they are trapped is to engage in a form of victim-blaming (Heglar 2019). When BP got environmentalists to start worrying about their own carbon footprint and judging others for theirs, they created a world in which most people have very few options, but then pretended as if choosing among those few options was the same thing as the power to change the world. As George Monbiot describes the strategy of getting individuals to blame one another for their meaningless choices within a system confined by structural players: "It is, we must admit, a brilliant con" (Monbiot 2019).

Individual ethics in an era of massive, collective threats, then, is a puzzle because what we do both seems to matter and not to matter at all. If I can compost my waste rather than put it in the landfill, it seems like I should. It's clearly better to compost. And yet, my composting won't make any meaningful difference to any of the various environmental problems stemming from waste disposal, and placing the responsibility for solving our problems with waste onto me seems unfair.

And unfortunately, climate change is not unique in raising this problem. The general structure that gives rise to the Puzzle is that a problem is so large and complex that it is insensitive to individual choice. But that replicates in many areas of life. Consider the case of choosing to eat plant-based meals for animal welfare reasons (rather than just for environmental reasons): the animal agriculture system is global in scale and involves trillions of animals, such that most of the meat we buy is from corporations that will not notice small changes in demand. Thus, although it might feel to those of us with animal welfare concerns as if we are contributing to suffering when we, say, order a meat dish or buy animal products from the grocery store, it is likely the case that refraining from such purchases is not going to have any meaningful effect on the suffering of any animals.

This point about animals makes clear that our consumer choices in general can have this structure. Buried in global supply chains for all sorts of products are terrible labor practices, such as child labor, exploitation, and even modern-day slavery. Indeed, one of the most important products in the modern world—lithium-ion batteries, which power everything from our computers and phones to the electric vehicles at the center of our green energy transition plans—is entangled in terrible human rights violations. This is because such batteries require cobalt, more than 70 percent of which is mined in the Democratic Republic of Congo, often under terribly exploitative conditions, sometimes by children (Kara 2023). So, should you stop buying all technology involving rechargeable batteries? Not only would that be incredibly difficult in the modern world, but, given the scale of the problem, you can rest assured that your protest would not make a difference to any individual in the Congo.

We can see how this form of problem continues to replicate. Any time it feels like perhaps we should withdraw support from a bad system, structure, or actor, but recognize that our individual actions won't make a difference, we have encountered a version of the Puzzle.

So what should we do?

Between a Purity Ethic and Nihilism

I think the Puzzle gets a grip on us through a bit of sleight of hand. It presents as if it's offering a dilemma: we must either embrace an ethic laser-focused on the moral purity of individuals, or we must accept moral nihilism about individual action in the face of problems like climate change. We either find a way to justify the view that individuals have a duty to change their behavior in the face of catastrophe, or we're left with the depressing conclusion that many of our actions don't matter.

Nihilism is awfully hard to accept. Although it seems true that there is something perverse about asking individuals to consume less when our individual choices are so insignificant, it also seems true that the ultra-wealthy shouldn't take private jets everywhere because they are not entitled to have carbon footprints that dwarf entire populations of poorer people. It seems like there is *something bad* about their lifestyle from an environmental perspective.

Moreover, those who seemed to be criticizing purity ethics as "deflections" and "victim blaming" aren't actually claiming that what individuals do doesn't matter morally. Rather, they are arguing that conscious consumerism shouldn't distract us from taking part in various collective actions—in trying to bring about meaningful change through advocacy and activism (Heglar 2019).

But of course, your contribution to advocacy might also not make a difference. Contributing to collective efforts to bring about change is not so dissimilar from withdrawing one's contribution to collective harms; in both cases, you are doing one very small piece of a much larger project, either by choosing *not* to do something (like emit GHGs) or by choosing *to do* something (like march in a protest or phone bank for a political candidate).

So those criticizing conscious consumerism don't actually seem to be supporting nihilism. They think that what each of us does matters morally; they just don't want us focusing on minimizing our carbon footprint or otherwise keeping our hands clean at the expense of more positive efforts to contribute to the good. But once we accept that our individual actions matter, why *shouldn't* we accept a purity ethic?

I think the best reason to avoid a purity ethic is that it is both unreasonable and unhelpful in the modern world. Given the number of catastrophes we face and the number of ways in which our individual actions can contribute to them, we are nearly constantly contributing to, participating in, and supporting bad structures, systems, or actors. A purity ethic commands us to withdraw such support, which means that we all need to spend an exorbitant amount of time trying to discover and disentangle ourselves from evil. This is unhelpful because it is paralyzing and therefore not action-guiding; and it's unreasonable because if we attempted such purity (despite the fact that we would almost certainly fail), we would have no time or energy for any other moral projects. Indeed, one way to reconstruct the criticism that focusing on purity is a deflection from collective action is to argue that individuals should have the moral freedom to combat climate change through, say, advocacy rather than purity. If my climate activism requires driving or flying around the country in order to speak, rally, or otherwise participate in the climate fight, a purity ethic would prohibit me from doing so, even if it might seem like that sort of travel is easily justified by the goal.

Thus, the Puzzle presents individual morality to us as if we must choose between the views that what we do doesn't matter at all, or that we are morally required to focus exclusively on purity. Since both of those options are unattractive, solving the Puzzle will require articulating a third way.

The Shift to Reasons

If the above is broadly on target, then we know a bit about what a satisfactory solution to the Puzzle will look like.

1. In order to avoid nihilism, it must offer a response to the argument from causal inefficacy. That is: it must explain how it can morally matter what one does, even when one's actions are unlikely to have a meaningful impact.

2. That explanation should not, however, imply a requirement of moral purity. That is, the solution to causal inefficacy should not prove *too much*.
3. In general, then: a solution to the Puzzle must navigate between the twin horns of being *too demanding* and *too lax*. Any solution that floats a bit too close to purity will fail on the first count, while straying too close to nihilism will fail on the second.

In what follows, I will argue that my preferred view of shifting from a focus on duty or obligation to a focus on reasons satisfies all these *desiderata*.

Duty and obligation are strict and invasive moral concepts. They carry the "moral must" of requirement: if I have a duty to tell the truth, I *must* do it, and so failing to do so is *wrong*. Often, I should be blamed for failing in my duty, perhaps even punished or otherwise held accountable (by, say, social pressure or falling in the esteem of my community). Some philosophers also believe that interpersonal duties correlate with rights, such that having a duty to do something implies that someone else, somewhere, has a right against me that I do it. My duty to tell the truth implies that someone has the right to my honesty, and they are thus *entitled* to it. According to the philosopher Stephen Darwall, this grounds a *standing to demand* that I comply with my duty (Darwall 2009). In short: duties are maximally strong, or weighty, normative concepts.

Duty and obligation (which I am here using interchangeably) are not our only normative concepts, however. There are much weaker ones, and I think a particularly important normative tool is that of a reason (Little 2013). A reason is simply a consideration that counts in favor of an action. It recommends the action or justifies it. But it need not require it. When I find a wild animal in some danger on my property, I typically try to free it to prevent its suffering or death. I think this is a good thing to do. But I do not believe that I have a general duty to rescue wild animals. Rather, the fact that a sentient being would suffer without my intervening seems to give me a reason to rescue it if I can. There is something good about such a rescue (since it relieves suffering), which justifies my action.

Reasons, then, come cheap. We have a reason to do something any time there is value in doing so, and a reason not to do something any time there is disvalue in doing so. We can thus easily explain the existence of reasons not to contribute to massive, structural harms, as doing so makes us a participant in that harm. It's bad to participate in harm, which grounds a reason to refrain. Similarly, it's good to invest in green technology, volunteer for the climate movement, or donate to environmental causes—not because you're likely to make a difference, but because it's good to participate in justice.

In a slogan: it's bad to be part of the problem, and good to be part of the solution (even when your part is very small).

We must remember, though, that these reasons are not in the business of requiring action, and so they do not generate duties. Thus, I have not solved the Puzzle of individual morality by figuring out how to justify a duty. Rather, I have tried to rescue the intuition that there is *something good* about taking small actions (like reducing our carbon footprint) without arguing that we are therefore obligated to take those actions. This, I want to suggest, provides a framework for avoiding an unreasonable purity ethic, but without reverting to nihilism. Because nihilism is the view that what you do doesn't matter; but your action does matter! It matters because some actions are recommended and others aren't, and some are better, and others are worse.

Unfortunately, my solution raises another problem, which is also daunting: if we have reasons to act in the face of catastrophe based on the value of participating in different structures and systems, then we have *a lot of reasons*. The environmental cost of animal-sourced foods generates reasons to reduce my intake of those foods by 10 percent; to become flexitarian; to become vegetarian; to become pescetarian; to become vegan; and almost certainly more. The treatment of migrant workers by some of the agricultural companies that provide our food gives me reason to buy my produce or meat from only some companies or some farms. The value of crop rotation, animal grazing, and regenerative farming gives me reason to buy meat from small, regenerative farms that sell animal products in order to pay for their work healing the land. And suddenly it is very difficult to know how I am supposed to respond to all of the reasons I face regarding my consumption (or not) of animals. Not to mention, of course, that this is only one facet of only one catastrophe, and I have reasons to participate (or not) in all sorts of structures.

I began this chapter by claiming that the goal of bioethics should include providing action guidance. So far, it looks like a reasons-based solution to the Puzzle fails on that account. What we need, then, is a way to organize and respond to our reasons that can justify our actions and lifestyles. This is the sort of work that may allow bioethicists to provide guidance in the realm of collective catastrophes like climate change in the same way that they do concerning more traditional bioethical concerns.

How to Make Progress

The first step in developing a framework for responding to an overwhelming influx of reasons is to propose heuristics, or rules of thumb, that provide action guidance in response to some set of reasons. So, for instance, the reasons that I have not to contribute to climate change justify many different heuristics. One would be, "Don't be wasteful." Waste, after all, is energy used for no good purpose; so, if we're trying to respond to the reasons commending reduced energy use, then this is a good start. It's not exactly specific, so we could further specify it: "Turn out the lights when you leave the room"; "don't buy groceries carelessly such that you end up regularly throwing food away"; "don't overheat or overcool your home or workplace"; and so on.

Reasons justify heuristics because they recommend without requiring. So, the sentence "don't be wasteful" in this context is not a duty-generating principle of the same form as "do no harm," but rather an organizing guideline. This makes them quite different from, say, the four principles of biomedical ethics (Beauchamp and Childress 2019). Principles are rules that imply duties: the principle of respect for autonomy can be specified into the particular duty for a clinician to ensure that their subject has given adequately informed consent prior to initiating an intervention. But a heuristic does not imply a duty; rather, it provides a general recommendation to do something based on the value of that action. Heuristics are helpfully efficient, allowing one to work out an appropriate response to value ahead of time and then set it and forget it. Leaving a room without turning off the light does not violate a duty. But there is a good justification for developing a habit of turning out lights, because leaving them burning is wasteful. And you have reason not to be wasteful.

Developing heuristics is helpful, but it's not nearly enough to provide all the action guidance we might want in the context of catastrophe. After all, we face many catastrophes, and the reasons they generate can justify many different heuristics.

So, the second step in developing a decision framework is to think about how we can organize our heuristics. I've proposed that in response to any catastrophe we face, we can organize candidate heuristics along two dimensions: first, according to what *kind* of reason justifies the heuristic in question; and second, whether the heuristic faces any significant competing reasons (and if so, how significant the competing reasons are). You can imagine using these two dimensions to arrange candidate heuristics along a 3×3 matrix (for a visualization of this matrix, see Rieder 2024).

Along the y-axis of such a chart, we can distinguish between different *kinds* of reasons. Taking the example of climate change, heuristics can be justified by at least three different kinds of reasons: purity reasons, social reasons, and structural reasons. Purity reasons are *negative* reasons, or reasons not to take some action. In terms of the discussion so far, these are the reasons to withdraw one's participation from some activity that is made morally problematic by its collective outcome. Social and structural reasons are *positive* reasons, or reasons *to do* some particular thing. Since not all positive reasons are the same, I've distinguished between reasons that commend a social activity (activities concerned with how we engage with others) and reasons that commend trying to change some structure through political or other collective action. Obviously, there can be overlap, as some social heuristics recommend actions that are also structural; but the distinction is helpful because in what follows, we will discuss the sorts of considerations that often lead individuals to be better or worse at responding to, or more or less inclined to respond to, various heuristics. And the social/structural distinction can often help to understand differences in these responses.

Along the x-axis, we can arrange heuristics by how much normative competition they face. So, for instance, we can distinguish between heuristics that face no competing reasons, those that face modest competing reasons, and those that face compelling competing reasons. When a heuristic genuinely faces no competing reasons, then it's the clearest case of something that one has particularly strong reason to do. Such heuristics might seem fairly rare, as most recommendations seem to face at least some minor competition from other considerations. But we likely can identify the occasional heuristic that faces no—or virtually no—normative competition, at least when specified in certain ways. The broad heuristic "Don't be wasteful" might start to face competing reasons if we try to define wasteful in terms of doing things we don't need; but if we just think of wastefulness as concerning actions that use resources for no good reason (like leaving lights on when we leave the room, or leaving water running), then we can identify versions of the principle that genuinely face no real competition (for this purpose, "I didn't want to move my arm to flip the lightswitch" wouldn't be taken seriously as a competing reason).

Even these heuristics that don't face meaningful competition don't carry the weight of the moral "must"; however, it's plausible to say that each of us *should* act on them, as such actions are definitionally recommended by reasons and not undermined by any other reasons. In addition to the purity heuristic of something like, "Don't be wasteful," we can posit social and structural heuristics that are similarly recommended by reasons and undermined by virtually none. Socially, I try to follow the heuristic, "Talk about climate change with others," since doing so costs me practically nothing, and it contributes to the collective effort to raise awareness. And structurally, I follow a heuristic to vote in all elections and to support environmental policy efforts when available. Here again, since I am an active citizen anyway, this recommendation faces virtually no opposition but is justified by the value of being part of important collective efforts.

Most heuristics, of course, face some normative competition, and in that case, it's helpful to think about whether that normative competition is modest or compelling. For example, I offer the heuristic "eat low on the food chain" as a climate-conscious food heuristic, which responds to the value of decreasing the energy use required to make one's food (but doesn't require strict adherence to, say, veganism, because it's a heuristic and not a duty). Although I love food and deeply value different food experiences, those interests don't seem like the most compelling reasons to, say, eat a lot of beef (which has a very high carbon footprint). They are reasons grounded by *mere interests*. Whereas a heuristic that advises me to, say, "minimize my carbon footprint" faces genuinely competing reasons, as following its recommendation would require an enormous amount of time, energy, and money. Truly minimizing my carbon footprint would be expensive, as it would require installing solar panels, driving an electric car, buying the most energy-efficient appliances, and so on. It might also be very difficult, as it might recommend walking or biking more than I want or have time to. Given where my family has chosen to live and how my partner and I have decided to commute in order to pursue our respective career goals, truly minimizing our carbon footprints might actually require changing jobs and/or moving. If we really took "minimizing" literally, perhaps we would be required to move off the grid and change all of our behaviors.

Thus, minimizing one's carbon footprint comes with very serious—morally real and weighty—trade-offs. Sure, I might not want to do these things because I like good food and whatnot; but I also would have to give up much that is genuinely valuable in order to pursue it.

When we imagine our candidate heuristics on this sort of matrix, I think we can start to notice a few things. The first is that we cannot respond to all of the heuristics that we could generate. What this means is that we will have to choose which ones to adopt, and that choice will allow subjectivity to enter the picture. Because heuristics are not duties, but recommendations, they allow for latitude—which is a good thing, considering the fact that we can't live up to all of them. That latitude, then, makes permissible the creation and organization of one's own matrix, and the adoption of some but not other heuristics.

How does one make such a decision? Since there is no single thing that anyone must do, I want to suggest that the choice of what moral features of the world to respond to is more akin to a lifestyle choice than a moral requirement. Some of us focus our efforts on the environment; others on animals; some are focused on relieving poverty or infectious disease burdens; and yet others place their efforts on responding to exploitation in the global supply chain. And within each project, some people are more drawn to purity, attempting to withdraw their participation from problematic practices, while others are activists, drawn toward organizing. Organizers might deride the purists for being overly precious. And purists might ask why organizing should be a substitute for not personally contributing to harm and injustice. But in my view, there is no objectively correct response to the threats of the world. There is much work to be done, and so we should recognize the moral latitude that allows people to follow their interests, passion, drive, skills, and privilege.

Indeed, on this last point: consider the difference in matrixes between someone with a lot of money, who can participate in the energy transition through installing solar panels, versus a young person with very few resources, but perhaps more time and energy. And this sort of consideration shows up in other places as well: those with more time and money will often be in a better position to research their food choices or the companies they buy from and spend more to ensure that they are getting an ethically produced product. Those with more education may find it easier to follow the policy and political discussions that allow for meaningful political action. And those with truly exceptional abilities and platforms will have opportunities to influence others in ways that most of us will not. In short: while it would be unreasonable to expect everyone to equally consider participating in the green energy transition through buying an electric car at a significant price premium, it is not as unreasonable for those with money to consider it a valuable way *for them* to participate in the collective effort.

More objectively, however, we can recognize that every moral lifestyle choice will face reasons of different strength. And so, each of us will need to decide how much of our moral resources (time, energy, financial) to give in responding to these reasons. Arguably, most of us should feel compelled to live up to heuristics that face no serious normative competition as we become aware of them. After all, there's no reason not to! But we will then start to feel the moral pressure pushing us in the direction of increasing moral ambition, with ever more heuristics asking, "Isn't there just a bit more you could do?" And the answer will almost always be, of course, "yes." There's more you could do, and it would be good if you did (even though you're not required to do so).

The moral work of facing catastrophe is thus never-ending. Although some people find relief in the idea that we are not duty-bound to respond to climate change or any other catastrophe in some particular way, that lack of duty comes at a cost. If we could identify the thing you must do, then you could do it, check it off your list, and be done with the moral work of facing that particular threat. But in the absence of duty, we're left facing a sea of values and recommendations, and we will always be left with the reality that we didn't do as much as we could.

This conclusion is likely to strike many as overwhelming, and that's understandable. But it's important to note what we gain in recognizing the reasons we face: we gain *meaning*. Recognizing the moral challenge of today is a rebuttal to nihilism, as it explains how it is that what we do matters, despite the insignificance of our own small contributions to problems and solutions.

So yes: everything you do matters. But that means you get to matter.

The Future of Bioethics

The work I have outlined here is only a sketch of a start of how we can live a justifiable life in the face of the many catastrophic threats of the twenty-first century. If the goal for bioethics is to be genuinely action-guiding, then there is much work left to be done. The promise of bioethics is to help us think through and resolve problems related to our existence as fragile beings—in the domains of medicine, public health, science, technology, and other fields that impact human (and planetary, some of us think) wellness. And so, we might hope and expect that bioethics is the field to guide us through a world in which so much is threatened by the large, structural forces we have built. But doing bioethics in a world on fire must recognize the gap between traditional individual ethics and traditional collective ethics and develop ways to provide guidance to individuals regarding collective threats that they cannot solve on their own. In closing, then, I want to make a few suggestions for how bioethics could make concrete contributions to the space of catastrophe ethics.

First, there are almost certainly many different ways to conceptualize the sort of moral framework I have offered, and it seems likely that some will be better for particular purposes. For instance: are there other ways to think about the different kinds of positive reasons one has? Are some reasons particularly salient for those who occupy a particular role (like, say, for healthcare workers)? The reasons and heuristics I have offered were for the purpose of drawing some very general lessons about catastrophe ethics, but there is no reason to think that I have found the best way to organize potential moral responses to the world.

Second, I have not yet offered any guidance on triaging one's moral response. I argued above that the lack of a strict duty to do any one thing suggests the latitude to adopt a moral lifestyle that suits one's strengths, interests, and privilege, but that doesn't mean that all moral projects are equally worthy of attention. Are there some threats to which virtually everyone should feel compelled to respond? Climate change seems a good candidate for such a threat, based on its scale and severity; but notice that other considerations also seem important. For instance, when Covid-19 emerged in early 2020, the acuity and time-sensitive nature of the outbreak seemed to demand that everyone respond immediately and aggressively to promote a public health good, and likely, during some time period, it was justifiable to prioritize one's moral efforts to combating Covid-19 rather than to thinking about climate change. Does this sort of example tell us anything about the circumstances under which individuals should feel especially compelled to adopt a moral project?

Finally, I want to close by going back to the idea that bioethics is supposed to guide action. Classically, bioethics could impact practice by engaging with a fairly limited audience, mostly composed of clinicians, scientists, and policymakers. And while communicating with these audiences is certainly a skill that requires training and development, it is relatively close to what most bioethicists are trained to do by their disciplinary education—they publish in peer-reviewed literature, write white papers, serve as expert witnesses or advisors, and so on. In short: they wear their expert hats to engage other experts and learn how to communicate in a way that is understandable to those experts.

Catastrophe ethics, however, is not an area of ethics that is aimed at some narrow class of experts. The questions it asks are questions for all of us, and so in order to be helpful—to be action-guiding—it needs to be communicated to, well, *everyone*. This is an argument that at least some bioethicists need to be able to speak not only to experts outside of their community but to the public at large. It's an argument for public bioethics, or on the model of science communication, for the development of a field of "bioethics communication" (Rieder, Hutchinson, and Kahn 2022). A particular question in bioethics communication for catastrophe ethics, then, is: How might we best help the public think through particular instances of the Puzzle that they are struggling with? The framework I've presented here is a general model that outlines a path; but just as a bioethicist might not engage with a doctor or researcher by giving them ethics frameworks, but rather by providing recommendations, arguments, or evaluations, we can expect that many people might want something more concrete than what I've developed here. The future of bioethics should, I'm suggesting, involve attempting to address the challenge of living ethically amidst catastrophe, provide concrete recommendations, and communicate those recommendations to the public in a way (and in a venue) that's accessible.

I'm sure there is much more that could be said, but hopefully these few words are sufficient to show that there is practical ethics work to be done in addressing a new kind of moral reality. There are still plenty of classic bioethics problems to be addressed and solved at the individual and collective level. But there is also a whole slew of questions to be addressed in the middle, as individuals attempt to respond ethically as individuals to collective threats. Bioethics, I think, can help them.

Bibliography

Allen, M. R., D. J. Frame, C. Huntingford, C. D. Jones, J. A. Lowe, M. Meinshausen, and N. Meinshausen. 2009. "Warming Caused by Cumulative Carbon Emissions Towards the Trillionth Tonne." *Nature*, 458: 1163–6.

Beauchamp, T. L., and J. F. Childress. 2019. *Principles of Biomedical Ethics*, 8th ed. Oxford University Press.

Broome, J. 2012. *Climate Matters: Ethics in a Warming World.* W. W. Norton & Company.

Cripps, E. 2013. *Climate Change and the Moral Agent: Individual Duties in an Interdependent World.* Oxford University Press.

Darwall, S. 2009. *The Second-Person Standpoint: Morality, Respect, and Accountability.* Harvard University Press.

Global Footprint Network. n.d. *Earth Overshoot Day.* March 24, 2023. https://www.overshootday.org.

Hale, B. 2011. "Nonrenewable Resources and the Inevitability of Outcomes." *The Monist*, 84 (3): 369–90.

Hedberg, T. 2018. "Climate Change, Moral Integrity, and Obligations to Reduce Individual Greenhouse Gas Emissions." *Ethics, Policy, & the Environment*, 21 (1): 64–80.

Heglar, M. A. 2019. "I Work in the Environmental Movement. I Don't Care If You Recycle." *Vox*, June 4, 2019.

Hourdequin, M. 2010. "Climate, Collective Action and Individual Ethical Obligations." *Environmental Values*, 19 (4): 443–64.

Kara, S. 2023. *Cobalt Red: How the Blood of Congo Powers Our Lives.* St. Martin's Press.

Kutz, C. 2000. *Complicity: Ethics and Law for a Collective Age.* Cambridge University Press.

Lamboll, R. D., Z. R. Nicholls, C. J. Smith, J. S. Kikstra, E. Byers, and J. Rogelj. 2023. "Assessing the Size and Uncertainty of Remaining Carbon Budgets." *Nature Climate Change* 13: 1360–7.

Liebow, N. K., and T. N. Rieder. 2022. "'What Can I Possibly Do?': White Individual Responsibility for Addressing Racism as a Public Health Crisis." *Bioethics*, 36 (3): 274–82.

Little, M. O. 2013. "In Defence of Non-Deontic Reasons." In D. Bakhurst, M. O. Little, and B. Hooker (eds.), *Thinking About Reasons: Themes From the Philosophy of Jonathan Dancy.* Oxford University Press.

Little, M. O., and C. Macnamara. 2022. "The Latitude-Preserving Nature of Commendatory Reasons." In Russ Shafer-Landau (ed.), *Oxford Studies in Metaethics*, vol. 17 Oxford University Press.

Mann, M. E. 2021. *The New Climate War: The Fight to Take Back Our Planet.* PublicAffairs.

Monbiot, G. 2019. "The Big Polluters' Masterstroke Was to Blame the Climate Crisis on You and Me." *The Guardian*, October 9, 2019.

Nefsky, J. 2015. "Fairness, Participation, and the Real Problem of Collective Harm." In Mark Timmons (ed.), *Oxford Studies in Normative Ethics*, vol. 5. Oxford University Press.

Nolt, J. 2011. "How Harmful are the Average American's Greenhouse Gas Emissions?" *Ethics, Policy, and the Environment*, 14 (1): 3–10.

Our World In Data. n.d.. United States: CO2 Country Profile. Retrieved August 27, 2025 from https://ourworldindata.org/co2/country/united-states.

Rieder, T. 2024. *Catastrophe Ethics: How to Choose Well in a World of Tough Choices.* Dutton.

Rieder, T. N., L. A. Hutchinson, and J. P. Kahn. 2022. "Why the World Needs Bioethics Communication." *Perspectives in Biology and Medicine*, 65 (4): 629–36.

Rieder, T., and J. Bernstein. 2020. "The Case for 'Contributory Ethics': Or How to Think about Individual Morality in a Time of Global Problems." *Ethics, Policy & Environment*, 3: 299–319.

Shotwell, A. 2016. *Against Purity: Living Ethically in Compromised Times*. University of Minnesota Press.

Sinnott-Armstrong, W. 2005. "It's Not My Fault: Global Warming and Individual Moral Obligation." In Walter Sinnott-Amstrong and Richard B. Howarth (eds.), *Perspectives on Climate Change: Science, Economics, Politics, Ethics*. Elsevier.

10

The Early Ethics of Planetary Health

Stephen M. Gardiner and Paul Tubig

Over the last decade, the concept of planetary health has risen to prominence on the public health landscape.[1] Planetary health holds promise as a way of motivating, articulating, and grounding a public health agenda in an era where global, intergenerational, and ecological challenges are intertwined. Its proponents constitute one branch of a wider movement which seeks to reorganize, and perhaps revolutionize, public health in response to global environmental problems, especially climate change. Planetary health is intended to serve an important practical need, as it calls for increased transdisciplinary approaches to the forces that shape public health. For many, the notion is also being introduced to fill a deeper conceptual need for a better understanding of public health itself. Thus, planetary health is sometimes "touted as the natural successor to public and global health" (Hill-Cawthorne 2019, 14).

Ethics is at the center of this push for transformation. As a conceptual frame, planetary health is of interest in part because it is one possible way of "environmentalizing" public health ethics and bioethics more generally (Gardiner 2022). In doing so, planetary health moves beyond narrower, more restrictive conceptions of bioethics—with their heavy focus on clinical ethics, healthcare provision, and health technologies (e.g., Schenck and Churchill 2021)—to embrace a broader vision of the subject. Thus, the pursuit of planetary health resonates with Van Rensselaer Potter's intent in introducing the term "bioethics," that the endeavor should transcend health care narrowly understood to become "the name of a discipline combining science and philosophy, with wisdom— 'knowledge of how to use knowledge' about human survival and flourishing—as its goal" (ten Have 2012; drawing from Potter 1970, 127). Given this, the planetary health movement might be seen as a "test case" for those interested in expansive visions of bioethics. Even if the effort itself falls short, there may be lessons to learn for that broader project.

Nevertheless, it is currently early days for planetary health ethics. Despite considerable enthusiasm for the basic idea, the core meaning, values, principles, and norms associated with the term require clarification and further exploration. This chapter aims to situate the discussion of planetary health through a critical engagement with how the concept is initially articulated in the early stages of the movement, and especially in its main foundational document, the Rockefeller-Lancet Commission (RLC) report (Whitmee et al. 2016). This engagement enables us to draw lessons for the ethical work needed to move forward, not just for planetary health as such, but for the wider project of environmentalizing both public health ethics and bioethics.

The Concept of Planetary Health

Context

Sometimes planetary health is described as a young concept, "first coined" as recently as 2013 or 2015, and established over the following decade (e.g., Rockefeller 2016). However, such claims are contentious. Some insist that the central motivating idea—roughly, that human health is deeply intertwined with and dependent on the larger environment, including planetary systems—is hardly new, and indeed has a long history. For one thing, it is "part of the traditional knowledge that has been passed on by Indigenous cultures since time immemorial" (Prescott et al. 2018, 31); for another, claims about interdependence are central to much environmental thinking, including in environmental ethics (e.g., Leopold, Callicott, Taylor, Norton). Experts say that even the specific term *planetary health* "re-emerged" from the environmental movement as long ago as the 1970s and was explicitly deployed in a public health context as early as 1980, in a proposal from Friends of the Earth to shift the World Health Organization's definition of health in a more expansive, ecological direction (Prescott et al. 2018, 31). Given this long history, some warn fellow enthusiasts for planetary health against "any claims of newness (or ahistorical assertions that marginalize ancestrally-rooted traditional perspectives)," in part because they fear that these "will only serve to magnify an unhealthy 'in-group' dominance and undermine the opportunities for high-level wellness" (Prescott et al. 2018, 31).

Against this backdrop, how should one characterize the recent rise to prominence of planetary health? First, it is perhaps best to say merely that "planetary health as a thing" gained a strong foothold in the public health discourse only a decade or so ago, as the result of a collaboration between two powerful actors, the Rockefeller Foundation and *The Lancet* (Drake 2021). Among other things, this collaboration produced the RLC report in 2015 and a new journal *The Lancet: Planetary Health* shortly thereafter. Second, it should be emphasized that planetary health did not ascend in a vacuum. Even in contemporary discussion, planetary health is but the latest member of a family of concepts being proposed to broaden the purview of public health beyond its traditional focus, with special attention to global and environmental factors. Close relations include One Health, EcoHealth, and Conservation Medicine (Hill-Cawthorne 2019). In short, placed in context, planetary health is not particularly exceptional, and its power might be seen as institutional as much as conceptual.

Nevertheless, there are reasons to pay attention to the notion of planetary health. Although the various revisionary concepts of public health (and bioethics more generally) could easily become positioned as rivals and compete for limited intellectual space and resources, so far this has not happened. Instead, a popular view among both proponents and practitioners appears to be that the new concepts complement one another in serving shared goals and being mutually reinforcing. For example, while a recent piece comparing One Health and Planetary Health identifies overlaps, confusion, and a need for clarity, it nevertheless concludes that "diversity should not be a reason to diverge or compete but to collaborate" and "our diversity will only make us stronger" (de Castañeda et al. 2023).

One reason for the stress on complementarity is political. Each concept is often said to have its own "convening power" in particular health communities that is helpful in advancing a broader, shared agenda. Indeed, this sense of common purpose is strong enough that sometimes even supporters of other concepts in the family suggest that planetary health might emerge to play a coordinating, leadership role.

Beyond its institutional reach, there may also be theoretical reasons to highlight planetary health. Some suggest that the term is a *natural extension* of earlier concepts, including One Health. For example, John Drake sketches a historical progression of narratives for how we should think about health. This progression begins with individual health, but then runs through public health, global health, and on to One Health. Drake says planetary health "takes this delocalization of health *another step further*" because it "recognizes the health of the planet as a system, and that even its non-living components are wrapped up in that state of well-being or disease" (Drake 2021, emphasis added). In such accounts, planetary health is positioned as the logical or ethical next step in a history of ever more expansive understandings of health. Notably, the framing is reminiscent of discussions of expanding circles of moral concern in ethics, typically from humans to animals to plants to ecosystems to the "land" (e.g., Singer, Taylor, Callicott).

Given this context, it is worth taking seriously the development of a shared understanding of planetary health as a concept. Early decisions about how to conceptualize a movement often have profound implications for how that movement evolves in ways that influence outcomes.

Surface Meaning

At first glance, the concept of "planetary health" appears straightforward and obviously attractive. On the surface, it simply joins together the words "planetary" and "health," so that "planetary health" is health seen from a planetary perspective. Understood just a little more strongly, planetary health represents "the idea that human health and the health of the environment are inextricably linked" (Cole 2019).

Nevertheless, even at the outset there is more going on. Medical labels like "health" and "disease" are not neutral terms but carry normative force. Partly, this is because "health" is a positive evaluative concept. Colloquially, it denotes something that should be protected and promoted. Given this, when "health" is invoked to describe social and ecological conditions—as it is in the simple phrase "planetary health"—this framing functions to shape our perceptions *in favor* of that agenda. Implicitly, we are invited to share the view that pursuing states of the world that align with the standard represented in the term "planetary health" is desirable, and uncontroversially so. For instance, someone who resists "planetary health" risks being portrayed as indifferent to, or even in favor of, the contrary—"planetary sickness" or "planetary disease." Thus, enthusiasm for the idea and movement is actively encouraged by the mere form of words "planetary health," and resistance actively discouraged.

Still, the normative loading of the "planetary health" concept through its surface-level meaning is hardly sufficient to ground the term or to make it sustainable in the long run. Catchy terms come and go. Moreover, even supporters of planetary health have noticed that discussions of it have already "become peppered with a series of phrases that seek to capture the zeitgeist of the approach but do not always contain much substance," such that "there is a danger that if we do not promote principles that define the ethics of how we look after the planet, the scientific evidence we gather on the harm being committed will have little impact" (Foster et al. 2019). In short, if the movement is to endure, the bare phrase "planetary health" must be interpreted, elaborated, and defended. Among other things, a deeper account would specify the following: the *standard* signaled by using the label "health" in relation to the planet; the kinds of planetary *states* or phenomena that the notion is meant to track; and the *norms* that should govern the pursuit of planetary health. More broadly, since planetary health is being put forward to address fundamental practical and conceptual needs in public health, clarifying those needs is central. Notably, the simple conjunction of "planetary" and "health" does not tell us the *purpose* for which the concept is being introduced into the public health lexicon and what drives the movement introducing it. Given this, we suggest pursuing the question, "What is planetary health?" in part by asking, "What is the planetary health movement trying to be?" (Gardiner 2022).

This chapter aims to elaborate on the planetary health agenda through an examination of the key early text of the planetary health movement, the Rockefeller Foundation–Lancet Commission report on planetary health (Whitmee 2016), supplemented by early framings provided by leading professional organizations, such as the Planetary Health Alliance (PHA). Interestingly, this approach reveals that early proponents may diverge in their interpretations of the key ideas of planetary health; moreover, these differences in vision illuminate some basic challenges for the planetary health agenda moving forward.[2]

Generic Meaning

A useful generic characterization of the planetary health movement is provided by the key journal, *The Lancet Planetary Health*, as featured on its website in 2018:

> Generic Definition: "[P]lanetary health *broadens health research* to include the *external systems* that *sustain or threaten human health.*" (Lancet 2018, emphases added)

This definition explicates the aim of planetary health, which is to expand health research beyond conventional public health boundaries to external, typically environmental and social systems. The idea is that a broadened research agenda is necessary if the public health community is to properly recognize the magnitude and complexity of the problems it seeks to address. On this understanding, the aim of the planetary health concept and its allied movement is: (1) to expand the usual areas of concern for the public health community (e.g., the discipline, its major institutions, etc.), (2) to include the underlying drivers of health, (3) as part of the research agenda, (4) with a special emphasis on environmental systems, since (5) this is necessary to properly address the fundamental goals of health policy, where (6) conventional understandings of public health have fallen short in achieving those goals, and (7) this failure is driven (at least in part) by conceptual shortcomings.

The generic understanding of "planetary health" is shared across the movement. Nevertheless, the concept can be further specified in distinct ways, and it is instructive to compare them. Notably, several key terms are subject to deeper interpretation, including "broadens," "health research," "external systems," and "health" itself. Consequently, the generic understanding of planetary health leaves its precise role, purview, limits, scope, and targets underdetermined. This implies that there are numerous possibilities for more concrete interpretations of planetary health. While this need not be a problem in itself, in practice, underdetermination obscures some fundamental differences in how the planetary health agenda might be understood.

To illustrate this, we will focus on two visions of planetary health that we take to be especially salient. Before doing so, let us emphasize two points. First, our "two visions" function merely as a heuristic. In reality, those advocating for planetary health are unlikely to be sharply divided into two distinct interpretative "camps"; indeed, in our judgment, it is more plausible to believe that views on the meaning of planetary health are dispersed along a spectrum that runs across both interpretations. Second, given our purpose, we characterize the two interpretations only loosely. The aim in identifying two visions is to present a picture of what is at stake in divergent attitudes to planetary health that is helpful in thinking about how to shape the movement, as well as public health and bioethics more generally, moving forward.

The Narrow Vision

The first vision offers a narrow (or descriptive, restrictive, or conservative) interpretation of planetary health. The first way in which this interpretation is narrow is in its approach. Planetary health is seen (strictly, or at least overwhelmingly) as an *empirical* project, driven by needs in the natural and social sciences. The project aims to address a critical knowledge gap that previous divisions of scientific work on public health fail to cover adequately or systematically. The central concern is with expanding research to account explicitly for the widespread effects of natural and social systems on human health, especially when they are disrupted or modified by human activity (Seltenrich 2018; Bansal 2020). Proponents of the narrow interpretation look to the sciences to fill the gap by examining the interplay of environmental and sociopolitical factors in generating human health impacts.

The second way in which the interpretation is narrow is its target or scope of concern, which is typically confined to human health, *narrowly and traditionally conceived* (e.g., as the proper or species-typical functioning of the human body). The motivation for the narrow vision is that existing ways of thinking about public health do not adequately capture central factors that drive *conventional* health problems, that this inattention results in institutional failures in addressing health needs, and that this results in worse health outcomes, conventionally understood. Thus, on the narrow interpretation, the planetary health movement and concept aim to correct a failure that is itself fully explicable in conventional terms.[3] Implicit in the background is the assumption that, while there is much empirical scientific work to be done, *the central values to be pursued are already more-or-less clear and given*, so that planetary health requires no new or updated ethical agenda *there*. Instead, the transformation needed is mainly in the realm of the sciences.

Significant evidence for the narrow vision appears in primary sources. In general, the PHA initially introduced the concept on its website, saying: "[P]lanetary health is a field focused on *characterizing* the *human health impacts* of human-caused disruptions of Earth's natural systems" (PHA 2018a, emphases added). Moreover, the bulk of the articles on planetary health published in the early years appear to signal a narrow approach.

More specifically, in many sources the emphasis appears to be on improving scientific knowledge in ways that suggest a strong, perhaps exclusive, focus on empirical science for understanding environmental impacts. For instance, the PHA's original mission statement stated its role as being to "forge collaboration across a broad array of *scientific* disciplines, as well as with decision-makers, movement builders, and local communities, *to build a rigorous evidence base* for *informing* policy solutions" (PHA 2018a, emphases added). In its more specific account of its remit, the PHA spoke of "facilitating the training of the next generation of *scientists*," "*communicating* planetary health *science*," and "*applying planetary health science* directly to inform policy and practice" (PHA 2018a, emphasis added; PHA 2020). Relatedly, in the welcome to its inaugural issue, *Lancet Planetary Health* stated: "Planetary health is an exciting opportunity for finding alternative *solutions* for a better and more resilient future. *The Lancet Planetary Health* invites you to submit the best (and *still missing) scientific evidence* that can strengthen the case for policy action and can help write a new narrative for planetary health" (Editors, *Lancet Planetary Health* 2017, emphases added).

Similarly, numerous early sources appear to imply that planetary health is ultimately concerned solely with *human* health. For example, the PHA's 2018 statement states: "[P]lanetary health is a field focused on characterizing the *human health* impacts of human-caused disruptions of Earth's natural systems" (PHA 2018a, emphasis added). Moreover, a prominent introductory book, edited by two leaders in the field, is entitled "*Planetary Health: Protecting Nature to Protect Ourselves*" (Myers and Frumkin 2020, emphasis added). A reviewer in *The Lancet* notes that this "is certainly an anthropocentric title," but takes this as "understandable, and reasonable" (Capon 2020). More recently, in featuring planetary health on its website, the United Nations characterizes the concept in exclusively human terms: "Planetary health is a new field, and one that needs ideas and solutions that span multiple sectors and disciplines to guide the creative stewardship of our planet to protect *our own health*. Planetary Health shows how communities are creating new ways to use the planet's resources wisely to protect *their* health" (UNFCCC 2023, emphases added).

Wide Vision

The second vision can be characterized as wide (or normative, expansive, or revisionist) since it takes a much more capacious view of planetary health. Its proponents accept the basic claim of the narrow vision—that orthodox approaches to public health are failing in protecting human health as conventionally understood—and therefore support the narrow vision's push for reform in the empirical domain. However, advocates of the wide vision wish to push beyond a narrowly scientific agenda toward explicitly normative, institutional, and potentially also political transformation. They propose that reform requires a *relatively comprehensive account of the objectives and organization of the social order itself*, globally, intergenerationally, and perhaps ecologically. Most prominently, on the wide vision, the normative concerns and foundations of PH are not restricted to the promotion of human health conventionally understood, but extend to addressing *a broad range of moral and social values, including human flourishing in general, inequality, intergenerational justice, and (sometimes) the welfare and interests of nonhuman species*, such as nonhuman animals, plants, and ecosystems.[4] In light of this expanded ethical vision, those endorsing a wide interpretation of planetary health tend to have a strong interest in normative research on values and institutions, in research that informs the process of social transformation they believe is necessary to promote an expanded set of values, and often also in activities that go beyond research, such as institution-building and various kinds of activism (e.g., through the activities of professional associations and academic institutions).

The upshot is that the wide vision of planetary health encourages a substantial *reorientation of the central role and goals of public health*, with potentially dramatic implications for institutions. Indeed, at the extreme, one might think that the planetary health agenda becomes *primarily* a call for a thorough rethinking of how global society should understand its central objectives and reform its institutions, *secondarily* an appeal for the public health community to play a major, perhaps leading, role in the necessary transformation, and perhaps only *thirdly* a call to change the ways in which public health professionals think about how to succeed in their traditional work of promoting human health, conventionally understood. This is very different from the narrow vision of planetary health.

Strikingly, the wide vision appears to dominate the early movement. Despite the prominent representations of the narrow vision noted above, there is both ample evidence for the wide vision in the early history of PH and reasons to take it as central. First, and most importantly, the foundational report from the RLC itself defines "planetary health" in explicitly wide terms:

> Rockefeller-Lancet Commission Definition: "Our definition of planetary health is the achievement of the *highest attainable standard of health, wellbeing, and equity* worldwide through judicious attention to the *human systems*—political, economic, and social—that shape the future of humanity and the Earth's natural systems that define the safe environmental limits *within which humanity can flourish.* Put simply, planetary health is the *health of human civilisation and the state of the natural systems* on which it depends." (Whitmee et al. 2016, 1978, emphases added)

Relatedly, the RLC repeatedly characterizes the policy goals of PH in terms of "[balancing] social progress, environmental sustainability and the economy" (Whitmee et al. 2016, 1973), rather than health alone (as traditionally understood).

Second, an early "manifesto" in *The Lancet* written by founders of the movement describes planetary health as "an attitude towards life and a philosophy for living," claims that "an urgent transformation is required in our values and our practices," and calls for "a powerful social movement based on collective action at all levels of society" (Horton et al. 2014). Similarly, an account of the history of the idea of planetary health describes planetary health as "a distinct formation of environmental health, a divergent configuration in which *environmental ethics on a planetary scale* productively meets human population health" (Dunk, Jame and Anderson 2020, 18, emphasis added).

Third, over time the PHA has also made more expansive claims about the remit of planetary health. By November 2020, for instance, PHA was calling for "massive collaboration across disciplinary and national boundaries" and "facilitating the training of the next generation of planetary health leaders" (PHA 2020) rather than focusing on science and scientists (as it did in 2018). By October 2021, PHA's initial characterization was also emphasizing that planetary health is a social movement, as well as a transdisciplinary field: "Planetary health is a solutions-oriented, transdisciplinary field and social movement focused on analyzing and addressing the impacts of human disruptions to Earth's natural systems on human health and all life on Earth" (PHA 2021). Perhaps most strikingly, PHA appears to embrace a wide interpretation in its "conference principles" for the 2018 meeting in Edinburgh. While its first principle reaffirms the interest in science,[5] its second principle explicitly declares a wide, *distinctively ethical* agenda: "We seek to reinforce the *foundational values* of planetary health, including *respect for the value of both human and non-human life*, the *human rights of all people*, and *distributive and intergenerational justice*" (PHA 2018b, emphasis added).

Fourth, more recently, *The Lancet Planetary Health* describes itself as "the pre-eminent journal for enquiry into *sustainable human civilisations* in the Anthropocene," and states: "we particularly favour work that contributes to our understanding of, and transition into, a *safe and just space for humanity*" and "we are interested in *all important aspects of societal development* and its interaction with the environment" (LPH 2024, emphases added).

In sources such as these, we see examples of various elements of the wide vision, including expansive accounts of "health" (e.g., "the health of human civilization"), an explicit recognition of a plurality of normative ends (including health, well-being, equity, human rights, distributive justice, environmental sustainability, intergenerational justice, social progress, the flourishing of humanity), and a central concern for social change at multiple levels (e.g., calls for societal development and powerful social movements). Notably, while there is substantial convergence, there is also some divergence, and this provides evidence that we should be thinking more in terms of a spectrum of views than rigid "camps." One prominent example is the issue of ethical anthropocentrism: the claim that only humans are worthy of direct moral consideration in their own right. While most sources speak as if only humanity, human civilization, and human health matter for their own sake, some sources claim that "respect for the value of non-human life" is a foundational value of planetary health.

Does It Matter?

One reason for identifying the two visions is that they encourage diverging accounts of the central ideals and objectives of the planetary health agenda. Recall the generic definition: "planetary health *broadens health research* to include the *external systems* that *sustain or threaten human health*" (Lancet 2018). Already we see a reason to broaden this definition to accommodate non-anthropocentric accounts of value that include nonhumans within the scope of concern of planetary health. Thus, we might adopt:

> Expansive Generic Definition: Planetary health broadens health research to include the external systems that sustain or threaten the health of relevant populations.

Importantly, the narrow and wide interpretations suggest different understandings of this project, including how one might see the *role* of planetary health (e.g., what kind of broadening is needed), the kinds of *activities* that the term "broadening" is trying to inform (e.g., empirical research only, institution building, normative theorizing), the *target* of those activities (e.g., human health conventionally understood, a broader set of values), and the fundamental *subjects* of moral concern (e.g., humans only, nonhumans as well). For illustrative purposes, we sketch a version of this divergence in Table 10.1.

Notably, each interpretation of planetary health has some features that seem initially appealing and others that are potentially unsettling. To begin with, the narrow vision can seem safer and less controversial. For one, its ethical basis is straightforward and likely to be readily accepted. Concern for human health, conventionally understood, is already directly rooted in the discipline of public health. For another, the concerns of the narrow vision are shared by everyone in the planetary health community (including proponents of the wide view), so that it constitutes a kind of "minimal core" of the planetary health agenda on which

Table 10.1. Narrow and Wide Visions of the Planetary Health Agenda
How to interpret: Planetary health broadens health *research* to include the external systems that sustain or threaten the *health* of *relevant populations*

	Generic statement	Narrow interpretation	Wide interpretation
Role	"broaden"	Expand public health to include work on natural and social systems, with an emphasis on empirical work in natural and social sciences related to impacts, to provide evidence base for policy	Expand public health to include work on natural and social systems, including values and institutions; strong interest in normative and prescriptive work, including conceptual analysis and innovation; expand empirical work in natural and social sciences beyond impacts
Activities	"research"	Pursue traditional empirical research on health but expanded to include natural and social systems	Pursue all research relevant to needed social transformation to address global, intergenerational, ecological problems (e.g., including normative, empirical); consider activities beyond traditional research, such as institution-building, activism (professional, academic, perhaps also social, political), etc.
Target	"health"	Human health, narrowly and traditionally conceived	Central values (e.g., well-being, equity, intergenerational justice, nonhumans?)—e.g., "health of human civilizations"
Subjects of ultimate concern	"relevant populations"	Humans only	Humans, probably also nonhuman animals, perhaps plants, ecosystems, and other entities

everyone can agree. On the other hand, the narrow vision risks seeming too modest and tentative to achieve the transformation that many advocates in the movement hope for and believe is ethically required. An overly restricted construal of planetary health may render it insensitive and unresponsive to important dimensions of public health problems. For instance, a narrow vision may prevent planetary health from serving important values that, though not traditional within public health, turn out to be essential to its effectiveness.

By contrast, for many, the wide vision has the advantage of seeming more enlightened in ways that help confront the problems facing us. For instance, it defines planetary health in ways that incorporate multiple ethical values, makes public health more sensitive to social and environmental justice concerns, and is open to the value of nonhuman aspects of nature. In this, it is bolstered by the prominence of other wide definitions of health, such as that of the World Health Organization (WHO 1946; for early criticism, see Callahan 1973). Given this, the wide definition makes planetary health seem radical in the traditional sense of "getting at the roots" of the challenges that confront humanity.

Nevertheless, there are notable risks. For one thing, too dramatic an expansion of the concept of health may obfuscate, and so undermine, the planetary health agenda (see below). For another thing, revisionist forms of planetary health may fail to attract a broad enough consensus to sustain a movement, both within public health and beyond, since they encompass values and commitments that may seem less intuitive and more contentious to some. For instance, some enthusiasts for planetary health insist that "we must be mindful of guarding against the movement slipping into a new form of eco-environmentalism and ensure that the language used remains attractive to policymakers, the business sector and economists" (Foster et al. 2019, 14). While others may balk at this suggestion, the issues it raises about the role of planetary health are important for the movement moving forward.

Given such concerns, it is important to understand more deeply the aims of the planetary health movement. In this spirit, the next section examines the wide vision further, using the RLC definition to explore some of the conceptual difficulties that arise. Our objective is to identify some central features of a research agenda that any adequate conception of planetary health should embrace.

Early Ethical Foundations of Planetary Health

As well as serving as a paradigm of the wide vision, the RLC's canonical definition of planetary health offers a specific instantiation of that vision.[6] Three features stand out. First, planetary health is defined in terms of three core values "*health, wellbeing, and equity* worldwide" (as we call them, "the triumvirate" (i.e., "three rulers") of the planetary health agenda). Second, planetary health is understood as a maximizing doctrine: the aim is "the achievement of the *highest attainable standard*" of health, well-being, and equity. Third, planetary health is ethically anthropocentric: "planetary health is the health of *human civilisation* and the state of the natural systems on which *it* [i.e., 'human civilization'] depends." All three aspects of the RLC definition are controversial in themselves and raise important questions for the planetary health agenda, some of which we have explored elsewhere (Gardiner and Tubig 2023; Gardiner 2022). In this section, we will highlight three points, and in the next, we identify lessons for moving forward.

Internal Structure of "Planetary Health"

Our first point is that the concept of planetary health requires a better structure and terminology. One way in which the RLC definition is unhelpful is that it forces the term "health" to do *double duty*. Early in the definition, "health" is deployed in a restricted sense that *contrasts* health with well-being and equity as one of the triumvirate ("Planetary health is the achievement of the highest attainable standard of health, well-being and equity worldwide"). This is presumably a traditional sense of health, related to proper or species-typical functioning of the human body. By contrast, later in the definition, "health" is used to *cover all three* values of the triumvirate (including health, conventionally understood), and then applied to natural and social systems ("planetary health is the health of human civilization and the state of the natural systems on which it depends").

This double usage of "health" is problematic. First, it undermines effective communication by introducing ambiguity. Second, it makes the concept of planetary health look more rooted in public health than it really is. Third, it serves to obscure the essentially ethical character of the enterprise. One way to see this is to highlight alternatives. For instance, the three core values that constitute the triumvirate are health, well-being, and equity. So, why pick the term "planetary health" to cover all three? If one must choose from among the three, why not "planetary equity" or "planetary well-being" instead? More importantly, why choose from among them at all? Doesn't it seem better to find a distinct, broader term under which to organize?

Elsewhere, we have suggested that a better higher-level concept might be "planetary *eudaimonia*" or "planetary flourishing" (or some similar notion) (Gardiner and Tubig 2023).[7] One advantage is that, as associated with Aristotle and the ancient Greek tradition, "flourishing" is a broader notion than "health," "equity," or "well-being," yet can include all of them and a wide range of other values too. Another advantage is that the concept of flourishing appears to be implicit anyway. For instance, the RLC definition already refers to "the safe environmental limits within which humanity can *flourish*"; moreover, it uses this to characterize the general idea.

In our proposal, "planetary health" becomes a nested concept. If one deploys the term "planetary flourishing" at the higher level, the term "planetary health" can then be reserved to refer only to the element of the triumvirate that focuses on a more specific conception of health, where health professionals and the public health community can be expected to play a distinctive and perhaps critical role. This could be health as traditionally understood but need not be so restrictive. Either way, the aim is that the term "planetary health" would not be so expansive as to attempt to cover the whole realm of ethical concern associated with planetary flourishing.

In summary, our first basic conclusion is that the planetary health concept requires a better structure and terminology. The RLC's definition renders planetary health internally confusing and potentially incoherent. To remedy this, our proposal is to clean up the double duty problem by deploying "planetary flourishing" (or a term like it) for the higher-level concept that describes the overall ethical framework within which the movement is embedded, and reserve "planetary health" for a more specific idea that is nested within that framework.

Scope

Our second point concerns the ethical scope of the RLC's definition. This seems limited in two ways: it includes only three core values and is restricted to concern for humans. Both limitations are likely to prove unpopular with many who sympathize with the planetary health agenda.

The first limitation (of including only three core values) invites the question of what to say about other values, such as (for example) autonomy, rights, justice, freedom (of various kinds), community, sustainability, and so on. Is the claim that the triumvirate should take precedence over them, in the sense that other values should always be sacrificed to the "big three"? That position seems in need of an argument, one that will likely be difficult to make.

Alternatively, a more plausible position may be to claim that the triumvirate absorbs or subsumes the other values, so that, say, justice and human rights are included under "equity," and community under "well-being." Still, the absorption strategy also has its own costs (Gardiner and Tubig 2023). For one thing, it threatens to stretch the meaning of "well-being," "equity," and "health" itself to their limits. For another thing, it merely postpones questions about how to prioritize or how to achieve a grand integration of values. For example, some enthusiasts for planetary health already observe that "exactly how concepts such as social equity and justice, responsible and sustainable development, and achievement of high standards of living for all can be made to fit together is not well-defined" (Foster et al. 2019). Moreover, this issue is especially pressing if one believes that a central role of planetary health ought to be to help humanity negotiate "difficult trade-offs" (Foster et al. 2019).

One reason to be concerned about such questions is the risk of vacuousness. Perhaps a critic may insist, part of the appeal of the planetary health concept is that it lacks a central meaning and so can be "everything to everyone." Occasionally, this worry is encouraged by leaders of the movement itself. For instance, Richard Horton, editor of the *Lancet*, once claimed that "we can choose what justice means to each one of us," and that "it was entirely right that we should have felt that radical liberty to choose last week at the annual Planetary Health conference" (Horton 2014). It is unclear what Horton meant by "radical liberty." One natural (but presumably uncharitable) interpretation is that it is *up to each of us as individuals to decide what justice is, according to whatever criteria we see fit*. Yet this position is highly controversial, since it appears to assume that there are no further considerations (e.g., reasons, moral facts, shared sentiments) to appeal to in making judgments about justice. That is, it reduces justice to a kind of moral relativism. Conventional moral and political philosophers largely reject this view. (Notably, Horton quotes the philosopher David Hume, but most philosophers would reject this reading of Hume.) Instead, they believe that ethical concepts like justice are sensitive to reasons and that these are accessible to public deliberation. In particular, they claim that individual judgments about justice can be better or worse, and therefore are subject to scrutiny by others.

One reason why this claim is so widespread is that it is not clear how the radical "up to you" view of justice could allow the concept to play the social role we expect justice to play. Suppose, for instance, that you and I disagree about a claim of justice. For example, you believe that the innocent should not be punished for crimes they did not commit, but I think they should. If there is nothing to appeal to beyond our individual claims about justice, it is not clear how the disagreement can be resolved. Indeed, it is not clear that it is a real disagreement. On the radical view, we might each agree that the other is correct according to her own conception of justice. The question of disagreement comes up only if we make further claims, such as that one conception of justice is better than the other, or ought to determine what happens to the innocent. But, of course, we do want to make such claims, partly because there is not much point in our employing the concept of justice if we cannot. Moreover, we routinely discuss justice in just this way. For example, we normally maintain that punishing the innocent is unjust, and that conceptions of justice that show no regard for this are thereby worse conceptions of justice. Philosophers then employ such constraints to fashion theories of justice that shape how we think about public life, including what law is, what principles it should respect, and how a legal system should function.

Given all this, a more charitable interpretation of Horton's claim that justice is "up to us to choose" (as individuals) is that each of us has a responsibility to assess the reasons relevant to claims of justice, including by paying attention to the positions, arguments, and theories of others. This position helps to diffuse the vacuousness objection. It is also widespread among theorists of justice and seems much more friendly to the evolution of the planetary health movement.

The second limitation suggested by the scope of the RLC definition concerns the thorny question of the status of nonhuman entities, including animals, plants, ecosystems, and so on. It is common to interpret the RLC's definition as being ethically anthropocentric, in the sense that its account of planetary health restricts its fundamental ethical concern to humans alone (e.g., planetary health is described as "the health of human civilizations").[8] Yet many enthusiasts for planetary health explicitly maintain that nonhumans matter independently, and so not only for the sake of human interests (e.g., Kiran, Sander, and Duncan 2022). One reason this difference is difficult to ignore is that many hold that anthropocentrism is a root cause of environmental degradation and so will resist any proposed "solution" that takes anthropocentrism as fundamental. Another reason is that, by contrast, accounts of One Health often seem overtly non-anthropocentric—they take the view that at least some nonhumans matter for their own sake—so that the RLC definition makes planetary health appear less like progress and more like a step backwards. Consequently, we propose that non-anthropocentrism should be taken as the natural default position for planetary health, so that there is a strong presumption against the RLC's account.

In summary, our second basic conclusion is that the RLC account of the ethics of planetary health is too limited in scope. On both issues—the triumvirate and ethical anthropocentrism—the restrictions implied by the RLC definition threaten the core project of planetary health and thus undermine the movement.

Maximization

Our third point concerns the RLC's commitment to maximization. One issue is that insisting that the goal of planetary health is to achieve "the highest attainable standard" of well-being, equity, and health obscures more than it reveals. There are, after all, three central values, and it is not clear that all three can be maximized at the same time. Again, this threatens the claim—strongly emphasized by some advocates—that a central advantage of planetary health is that it allows us to focus on trade-offs between different objectives (Foster et al. 2019). It is not clear that the RLC's interpretation allows for this, especially given the attractiveness of the absorption strategy and the threat of vacuousness (as mentioned above).

Another issue is that maximization is a controversial objective within ethics. One concern is that theories that embrace it often appear too ready to sacrifice individuals for the sake of some "greater" social good (e.g., simple, direct versions of utilitarianism). Another concern is that in many contexts, lower standards than maximization seem at least acceptable and sometimes preferable, such as generous, decent, adequate, or sustainable provision of certain kinds of health or health care. A third concern is that maximizing achievement of the triumvirate would appear to crowd out other values. Arguably, the big three are so pervasive that achieving the maximum with respect to them seems likely to preclude the pursuit of any other social objectives, such as knowledge, beauty, freedom, community, and others mentioned above. This concern is especially pronounced if one adopts ethical anthropocentrism, as the RLC appears to do.

In summary, our third basic conclusion is that, under the RLC's definition, planetary health risks becoming an unattractive ethical ideal. Though superficially appealing, the RLC's appeal to maximization risks making the notion obscure, controversial, and overly demanding, in the sense that it overwhelms all other endeavors. At the very least, the RLC's pursuit of the "highest attainable standard" requires a serious, deeper defense. For instance, is there something about the "big three" values picked out by the definition that makes maximizing appropriate? If so, the rationale should be made explicit.

Taken together, our three basic conclusions suggest the need for a central debate within the wide vision of planetary health. The aim of the next section is to suggest pathways forward.

Lessons: Toward a Satisfactory Ethics of Planetary Health

Initially, the planetary health concept provides a powerful touchstone from which to begin to imagine a different world, including a new ethics of public health. Nevertheless, there are many possible paths forward, and the first steps are vital. We have argued that for planetary health to be a coherent ethical project that shapes research agendas and social actions, it needs greater analytical precision. We have investigated early framings of the planetary health concept and some of the motivations behind the movement to identify ambiguities and gaps in the basic vision. In conclusion, we will summarize the lessons learned by suggesting an agenda for the way forward.

The first item on our agenda is that a satisfactory account of planetary health *should clearly specify its central values* in order to better organize research and other activities. Key questions include:

- Should the movement embrace a narrower or wider conception of planetary health?
- What values should the chosen vision embrace, and how should these be understood?

Our initial suggestions are:

1. The movement should continue to embrace a fairly wide vision of planetary health, in keeping with the RLC definition but pushing beyond it.
2. The movement should shift to characterizing its overarching normative concept in terms of a broader ideal, such as planetary flourishing, while rendering planetary health an essential but subsidiary component.
3. While the early triumvirate of health, well-being, and equity remain important, these values require further articulation and should be understood in ways that do not arbitrarily exclude other values.
4. The movement should address central comparative ethical questions, such as:
   a. Should certain values be central while others be secondary or marginal?
   b. Should the central values be maximized?
   c. How should these values be balanced or integrated with respect to each other?
   d. Should planetary health be anthropocentric or non-anthropocentric?

Moving forward, we would also suggest a second agenda item: the planetary health movement should seek a better understanding of *the challenges it intends to confront* and *how responsive its efforts are likely to be to those challenges*. Some key questions are:

- How does the planetary health movement understand global environmental change and the challenges it exposes, especially the ethical challenges?
- How and to what extent do these challenges require a rethinking of conventional concepts that are important to public health and bioethics, and the possible extension, revision, or replacement of such concepts?
- Should the movement be focused primarily on change within the public health and bioethics communities, or should it pursue a broader activist agenda as part of its professional responsibility?
- How should the planetary health movement reach out to, and seek to align or integrate its efforts with other agents, including academic disciplines, institutions, and organizations? How far might this require pushing for new structures, or the reconfiguring or evolution of existing structures?

Naturally, this simple agenda is only a first step (see also Baeroe, Bhopal, and Gundersen 2024). So, we close with the simple thought that the evolving literature in climate ethics, environmental ethics, global justice, and intergenerational ethics should prove useful in moving forward.[9] One of us has made a start in the context of the perfect moral storm framework (Gardiner 2022, 2011). We encourage others to embark on similar projects. Such endeavors should enrich not only planetary health, but also the wider enterprise in which it is embedded, of environmentalizing bioethics in general and public health ethics specifically. Even if planetary health is not the right concept and ultimately fades, we should learn from it, since the overall project must continue.

Notes

1 The authors are grateful to audiences at the Center for Bioethics and Health Law at the University of Pittsburgh, the Joint Centre for Bioethics at the University of Toronto, and the University of Washington. We especially thank Erika Blacksher, Larry Churchill, Jeffrey D'Sousa, Rob Figueroa, Carina Fourie, Jeremy Hess, Paul Kelleher, Elizabeth Lanphier, Lisa Parker, and Ross Upshur. For related material, see Gardiner (2022) and Gardiner and Tubig (2023).

2 When we speak of "early," we are focused primarily on the RLC report and its immediate aftermath. Since then, the PH movement has continued to evolve. We believe both that the history is of interest in its own right, and that the early framings remain influential (e.g., Drake 2021). However, we will not defend the latter view in this short chapter.

3 To illustrate this, consider a summary graphic from the *Lancet* (Lancet 2018), where the human body is placed at the center of a network of influences. These are mainly natural drivers such as climate, water, agriculture, soil, air, oceans, land, weather, and so on, though they also include some social drivers, such as the economy, industry, migration, and politics. The basic thought of the narrow interpretation is that public health research must take such factors into account, and especially the overtly environmental ones, if it is to succeed in furthering *conventional* public health aims.

4 Exactly how to specify the relevant scope of concern is a topic worth investigating and is already central in other areas, particularly contemporary environmental ethics (see footnote #5 below).

5 "We aim to advance the science of planetary health from the global to the local scales, including understanding of threats to both human and ecosystem health and evidence-based strategies to prevent and reduce these threats."

6 The portion of this chapter Early Ethical Foundations of Planetary Health is based on Gardiner and Tubig, 2023.

7 Cf. Sen (1999), Nussbaum (2000), and Schlosberg (2012). We are open to other concepts that may play this role and offer PF mainly as an example of one that does so better than PH.

8 A complication here is that often key sources appear ambiguous on this point. In some places, they appear to display an exclusive concern for human health, but in others, they assert (or come close to asserting) that we should value nonhuman entities for their own sake. An additional interpretive difficulty is that it is possible to adopt a form of ethical anthropocentrism whereby humans should value some nonhuman entities for their own sake, but only because such valuing would ultimately promote human interests. Interestingly, some PH sources can be read in this way.

9 As gateways into this literature, we suggest Brooks (2023), Gardiner and Obst (2023), Gardiner and Thompson (2016), Gardiner (in press), Jamieson (2014), McKinnon (2022), Shue (2022), and Williston (2023).

Bibliography

Baeroe, Kristine, Anand Singh Bhopal, and Torbjorn Gundersen. 2024. "Towards an Environmentally Sensitive Healthcare Ethics: Ten Tasks and One Model." *Journal of Medical Ethics*, 50 (6): 382–3.

Bansal, Aarti. 2020. "Planetary Health Underpins an Economy of Wellbeing." *BMJ: British Medical Journal*, 370: 1.

Brooks, Thom, ed. 2023. *The Global Justice Reader*, revised ed. Wiley-Blackwell.

Callahan, Daniel. 1973. "The WHO Definition of 'Health.'" *Hastings Center Studies*, 1 (3): 77–87.

Capon, Anthony, 2020. "Planetary Health: Protecting Nature to Protect Ourselves." *The Lancet* 396 (10249): 95. October 24, 2020. https://www.thelancet.com/journals/lancet/article/PIIS0140-6736(20)31406-6/fulltext.

de Castañeda, Rafael Ruiz, Jennifer Villers, Carlos A. Faerron Guzmán, Turan Eslanloo, Nicole de Paula, Catherine Machalaba et al. 2023. "One Health and Planetary Health Research: Leveraging Differences to Grow Together." *The Lancet: Planetary Health*, 7 (2): E109–E111.

Cole, Jennifer. 2019. *Planetary Health: Human Health in an Era of Global Environmental Change*. CABI.

Drake, John. 2021. "What is Planetary Health?" *Forbes*, April 22.

Dunk, James and Warwick Anderson. 2020. "Assembling Planetary Health: Histories of the Future," in *Planetary Health: Protecting Nature to Protect Ourselves*. Edited by Samuel Meyers and Howard Frumkin, 17–36, Washington, D.C.: Island Pres.

Editors of the *Lancet Planetary Health*. 2017. "Welcome to The Lancet Planetary Health." *The Lancet Planetary Health*, 1: 1.

Foster, Alexander, Jennifer Cole, Andrew Farlow, and Ivica Petrikova. 2019. "Planetary Health Ethics: Beyond First Principles." *Challenges*, 10: 14.

Foster, Alexander, Jennifer Cole, Ivica Petrikova, Andrew Farlow, and Howard Frumkin. 2020. "Planetary Health Ethics." In Samuel Myers and Howard Frumkin (eds.), *Planetary Health: Protecting Nature to Protect Ourselves*. Island Press.

Gardiner, Stephen M. 2011. *A Perfect Moral Storm: The Ethical Tragedy of Climate Change*. Oxford.

Gardiner, Stephen M. 2022. "Environmentalizing Bioethics: Planetary Health in a Perfect Moral Storm." *Perspectives in Biology and Medicine*, 65 (4): 569–85.

Gardiner, Stephen M., ed. 2025. *The Oxford Handbook of Intergenerational Ethics*. Oxford.

Gardiner, Stephen M., and Arthur Obst. 2023. *Dialogues on Climate Justice*. Routledge.

Gardiner, Stephen M., and Allen Thompson, eds. 2016. *The Oxford Handbook of Environmental Ethics*. Oxford.

Gardiner, Stephen M., and Paul Tubig. 2023. "Climate Change, Global Health and Planetary Health." In Gianfranco Pellegrino and Marcello Di Paola (eds.), *Handbook of Philosophy of Climate Change*, 799–819. Cham: Springer.

Hill-Cawthorne, Grant A. 2019. "One Health/EcoHealth/Planetary Health and their Evolution." In Merrilyn Walton (ed.), *One Planet, One Health*. Sydney University Press.

Horton, Richard, Robert Beaglehole, Ruth Bonita, John Raeburn, Martin McKee, and Stig Wall. 2014. "From Public to Planetary Health: A Manifesto." *The Lancet*, 383: 847.

Jamieson, Dale. 2014. *Ethics in a Dark Time*. Oxford.

Kiran, Dilara, William E. Sander, and Colleen Duncan. 2022. "Empowering Veterinarians to Be Planetary Health Stewards Through Policy and Practice." *Frontier Veterinary Science*, 9: 775411.

Meyers, Samuel and Howard Frumkin (eds.) 2020. *Planetary Health: Protecting Natural to Protect Ourselves*. Island Press.

The Lancet. 2018. "Planetary Health: A New Discipline." https://www.thelancet.com/infographics/what-is-planetary-health (accessed November 12, 2020).

The Lancet Planetary Health (LPH). 2024. "About the Lancet Planetary Health." LPH Website. https://www.thelancet.com/lanplh/about (accessed February 16, 2024).

McKinnon, Catriona. 2022. *Climate Change and Political Theory*. Polity.

Nussbaum, Martha. 2000. *Women and Human Development: The Capabilities Approach*. Cambridge University Press.

Planetary Health Alliance (PHA). 2018a. "Planetary Health." *Planetary Health Alliance Website*. https://www.planetaryhealthalliance.org/planetary-health (accessed November 26, 2020; October 21, 2021).

Planetary Health Alliance (PHA). 2018b. "The 2018 Planetary Health Annual Meeting." Department for Social Responsibility and Sustainability at the University of Edinburgh, *The University of Edinburgh Global Environment & Society Academy Events Page*. https://www.ed.ac.uk/global-environment-society/news-events/events/planetary-health (accessed November 26, 2020).

Planetary Health Alliance (PHA). 2020. "An Anthology of Solutions." *Planetary Health Alliance*. June 18, 2020. https://planetaryhealthallinace.org/planetary-health-textbook/case-studies-anthology/.

Planetary Health Alliance. 2020. "Planetary Health Newsletter: November 2020." Accessed August 25, 2025. https: mailchi.mp/harvard/planetary-health-newsletter-november-2020.

Planetary Health Alliance, 2021. "Planetary Health Newsletter: October 2021." Accessed 25, 2025. https://mailchi.mp/harvard/planetary-health-newsletter-october-2021.

Potter, Van Rensselaer. 1970. "Bioethics, the Science of Survival." *Perspectives in Biology and Medicine*, 14 (1): 127–53.

Potter, Van Rensselaer. 1988. *Global Bioethics: Building on the Leopold Legacy*. Michigan State University Press.

Prescott, Susan et al. 2018. "The Canmore Declaration: Statement of Principles for Planetary Health." *Challenges*, 9 (2): 31.

Rockefeller, David. 2016. "The Role of Foundations: Rockefeller Foundation." *Public Health Reviews*, 37: 32.

Schenck, David, and Larry Churchill. 2021. "Ethical Maxims for a Marginally Inhabitable Planet." *Perspectives in Biology and Medicine*, 64 (4): 494–510.

Schlosberg, David. 2012. "Climate Justice and Capabilities: A Framework for Adaptation Policy." *Ethics & International Affairs*, 26 (4): 445–61.

Seltenrich, Nate. 2018. "Down to Earth: The Emerging Field of Planetary Health." *Environmental Health Perspectives*, 126 (7): 072001. https://doi.org/10.1289/EHP2374.

Sen, Amartya. 1999. *Development as Freedom*. Knopf.

Shue, Henry. 2022. *The Pivotal Generation*. Princeton.

ten Have, Henk. 2012. "Potter's Notion of Bioethics." *Kennedy Institute of Ethics Journal*, 22 (1): 59–82.

UNFCCC (United Nations Framework Convention on Climate Change). 2023. "UN Global Climate Action Awards: Planetary Health." UNFCCC.
Whitmee, Sarah, Andy Haines, Chris Beyrer, et al. 2016. "Safeguarding Human Health in the Anthropocene Epoch: Report of The Rockefeller Foundation–Lancet Commission on Planetary Health." *The Lancet*, 386 (1007): 1973–2028.
Williston, Byron. 2023. *The Ethics of Climate Change: An Introduction*, 2nd ed. Routledge.
World Health Organization. "Preamble to the Constitution of the World Health Organization as adopted by the International Health Conference, New York, 19–22 June, 1946; signed on 22 July 1946 by the representatives of 61 States (Official Records of the World Health Organization, no. 2, p. 100) and entered into force on 7 April 1948.

11

Can Ethical Input into Policy Advance Environmental Sustainability?

Cheryl C. Macpherson and Katharine Wright

The central question of this chapter is whether bioethics input into public policy may prompt more effective policy responses to the production of greenhouse gas emissions. To answer this question, the chapter reviews bioethics perspectives on climate change and the scale of emissions that cause it, discusses reasons for assigning responsibility to certain types of individuals (including bioethicists) and to certain entities (primarily governments and also industries and multinational corporations), and highlights ways in which bioethics is beginning to influence public policy. The routine activities of governments and the built environments in which they function contribute directly to the scale of emissions-production that causes climate change. Indirectly, governments contribute by facilitating emissions-production by industries and corporations rather than implementing penalties on emissions-production and incentives for emissions-reduction. Industries and multinational corporations produce disproportionately large volumes of the greenhouse gases that have altered, and are altering, earth's atmosphere and worsening climate change (Jamieson 2015; Jamieson 2014; Macpherson 2019).

Public policy could have a significant impact on the largest global emitters; hence, our attention to governments, their leaders, and their respective responsibilities. To advance public policy for global emissions-reduction by the largest global emitters, we discuss the potential for bioethics input to help governments, and perhaps government and other leaders, to accept and act on their responsibilities for their direct and indirect emissions-production. We focus on present day emissions-production (not historic emissions-production) because responsibility for climate change has evolved and continues to evolve with geographic, socioeconomic, national, and other circumstances; this makes it difficult to equitably apportion responsibility (Jamieson 2015). The morass of how to apportion responsibility for historic emissions has long deterred consensus and progress on emissions-reduction and building resilience.

In several ways, bioethics has the potential to direct attention to the urgent need for the world's largest emitters to reduce their emissions-production. In clinical and other realms, bioethicists offer ways in which to discuss and understand responsibilities. They routinely help to illuminate values that are otherwise overlooked, including during risk and benefit analyses. Their participation in public policy and engagement could also do this, and also inform policy and practices that bear on the global scale of emissions-production.

Bioethics Perspectives on Emissions-Production

Industrial emissions-production has disrupted a balance of atmospheric gases that endured for thousands of years (NOAA 2022). The multitude of interlinked and dynamic causes and impacts creates a perfect moral storm with far-reaching and devastating, but amorphous, impacts on human, animal, and planetary health in ways that challenge the assignment of responsibility (Gardiner 2022; Jamieson 2015). Consequently, earth's populations are experiencing globally rising sea and air temperatures, sea levels, and polar melting; declining diversity of plants, insects, amphibians, birds, and fish; migration of disease-carrying vectors into new geographic locations where they infect previously unexposed populations; and frequent extreme weather events (Abbasi et al. 2023; Romanello et al. 2022). At the time of writing, record high global temperatures have been reported by mainstream news outlets for two consecutive years with consequent record-breaking forest fires in the United States and Canada in terms of sizes, damages, and numbers so early in the fire season.

Each such consequence directly or indirectly harms health, deepens existing socioeconomic determinants of health, and worsens structural injustices—with the greatest harm on those least well off and least able to protect themselves (Ray and Cooper 2024; Pratt 2023; Dwyer 2020; Resnik 2022). This is an ethical problem because the annual global volume of emissions-production varies with human activities, policies, and practices (Macpherson 2022a). When industrial levels of emissions-production began in the 1850s, the policies and practices adopted made possible today's levels of emissions-production and climate change. The harm was presumably unintentional in the 1850s but today's steadily rising emissions-production continues intentionally—with knowledge of the harm caused—and based on trade-offs by government and other leaders who support and facilitate status quo policies and practices. These policies and practices can and should be redesigned to provide goods and services in environmentally responsible ways (Macpherson 2016, 203–10; Macpherson 2022a). The relatively small role and influence of consumer behavior in global emissions-production is discussed briefly below.

Those best placed to reduce emissions at the necessary scale are those with influence over government policies and practices (and over those of industries and corporations that include governments). With respect to global emissions-production and climate change, "intervention-responsibility" says that those best placed to intervene and reduce emissions have a greater responsibility to do so than others (Jamieson 2015). Five corporations (Chevron, ExxonMobil, Saudi Aramco, BP, and Gazprom) are presently and were historically the greatest emitters and have the greatest potential to reduce global emissions-production (Jamieson 2015). Those corporations and eighty-five others produced more than 60 percent of global emissions between 1854 and 2010 and, remarkably, governments partly own or run forty of these corporations (Frumhoff, Heede, and Oreskes 2015).

The countless benefits and co-benefits of global emissions-reduction will have economic and other short-term costs for governments and other large emitters. These entities and their leaders can, however, afford the costs. Consider that corporations today pay their leaders 200 hundred times more than they pay their average workers—up from fifteen times more in the 1960s (Krugman 2023). Instead, that money could be allocated by high-income governments and other large emitters to create markets for environmentally sustainable products and leveraged as purchasing power for emissions-reduction (Gates 2024). The costs, risks, and harms of emissions-production can and should be integrated into risk-benefit analyses and public policy negotiations (Singh 2012).

Impediments to such actions include leaders and senior advisors who prioritize short-term economic growth, political gain, and ideological interests over long-term fiscal and civic stability. Additionally, globalization hinders emissions-reducing policy negotiations by permitting industries and corporations to determine what goods and services are manufactured and sold, at what cost, and to what consumer market (Ortiz-Millán 2022). With tacit government acceptance, industrial and corporate actors determine what seeds are sold to farmers, and thus what crops they grow, and what products and brands are sold in supermarkets (Patel and Rudolph 2023; Mialon et al. 2020). Even collectively, consumer influence over the goods and services available to them is small. While informed by their preferences and household needs and resources, consumer choices and decisions are determined by what is available (Nielson et al. 2024). Intervention-responsibility indicates that even collectively, consumers have far less influence and responsibility for global emissions-production than governments.

The governments of low- and middle-income countries (LMICs) have lower levels of socioeconomic development and less power and capacity than other countries in climate and other negotiations. Some high-income countries and LMICs do, in some ways, advance environmentally sustainable policies and practices. Others are swayed by industries and corporations and either ignore or reject emissions-reduction as expensive, unnecessary, and incompatible with providing public services and meeting consumer demand (Shue 2022). That consumer demand is greatly influenced by marketing is clear across the food and agriculture industries which could choose instead to be exemplars for emissions-reduction (Patel and Rudolph 2023). The wealth and influence of industries and corporations give them power with which to successfully negotiate tax breaks and unrestricted use of public infrastructure and resources. Governments seem generally unwilling or underprepared to negotiate emissions-reduction with these entities. Governments, industries, corporations, and their leaders are easily swayed by hope for technological rescue regardless of financial cost, likelihood of failure, or probability of causing more harm than benefit. Bioethicists and others might help them to acknowledge that the only safe and reliable way to reduce the global emissions causing climate change is to simply reduce emissions-production by the largest emitters.

Government Responsibility

Industries knew in the 1980s that their emissions-production was causing global warming but chose to continue, and governments permitted them to do so, while today, governments and the largest global emitters have access to an abundance of evidence, with global atmospheric concentrations more than 150 percent higher than ever before (UN 2021; EPA 2022; Ritchie, Rosado, and Roser 2020). These entities should accept responsibility for their current emissions-production and adopt policies and practices to stop it. The most successful emissions-reduction policies and practices will be responsive to contextual factors. Financial disincentives, for example, can deter individuals from driving cars into congested areas and thus improve air quality but are unfair burdens on those who cannot afford to pay to drive through these locations, particularly so if their families and livelihoods rely on them doing so.

Many leaders and other stakeholders overlook the role of values in emissions-related policy-making and implementation. Bioethicists invited to participate in such work could help identify and offer insight into competing needs and values at stake and facilitate dialogue about how best to balance approaches and responses. Bioethics is not alone in its ability to do this, but bioethicists routinely conduct such work in public health, clinical, and research contexts. They might help government leaders more willingly acknowledge responsibility for, and willingness to reduce, their direct or indirect emissions-production. Government and other leaders should invite bioethicists to participate meaningfully in emissions-related deliberations, and bioethicists should eagerly engage. This would likely advance the identification and investigation of key issues, values, and perspectives about emissions, and perhaps help build consensus on the need for emissions-reduction by those best placed to stop their production and to rectify the harm.

When one's actions cause harm, it is generally expected that the actor will apologize and make a viable attempt to rectify the harm. Many parents teach their children to be responsible when they cause harm, even unintentionally. Not doing so is a moral problem. This moral expectation of apologizing and rectifying a harm one is complicit in seems equally applicable for the leaders and advisors employed by governments, industries, corporations, and large organizations and institutions. These individuals are well-positioned to advocate for and advance emissions-reduction and arguably have a professional, civic, and moral responsibility to do this based on the profound, if indirect, harm their emissions-production causes. Intervention-responsibility accentuates this.

Most governments have policies and programs that aim to protect and promote health, deliver healthcare, and regulate healthcare institutions, practices, and practitioners. With their capacity and influence, governments should advance emissions-reduction through policy dialogue, host public engagement activities, and respond positively to individual and collective actions that signal social acceptance of emissions-reducing laws and regulations (Jamieson 2015; Singh 2012). Contrasted with high-income country governments, LMIC governments are disadvantaged in policy dialogue by power differentials and legacies of structural and epistemic injustices that worsen health disparities, hinder representation of marginalized populations, and contribute to misappropriation and misuse of resources (Pratt 2023). High-income country governments thus have more capacity and responsibility for emissions-reduction than LMICs.

Despite this, LMICs do bear at least some responsibility for their own emissions-production (Garvey 2008, 73–6). Some reject this and attempt to justify their inaction on the grounds that high-income countries are larger emitters with greater capacity for emissions-reduction and benefit more from their emissions-production than do LMICs. Another perspective, however, draws from the global South and African moral theory to hold that (1) harming environments is wrong because it disrupts harmonious relationships between living things that inhabit or interact with environments; (2) those who cause environmental damage should take reparative and reconciliatory actions toward restoring those harmonious relationships; and (3) that the impacts of LMIC's taking reparative and reconciliatory responses to emissions-production may entice high-income countries to act similarly (Behrens 2021).

The healthcare industry and its corporations, organizations, and institutions warrant special attention because their work is to protect and advance health. Governments should therefore regulate their emissions-production. Healthcare entities that prioritize public over commercial interest would naturally be eager to protect health by implementing emissions-reductions, and governments could offer incentives for doing so. Commercial healthcare entities, however, function within and profit from social structures that worsen health disparities, and thus have a responsibility to refrain from worsening existing injustices (Danis and Sepinwall 2002). Moreover, their priorities are influenced by conflicts of interest involving financial gain and public service, and by conflicts of commitments to shareholders, patients, and other stakeholders. Emissions-reduction is a low priority for many healthcare entities, but some have prioritized and advanced it with simultaneous increase in revenue and profit and no compromise to clinical standards or patient satisfaction (Macpherson 2022a,b).

Individual Responsibility

Individuals vary in their characteristics, circumstances, knowledge, and experience. Some are more vulnerable than others to climate change. Others are better placed to advance emissions-reduction through research, education, advocacy, or other means. Individual responsibility varies with employment, socioeconomic status, and other factors. How much responsibility an individual bears for their emissions-production depends on (1) what share they take of a public good or resource, (2) the extent of consequent harm, (3) their wealth and social privilege, (4) the extent of their harm to those with less wealth and privilege, and (5) their ability to use a smaller share of public goods to maintain their lifestyle (Jamieson 2014, 148). These factors are generally larger for senior leaders and advisors to governments and industrial and corporate entities. They thus have more responsibility for emissions-production than those with less. Their influence over emissions-production accentuates this responsibility.

Likewise, physician responsibility to advocate for emissions-reduction involves these factors and is accentuated by their inherent and historic commitment to patients and public trust. Additionally, professionals and others with greater wealth than average citizens attain their income and status through social structures that disadvantage average citizens and thus bear more responsibility for emissions-production (Dwyer 2020). As professionals with comfortable incomes, bioethicists bear a larger share of responsibility for emissions-production than average citizens and others with less, particularly within the entities that educate and employ them (Macpherson 2022a; Dwyer 2020).

Bioethicists are diverse in background, expertise, and type and approach to their employment. Some work exclusively in clinical settings and others in academic, research, or other roles. Their income varies with location, institution, and position, as does their influence on emissions-production. But they are all equipped to articulate and nurture thought and discourse about emissions-production by hosting seminars, teaching, publication, and advocating within their own institutions and, as we discuss below, engaging with public policy. Additionally, bioethicists can help students and colleagues learn that autonomy exists within, and is not separate from, environments; and help administrators, policymakers, and the public understand the value of iterative evidence about emissions and their consequences (Macpherson 2022a). As an integrative field concerned primarily with health, and based on their privileged social positions, bioethicists have a responsibility to advance emissions-reduction. If accomplished successfully within the field of bioethics, emissions-reduction would become a norm within healthcare-related academic, clinical, and research entities and, arguably, match the value of making autonomy a norm across healthcare (Macpherson 2022a).

A better-informed public, and better-informed policymakers, might lead to stronger democracies, emissions negotiations, and regulatory environments, and thus global emissions-reduction that advances healthy environments (Solomon 2021; Solomon and Jennings 2017). Public deliberation and public engagement are one means of informing citizens and policymakers about the value trade-offs that pervade all policy including that involving emissions. Public engagement is a two-way process that includes informing and learning from the public; it can increase trust, generate action, ensure representation, defuse conflict, and test policy arguments (Climate Citizens 2022).

Ethical Input into Public Policy

We touched briefly on the role that bioethicists can play in seeking to have an impact on emissions-related policy, through influencing the policy and actions of their own organizations, their choice of research topics, and their teaching and personal advocacy.

As we have argued, such actions are important in themselves and can be influential, particularly where bioethicists working within the health sector can influence the direction of their own institution or have leading roles within wider professional networks. However, these acts will never be enough in themselves because of the profoundly structural nature of the problems that confront us. Individual responses to emissions and climate change will never be sufficient because the public, bioethicists, and government and other leaders all operate within systems that are blind to, or actively incentivize, climate-harming actions.

This then raises the question of how bioethicists could or should seek to influence the actions of governments (leaving aside any exercise of their own democratic rights as individual citizens). The question of *whether* bioethics should be an "activist" field has been strongly argued by others (Rogers and Scully 2021; Rogers 2019) and we limit ourselves to noting our agreement with the claim that "bioethics is inescapably partisan; bioethical deliberation is based on trying to determine morally relevant features of situations and morally justifiable outcomes" (Rogers and Scully 2021, 32). Moreover, we have already laid out our justification for why governments, industry, and corporations have a responsibility to act in response to the particular threats of climate change. Below we focus on the "how" those working in the sphere of bioethics might engage in public policy in connection with this duty.

On an individual basis, bioethicists and others with ethical expertise from a wide range of academic disciplines may have the opportunity to directly influence public policy through membership on national, regional, or global advisory committees—as for example was seen through the plethora of such bodies established to provide advice on the unprecedented public policy challenges of the Covid-19 pandemic. It is important to recognize, however, that the extent to which the contributions of ethicists through these means was attended to by decision-makers was highly variable.

Perhaps the most obvious example of more formal ethical influence in public policy at the national level (or more accurately *opportunity* for ethical influence, depending on the willingness of those in power to respond) is that of the National Ethics Committee (NEC), or similarly named body (e.g., National Bioethics Committee, National Ethics Commission). The Health Ethics and Governance Unit of the World Health Organization provides the secretariat for a biennial global summit of these bodies (Hummel, Littler, and Reis 2023), and as of 2018, committees from 146 countries were included in the database maintained by WHO (Köhler, Reis, and Saxena 2021).

The 2018 Global Summit of NECs, held in Dakar, Senegal, resulted for the first time in a shared "call for action," endorsed by the WHO (WHO 2018). Agreed by representatives from seventy-one countries and all continents, this statement set out NECs' own vision of their role, that of:

> Aspiring to advance the application of ethical principles and relevant international instruments in order to guide reflection and help answer ethical questions among different value systems and cultures, and to provide all stakeholders, including healthcare professionals, research scientists, citizens, community leaders, patients and families, ethics/bioethics committees and governmental policymaking bodies

> in healthcare, biotechnology, environment, population and related fields with guidance and tools to support them in carrying out their responsibilities. (12th Global Summit of National Bioethics/Ethics Committees 2018)

Presciently, in light of the forthcoming global threat posed by Covid-19, NEC representatives further stated that they

> Agree[d] that ethically informed and integrated systems should be developed and maintained that support the protection of populations through the preparedness for, and response to, health emergencies; that states should be encouraged to work together to facilitate coordinated and effective national and international responses and support; and that particular attention needs to be given to those who are made most vulnerable by health emergencies. (12th Global Summit of National Bioethics/Ethics Committees 2018)

The relevance of this statement to the climate change emergency cannot be overstated. In October 2023, coordinated editorials in more than two hundred health journals called on the World Health Organization to designate the current climate and environmental crisis as a "public health emergency of international concern" (Abbasi et al. 2023), highlighting the need to harness the same urgency of approach in response to the threat posed by climate change as to pandemics. The next in the series of global summits of NECs, held in San Marino in April 2024, was framed explicitly around "contributions and challenges of national ethics committees in a world of uncertainty" in the context of the "increasingly intense consequences of global warming on our world, and the resulting disruption to our societies" (Republic of San Marino n.d.).

Following up on the theme from 2018 of the need for particular attention to be paid to those who are made most vulnerable in health emergencies, the 2024 NEC summit program included sessions on the policy implications of responding to resource shortages, including people with disabilities in emergency preparedness, and equity of access to medical innovations. Individual NECs (whose work provides the basis for the discussion at the global summits) are also beginning to undertake specific explorations of the ethical implications of climate change and climate action with the aim of developing supportive guidance for policymakers (e.g., Deutscher Ethikrat n.d.). Some factors that influence how NEC members engage with and respond to the climate threat are outlined below and it remains to be seen what influence NECs will have in climate-related public policy.

Interrogating the Role and Status of National Ethics Committees

In making the claim that NECs provide an important opportunity for ethical reflection to inform and influence public policy at both national and global levels, it is, of course, important to scrutinize both their composition (who is given the opportunity to serve on such committees and the breadth of expertise they bring) and the status that their advice is afforded. Both the composition and the status of NECs vary substantially from country to country. Most are established by government with a specific remit to offer advice within defined boundaries. As a WHO survey published in 2021 outlines, the membership (and hence degree of ethical expertise), and also the funding and other support available to committees (an important constraint on their effectiveness), varies substantially:

> The 84 countries [of 146 surveyed] covered were in all World Bank income categories and all World Health Organization regions. Many national ethics committees lack resources and face challenges in several domains, like independence, funding or efficacy. Only 40.2% (35/87) of committees expressed no concerns about independence. Almost a quarter (21/87) of committees did not make any ethics recommendations to their governments in 2017, and the median number of reports, opinions or recommendations issued was only two per committee. Seventy-two (82.7%) national ethics committees included a philosopher or a bioethicist. (Köhler 2021, 138)

The authors went on to recommend:

> Particularly in times of great uncertainty, such as during the current coronavirus disease 2019 pandemic, governments would be well advised to base their actions not only on technical considerations but also on the ethical guidance provided by a national ethics committee. We found that, *if the advice of national ethics committees is to matter, they must be legally mandated, independent, diverse in membership, transparent and sufficiently funded to be effective and visible.* (Köhler 2021, emphasis added)

Despite these recognized constraints, there are many examples of how national ethics bodies can have an impact on public policy (Nuffield Council on Bioethics 2023), and there is growing interest at WHO in enhancing understanding of how ethics bodies, in various forms, can better influence policy, as explored in the first "ethics to policy summit" convened in December 2021 (WHO 2022). This summit brought together representatives of NECs, along with ethicists who had been involved in other ways in advising on the pandemic response (e.g., leading academics who had been members of Covid-specific advisory committees at both governmental and intergovernmental levels) to explore "what worked" in terms of ethical input into policy during Covid-19, and how ethical considerations could be better integrated into policy in the future. A second ethics to policy summit is planned for 2024, focusing specifically on ethical input into climate change policy (Katherine Littler, email to author, April 20, 2024).

A further important question relating to the role of NECs in influencing public policy is that of their *legitimacy*: not only in terms of their membership (which tends to include a wide range of disciplines) but also in terms of the way that they source evidence and take account of wider public perspectives in the guidance that they offer. There is an increasing awareness within NECs that their role cannot simply be one of a "group of experts" relying on their own areas of expertise: it is crucial that the beliefs, experiences, and preferences of those who will be affected by the area of public policy in question inform that ethical deliberation, for example through consultative approaches that ensure committees are alerted to a range of perspectives and are prompted to challenge their own biases and assumptions. The extent to which such consultations and discussions are conducted will be influenced by a NEC's level of expertise and funding.

The 2018 Dakar call for action set out the need for such public engagement clearly, stating that

> National Ethics/Bioethics Committees should seek to ensure that the views and interests of all members of society are considered and represented; that this must involve the engagement of all areas of civil society in their work as well as the promotion of public discussion of issues in the life sciences, social and environmental sciences and biotechnologies that have implications for the health and wellbeing of all citizens and groups; and that whilst engagement strategies are still needed, and will vary, lessons should be shared about effective approaches to such engagement. (12th Global Summit of National Bioethics/Ethics Committees 2018)

In this spirit, one of the four "pillars" of the San Marino summit in April 2024 was concerned with the role of NECs in promoting public engagement, dialogue, and trust in public health and welfare (Republic of San Marino n.d.).

Ethical Influence at Intergovernmental Level: The Role of WHO

In addition to supporting global collaboration between members of NECs, the Health Ethics & Governance Unit at WHO provides an important focal point both for the examination of ethical issues raised by activities within WHO itself and in supporting member states in addressing ethical issues that arise in their own countries. This work is supported by individual academics from across the world, through a global network of WHO Collaborating Centres for Bioethics (WHO n.d.), and through the establishment of ad hoc expert committees to produce guidance on issues of developing concern. In 2023, a new workstream was established by the unit with the specific remit of "deliver[ing] a range of supporting tools and materials to help navigate ethical issues across the health (and health research) and climate change field and embed them effectively in relevant policies." This work is ongoing at the time of writing, with a Technical Advisory Group on embedding ethics in health and climate change policy established in December 2023 to support the development of actionable guidance and tools for policymakers (WHO 2023).

Roles for Those with Ethics Expertise

We have argued that individual bioethicists, as privileged and influential individuals, have professional and other types of responsibility to advance emissions-reduction within their affiliated institutions and organizations, and sketched several actions that they might take to fulfill these. We showed that governments, industries, and large corporations are among the largest global emitters and produce disproportionately high quantities of emissions, and that their senior leaders and advisors have significantly more responsibility and capacity for emissions-reduction than many other stakeholders. We also described the potential for national and international influence by NECs and their members on emissions-related public policy.

Collective actions by individual bioethicists and other ethicists, particularly in multidisciplinary collaboration, may have a more impactful influence on emissions than individual actions. As noted, collective actions can help signal to governments, industries, and corporations that emissions-reducing policies and practices are publicly and morally acceptable and desirable. Collective actions may be more visible and influential than others and nurture enthusiasm. Among the most important actors are governments, industries, corporations, national and international organizations like the WHO, and many others who can and should invite bioethicists and other ethicists to participate in policy dialogue and public engagement and consultations. These entities should allocate funds for such participation and engage thoughtfully with the ethical questions and concerns brought forward. Doing so would bring more objective and ethical perspectives to public policy and enhance implementation and public acceptance of emissions-related policy.

Carbon neutrality is advancing in countless locations and contexts despite well-funded "greenwashing" campaigns and increasingly populist politics challenging numerous democracies. For example, the United Kingdom's National Health Service has demonstrated decades of progress in emissions-reduction and, under the current administration, US policy for emissions-reduction has strengthened. The health and economic damages experienced in 2024 indicate that much more such work and policy is needed globally. One of many ways forward is for bioethicists and NECs (and others) to explore the value of prioritizing emissions-reduction in healthcare and public policy; and for governments to invite bioethicists, and members of bodies such as NECs to contribute their expertise to policy-making and take seriously the insights and perspectives they offer.

Conclusion

We have made the case in this chapter for the importance of identifying the moral and practical responsibilities borne by governments in responding to the climate crisis. Individual and collective input into public policy is needed, but government responsibilities cannot be offloaded to individuals because of the collective and structural nature of the systems that contribute to spiraling emissions and the limitations of individual action. Some working in bioethics make valuable contributions as individuals, advancing climate action through their scholarship and teaching and through their influence within their institutions. Given the nature of the ethical challenges inherent in climate policy, from analyzing the ethical trade-offs between different courses of action to making the case for policy to put concerns of equity center stage, there is also a need for bioethics engagement at the level of national and global policy.

Such engagement requires invitations and support from governments through their NECs and other avenues, and from bodies like the WHO and other leading health organizations. This does not negate the responsibility of industries, corporate entities, and other influential organizations, associations, and societies to seek ethical input and reduce their emissions. Instead, it accentuates the responsibility of governments to more actively regulate emissions-production. Many aspects of public policy, including both regulation and incentivization, have an important role to play in the large-scale global emissions-reduction that scientific and clinical evidence shows is essential to health. Governments should prioritize such policies for emissions-reduction and consult bioethicists in the process.

Bibliography

Abbasi, Kamran, Parveen Ali, Virginia Barbour, Thomas Benfield, et al. 2023. "Time to Treat the Climate and Nature Crisis as One Indivisible Global Health Emergency." *British Medical Journal*, 383: 2355.

Behrens, K. 2021. "African Relational Environmentalism on Greenhouse Gas Emissions." *Ethical Perspectives*, 28 (2): 129–47.

Climate Citizens. 2022. "The Role of Deliberative Public Engagement in Climate Policy Development." https://www.theccc.org.uk/wp-content/uploads/2022/09/The-role-of-deliberative-public-engagement-in-climate-policy-development-University-of-Lancaster.pdf (accessed April 19, 2024).

Danis, Marion, and Amy Sepinwall. 2002. "Regulation of the Global Marketplace for the Sake of Health." *Journal of Law, Medicine & Ethics*, 30 (4): 667–76.

Deutscher Ethikrat. n.d. "Climate Ethics." https://www.ethikrat.org/en/topics/current-ethics-council-topics/climate-ethics/ (accessed December 21, 2023).

Dwyer, J. 2020. "Environmental Migrants, Structural Injustice, and Moral Responsibility." *Bioethics*, 34 (6): 562–9.

Environmental Protection Agency (EPA). 2022. "Climate Change Indicators: Atmospheric Concentrations of Greenhouse Gases." https://www.epa.gov/climate-indicators/climate-change-indicators-atmospheric-concentrations-greenhouse-gases (accessed November 13, 2023).

Frumhoff, P. C., R. Heede, and N. Oreskes. 2015. "The Climate Responsibilities of Industrial Carbon Producers." *Climatic Change*, 132: 157–71.

Gardiner, Stephen M. 2022. "Environmentalizing Bioethics: Planetary Health in a Perfect Moral Storm." *Perspectives in Biology and Medicine*, 65 (4): 569–85.

Garvey, James. 2008. *The Ethics of Climate Change*. Continuum Press.
Gates, Bill. 2024. "How I Invest My Money in a Warming World." *New York Times*, December 1, 2023. https://www.nytimes.com/2023/12/01/opinion/bill-gates-climate-change-cop28.html.
Hummel, P., K. Littler, and A. Reis. 2023. "Health Ethics & Governance at WHO: The importance of the Global Summit of National Ethics Committees." In M. D. C. Patrão Neves (ed.), *The Kaleidoscope of Global Bioethics*. Conselho Nacional de Ética para as Ciências da Vida (CNECV).
Jamieson, Dale. 2014. *Reason in a Dark Time: Why the Struggle Against Climate Change Failed – and What It Means for Our Future*. Oxford University Press.
Jamieson, Dale. 2015. "Responsibility and Climate Change." *Global Justice: Theory Practice Rhetoric*, 8 (2).
Köhler, Johannes, Andreas Alois Reis, and Abha Saxena. 2021. "A Survey of National Ethics and Bioethics Committees." *Bulletin of the World Health Organization*, 99 (2): 138–47.
Krugman, Paul. 2023. "Autoworkers Strike a Blow for Equality." *New York Times*, October 30, 2023. https://www.nytimes.com/2023/10/30/opinion/columnists/uaw-autoworkers-strike-union.html.
Macpherson, Cheryl C, ed. 2016. *Bioethical Insights Into Values and Policy: Climate Change and Health*. Springer.
Macpherson, Cheryl C. 2019. "Energy, Emissions, and Public Health Ethics." In A. Mastroianni A, N. Kass N, and J. Kahn (eds.), *Oxford Handbook of Public Health Ethics*. Oxford University Press.
Macpherson, Cheryl C. 2022a. "Can Bioethics Do for Our Planet What It's Done for Autonomy?" *Perspectives in Biology and Medicine*, 65 (4): 548–58.
Macpherson, Cheryl C. 2022b. "Global Bioethics: It's Past and Future." *Global Bioethics*, 33 (1): 45–9.
Mialon, M., C. Corvalan, G. Cediel, F. B. Scagliusi, and M. Reyes. 2020. "Food Industry Political Practices in Chile: The Economy Has Always Been the Main Concern." *Globalization and Health*, 16: 1–12.
Nielsen, K. S., V. Cologna, J. M. Bauer, et al. 2024. "Realizing the Full Potential of Behavioural Science for Climate Change Mitigation." *Nature Climate Change*, 14: 322–30.
NOAA. National Oceanic Atmospheric Administration. 2023. "Greenhouse Gases Contributed to Increase Rapidly in 2022." April 5. https://www.noaa.gov/news-release/greenhouse-gases-continued-to-increase-rapidly-in-2022 (accessed November 13, 2023).
Nuffield Council on Bioethics. 2023. "Impact report: 2018–2023." https://www.nuffieldbioethics.org/assets/pdfs/NCOB-Impact-Report-A4-portrait-V1.5.pdf.
Ortiz-Millán, G. 2022. "Bioethics, Globalization and Pandemics." *Global Bioethics*, 33 (1): 32–7.
Patel, Lisa, and Linda Rudolph. 2023. "Supporting Climate, Health, and Equity Under the Farm Bill." *New England Journal of Medicine*, 389 (17): 1541–3.
Pratt, Bridget. 2023. "Expanding Health Justice to Consider the Environment: How Can Bioethics Avoid Reinforcing Epistemic Injustice?" *Journal of Medical Ethics*, 49 (9): 642–8.
Ray, Keisha, and Jane Fallis Cooper. 2024. "The Bioethics of Environmental Injustice: Ethical, Legal, and Clinical Implications of Unhealthy Environments." *The American Journal of Bioethics*, 24 (3): 9–17.

Republic of San Marino. n.d. "Crisis, Evolution, Growth: Contributions and Challenges of National Ethics Committees in a World of Uncertainty." https://14globalsummitsanmarino.com/programme (accessed 21 December 2023).
Resnik, David B. 2022. "Environmental Justice and Climate Change Policies." *Bioethics*, 36 (7): 735–41.
Ritchie, Hannah, Pablo Rosado, and Max Roser. 2020. "Greenhouse Gas Emissions." OurWorldInData.org. Retrieved from: https://ourworldindata.org/greenhouse-gas-emissions [Online Resource]. https://ourworldindata.org/greenhouse-gas-emissions (accessed April 19, 2024).
Rogers, Wendy. 2019. "Bioethics and Activism: A Natural Fit?" *Bioethics*, 33 (8): 881–9.
Rogers, Wendy A., and Jackie Leach Scully. 2021. "Activism and Bioethics: Taking a Stand on Things That Matter." *Hastings Center Report*, 51 (4): 32–3.
Romanello, M., C. Di Napoli, P. Drummond, C. Green, H. Kennard, P. Lampard, and A. Costello. 2022. "The 2022 Report of the Lancet Countdown on Health and Climate Change: Health at the Mercy of Fossil Fuels." *The Lancet*, 400 (10363): 1619–54.
Shue H. 2022. "Unseen Urgency: Delay as the New Denial." *Wiley Interdisciplinary Reviews: Climate Change*, 14 (1): e809.
Singh, Jerome A. 2012. "Why Human Health and Health Ethics Must Be Central to Climate Change Deliberations." *PLoS Medicine*, 9 (6): e1001229.
Solomon, Miriam. 2021. "Trust: The Need for Public Understanding of How Science Works." *Hastings Center Report*, 51: S36–9.
Solomon, Mildred Z., and Bruce Jennings. 2017. "Bioethics and Populism: How Should Our Field Respond?" *Hastings Center Report*, 47 (2): 11–16.
United Nations. 2021. "'No Time to Lose' Curbing Greenhouse Gases: WMO." https://news.un.org/en/story/2021/10/1103892 (accessed November 13, 2023).
World Health Organization. 2018. "The Global Summit of National Bioethics Committees." https://www.who.int/news-room/events/detail/2018/03/22/default-calendar/the-global-summit-of-national-bioethics-committees (accessed December 21, 2023).
World Health Organization. 2022. "Bridging the Gap Between Ethics and Decision-making in Pandemics." https://iris.who.int/bitstream/handle/10665/365374/9789240065079-eng.pdf?sequence=1 (accessed December 21, 2023).
World Health Organization. 2023. "New Technical Advisory Group on Embedding Ethics in Health and Climate Change Policy (TAG-Ethics & Climate Health)." https://www.who.int/news/item/11-12-2023-creation-of-technical-advisory-group-on-embedding-ethics-in-health-and-climate-change-policy (accessed December 21, 2023).
World Health Organization. n.d. "Global Network of WHO Collaborating Centres for Bioethics." https://www.who.int/groups/global-network-of-who-collaborating-centres-for-bioethics (accessed December 21, 2023).
12th Global Summit of National Bioethics / Ethics Committees. 2018. "Bioethics, Sustainable Development and Society: Call for Action." https://cdn.who.int/media/docs/default-source/ethics/dakar-statement-of-gsnec2018.pdf?sfvrsn=1849d56_4.

12

The Necessity of Fusing Bioethics and Geoethics

An Ecointersectional Approach

Nancy Tuana

My first teaching position was in a college close to Marysville, California. It was a small, sleepy town with a population of less than 8,000 people. But the history of Marysville is long and complicated. The town is located on the ancestral land of the Maidu, an area untouched by colonialism until 1828 when the explorer Jedediah Smith led trappers from the Hudson Bay Company into the region. It did not take long for colonialism to take root. Livestock farmers were the first to appropriate the land. The city of Marysville was incorporated in 1851, less than three decades after the Hudson Bay expedition. But it was the California Gold Rush that would transform the land as well as those living on it. Marysville became known as the gateway to the gold fields, the stopping point for the riverboats from San Francisco and Sacramento that brought prospectors hoping to strike it rich. Within less than a decade, Marysville became one of the largest cities in California, a city formed through exchanges between humans and land.

When we think of those prospectors mining gold, we envision bearded men in wide-brimmed hats bending down, holding their gold pan at an angle, rotating it in a gyrating fashion in order to remove the lighter material in the hope that they will discover gold at the bottom. But in the region around Marysville, excavating gold by hand gave way to hydraulic mining. This form of mining used water monitors, nozzles the size of a small cannon that channeled water at very high pressures to break up boulders, gravel deposits, and dirt to access gold buried beneath. Some monitors were 8 inches in diameter and could eject 185,000 cubic feet of water per hour (that's an astonishing 1,383,896 gallons) at a velocity of 100 miles per hour (Melosi 2022). The resulting debris was washed through sluices so that the heavier gold particles would settle behind riffle boards while the remainder would be washed into streams and rivers. Hydraulic water monitors blasted 1.5 billion cubic yards of rock and soil from the hillsides, filling streams and rivers with debris and changing the landscape of the area. Some of the debris was carried downstream by rivers like the Yuba, Sacramento, and Feather River where it inundated farmlands, burying fertile soil in mining debris.

Massive flooding became commonplace, ruining thousands of acres of farmland and open fields, and killing livestock and wildlife. Acres of forests were logged to supply the large amounts of wood required for building canal systems and for fuel. Streams once teeming with life were buried under the debris. Salmon runs relied upon by the Maidu and other Indigenous people[1] were ruined.

Carleton Watkins's prints of hydraulic mining made clear the geological devastation. Samuel Bowles, a leading journalist, painted a corresponding image in a news story when he reported that

> Tornado, flood, earthquake and volcano combined could hardly make greater havoc, spread wider ruin and wreck, than are to be seen everywhere in the track of the larger gold-washing operations. None of the interior streams of California, though naturally pure as crystal, escape the change to a thick yellow mud, from this cause, early in their progress out of the hills. The Sacramento River is worse than the Missouri. Many of the streams are turned out of their original channels, either directly for mining purposes, or in consequence of the great masses of soil and gravel that come down from the gold-washings above. Thousands of acres of fine land along their banks are ruined forever by the deposits of this character. (Bowles 1869, 422–3)

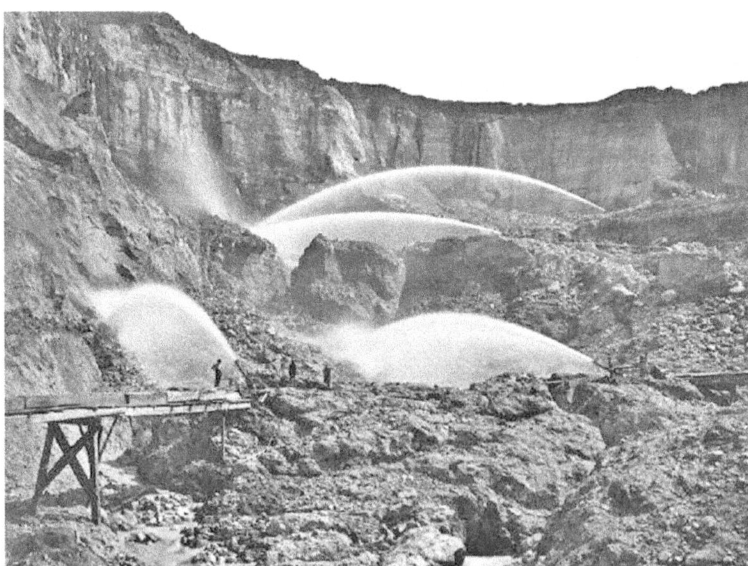

Figure 12.1 *Carleton Watkins's prints of hydraulic mining made clear the geological devastation.* U.S. Geological Survey Scientific Investigations Report 2009-5269, public domain.

The geological impact of hydraulic mining is literally etched in the mountains, valleys, and waterways. However, the geological impacts cannot be separated from the biological impacts. The gravel, sand, and soil particles filling the streams and waters negatively impact vegetation and aquatic populations alike. Sediment, for example, can clog fish gills and in doing so make fish more susceptible to disease; it also affects egg and larvae development. Suspended particles block light and affect growth of aquatic plants. Humans, the Maidu and the colonizing settlers alike, are impacted as food sources from waterways become scarcer and drinking water is affected.

Such geological impacts are heightened by the fact that gold mining deploys liquid mercury to concentrate gold particles in order to increase gold recovery. Hydraulic mining in the state of California alone from the 1860s to the early 1900s resulted in an estimated 10 million pounds of mercury being transported along with the gravel and dirt, the majority of which contaminated the Sierra Nevada region (Alpers et al. 2005, 2). Ten million pounds of mercury in waterways and soils. Bacterial processes convert the inorganic mercury used to secure gold into organic mercury, methylmercury, which bioaccumulates in the flesh of fish that live in the polluted waters, the plants that absorb those waters, the birds and insects that live in the region, and the animals, including humans, who drink from the water or eat plants and animals so contaminated. Methylmercury travels in the bloodstream and is distributed across the tissues of the body. It can cross the blood-brain barrier and affect the brain. Animals exposed to methylmercury, including humans, can experience reproductive issues, including central nervous disturbances and developmental disorders in fetuses. It can also result in cardiovascular diseases, as well as having negative cognitive impacts (Hong, Kim, and Lee 2012).

Those 10 million pounds of mercury still circulate in soils and flesh. Globules of mercury can still to this day be found in the streams and creeks that were fed by the hydraulic mining over a century ago. Those still wishing to pan for gold in the waterways of the Sierra Nevada risk exposure. But one need not pan for gold to be so exposed. Methylmercury remains in the soil for decades. It is carried by snowmelt and rain, and moves through waterways long distant from the original mining locations.

Human exposure to mercury can happen through air, food, drink, and even dental fillings. But most of the mercury accumulated in humans is ingested through eating seafood. Fish and shellfish contain much higher quantities of mercury than other foods and 90 percent of mercury in fish and shellfish exists in the form of methylmercury (Hong, Kim, and Lee 2012). But the burdens of mercury contamination are not equally distributed. Those people whose diet is higher in fish have higher blood mercury levels. Both economic reasons and cultural practices contribute to the finding that in the United States, Pacific Islanders and other Indigenous populations have a higher prevalence of elevated blood mercury than other groups (Hightower, O'Hare, and Hernandez 2006). Traditional foods of Indigenous people from Turtle Island are an important cultural component of Indigenous lifeways, yet the impacts of mercury contamination mean that these lifeways can put Indigenous communities at risk. The International Indian Treaty Council in San Francisco in collaboration with the Pit River Nation created the Mercury Tribal Health and Environmental Justice Program in order to help Native Californian communities balance health and cultures and traditions that define them (Cultural Survival 2004).

Fusing Bioethics and Geoethics— Apprehending Ecological Indifference

The story of the Gold Rush is just one illustration of the *inextricable intertwining of geos and bios*. It is a well-worn adage that healthy environments, ones in which all people have good air quality, safe drinking water, and uncontaminated food, are inextricably linked to positive human health outcomes. According to a recent report from the World Health Organization, "one quarter of the global burden of disease is attributable to avoidable environmental risk factors such as the chemical, radiological and biological contamination of air, food, water and soil" (World Health Organization 2022–3). This recognition combined with acceptance of the fact that human activities are having potentially catastrophic impacts on earth systems in the age currently dubbed the Anthropocene, and the stage is set for uniting bioethics and geoethics. While my insistence that these fields be united is arguably not unique, *what matters is how the uniting occurs*.

Too often the ethical concern—whether it be in bioethics or geoethics—focuses on human health and on what is good for human well-being. Consider just one of myriad examples. In a recent paper, "The bioethics of environmental injustice: ethical, legal, and clinical implications of unhealthy environments," Keisha Ray and Jane Fallis Cooper argue that it is essential that bioethics prioritize environmental health, and in doing so, address environmental injustices. As they phrase it, "we argue that if bioethicists take the project of health justice as seriously as our core professional principles purport, then we have to address environmental injustices and the threats they pose to our bioethics principles, health equity, and clinical care . . . to do this bioethicists must prioritize and advocate for a legal right to a healthy environment" (2023, 10). What becomes clear in this essay, indeed in many efforts to link bioethics and environmental ethics or geoethics, is that the concern for environmental justice is a concern to protect the health and well-being of current and future people. "Calling for stronger legislation to protect our environment's health underscores a commitment to justice. This includes righting past and current injustices, protecting social groups who have been politically taken advantage of by corporations and lawmakers, and protecting the environment for future peoples" (Ray and Cooper 2023, 10). Too often, the term "environmental injustice" refers not to impacts on the environment—to the harms done to myriad lifeforms and life ways—but rather to how those impacts disproportionately advantage or disadvantage certain groups of humans.

What such analyses fail to appreciate is the ways in which environmental injustice approaches are informed by a sensibility that is itself a core component of the very injustice these analyses are designed to reveal. Too often, efforts to link bioethics to issues of the environment are accomplished through theories and beliefs animated by a centuries-long separation of humans from nonhumans and the assumption that only humans have intrinsic value; that is, have moral standing. I have developed the phrase *ecological indifference* to refer to this sensibility (Tuana 2023). Ecological indifference signals the disposition of perceiving animals, plants, and/or ecosystems they are part of as resources for human consumption and well-being—usable, fungible, disposable, without intrinsic worth or moral standing. It involves the unquestioned conviction that the "nonhuman" world has value only instrumentally, that is, a value that is to be measured primarily by its usefulness for humans.[2] Indeed, this is exactly the conception we see in the Sierra Nevada during the Gold Rush. Mountains, rivers, and land are valued only for what they can produce that is of value to humans. If gold is to be desired, mountains can be washed away. Ecological indifference is a sensibility that cleaves a divide between humans and the nonhuman and views the latter as essentially lacking inherent value.[3] The farmers objected to hydraulic mining not because of the intrinsic value of the lives flourishing in the fields or streams but because of the damage to their crops, crops grown because of the value they have for human consumption.

Ecological indifference fuels and is fueled by the resource-extractive practices of capitalism and colonialism. A focus on consumption and conquest is grounded in a sensibility that separates the human from nature and sees the latter as having at best only use-value. This is a sensibility that has led to what Steve Lerner (2010) refers to as *sacrifice zones*. Sacrifice zones include areas of the environment that have been stripped of the resources viewed as valuable—logged-over forests, spent or abandoned uranium mines, the remains of mountaintop removal from coal extraction—or have been designated as repositories for the unusable by-products of consumption—the landfills, waste dumps, injection wells, and Superfund sites. These sacrifice zones include all the inhabitants, including the human inhabitants, who are relegated to living in what have often become toxic environs and who have thus been sacrificed along with the forests, mountains, and waterways. As Lerner explains, using the term sacrifice zone "dramatizes the fact that low-income and minority populations, living adjacent to heavy industry and military bases, are required to make disproportionate health and economic sacrifices that more affluent people can avoid." He argues that "this pattern of unequal exposure constitutes a form of environmental racism that is being played out on a large scale across the nation" (Lerner 2010, 3).

Lerner's account, like many who attempt to link environmental issues with bioethical issues, while making clear the injustice of unequal exposures and their differential impacts, overlooks the ways in which *the formation and tolerance of environmental sacrifice zones and the creation and acceptance of people and other lifeforms who are sacrificable are interdependent and mutually reinforcing*. The ecological indifference that undergirds sacrifice zones signals a form of indifference that often goes beyond the human/nonhuman divide, for this is a troubled divide in which some humans have historically been seen as less than fully human. Systemic racism and sexism both trouble this divide, carving the world up into types of humans who are seen as less civilized and thus less worthy of full moral standing. This creates a basis for treating some humans with an analogous indifference—as fungible and disposable. Understanding the various beliefs, habits, practices, dispositions by which systemic racisms reinforce and are reinforced by environmental degradation is an important and often missing component of the environmental justice literature. As Hop Hopkins (2020), with the Sierra Club, phrased it in the context of climate justice, "You can't have climate change without sacrifice zones, and you can't have sacrifice zones without disposable people, and you can't have disposable people without racism." Even if we succeed in uniting bioethics and geoethics, if the resulting approaches remain focused on the human and unjust differential impacts on groups of humans, they miss a more fundamental linkage between viewing environments as exploitable and seeing certain groups of people as exploitable. In short, they risk missing a fundamental interconnection between systemic racism and environmental indifference.

We see this entwining of systemic racisms and ecological indifference in the treatment of Indigenous communities during the Gold Rush. The impact of the Gold Rush is not only etched into the mountains of the Sierra Nevada; it was etched into the Indigenous communities who lived there. As thousands of miners moved into the region, a land that was once plentiful in elk, fish, and other wildlife, the food sources Indigenous communities had thrived on for centuries became scarce as miners hunted wildlife for their sustenance and their mining activities ruined the abundance in the rivers and streams. The miners also brought with them diseases that killed many Indigenous people. But the deaths of Indigenous people happened not only through illness and starvation. Private militia financed by the state of California were charged with killing Indigenous people to clear the land for settlers and to ensure access to gold found on ancestral land. State-sanctioned genocide was incentivized by paying bounties for scalps or even severed heads. There had been mass killings of Indigenous people in the land that is now known as California prior to 1848 (Madley 2016), but the gold rush triggered an avalanche of mass murders. Vigilantes and US Army soldiers alike murdered Indigenous people in Northern California. As the historian Benjamin Madley, author of *An American Genocide: The United States and the California Indian Catastrophe, 1846–1873*, explained:

> California governors called out or authorized no fewer than twenty-four state militia expeditions between 1850 and 1861, which killed at least 1,342 California Indians. 39 State legislators also passed three bills—in 1851, 1852, and 1857—that raised up to $1.51 million to fund these operations. By demonstrating that the state would not punish Indian killers, but instead reward them, militia expeditions helped inspire vigilantes to kill at least 6,460 California Indians between 1846 and 1873. Meanwhile, the state built an arsenal donated by the federal government. And Congress passed two bills—in 1854 and 1860—allocating up to $1,324,259 to reimburse California for past militia expeditions, retrospectively endorsing them, financially supporting them, and thus fueling genocidal campaigns. (Madley 2016, 455)

In the words of Peter Burnett, governor of California from 1849 to 1851, "that a war of extermination will continue to be waged between the races until the Indian race becomes extinct must be expected. While we cannot anticipate this result but with painful regret, the inevitable destiny of the race is beyond the power or wisdom of man to avert" (Burnett 1851).

In addition to state-sanctioned murder, California legislators passed bills allowing for Indigenous prisoner leasing and white custody of Indigenous minors, effectively legalizing unfree labor and servitude. Many of those sentenced to unfree labor were forced to work in the gold mining camps. Death due to malnourishment and neglect was common. Those people who were not murdered or enslaved were relocated to reservations. Indigenous children were forcibly placed into government or church-run boarding schools where they were often required to work in homes or farms.[4] It is estimated that in just twenty years following the start of the gold rush, 80 percent of California's Indigenous people had died (Blakemore 2023). During this period, the Maidu population dropped from 10,000 to 330 (Feather River Tribal Health n.d.).

The ecological indifference that resulted in the destruction of aquatic and terrestrial ecosystems alike in the Sierra Nevada area was inextricably interlinked with an analogous indifference toward the Indigenous people who lived with the land. To separate these two phenomena is to miss the ways that beliefs and practices that result in the types of disproportionate advantages or disadvantages that are at the heart of most environmental or climate justice frameworks are intertwined with the beliefs and practices that result in the very forms of harm to ecosystems and environments that are the reason for those differential impacts. As I have previously argued, ecological indifference and environmental or climate injustice are two sides of the same coin (Tuana 2023).

Ecointersectional Analyses

The example of the California Gold Rush is one of the myriad illustrations of the importance not only of seeing the interconnections between bioethics and geoethics, but also the reason it is essential to approach this work from what I've labeled an *ecointersectional analysis* (Tuana 2023). Ecointersectional analyses reveal the complex ways that environmental degradation and systemic oppressions are mutually constitutive. My approach is indebted to the work of US Black feminist thinkers such as Francis Beal (1969), Patricia Hill Collins (1990, 2019), the Combahee River Collective (1979), Anna Julia Cooper (1892), Kimberlé Crenshaw (1989, 1991), and many others who made evident the double jeopardy of being Black and being a woman. Intersectionality offers an "analytic sensibility" through which to examine "sameness and difference and its relation to power" (Cho, Crenshaw, and McCall 2013, 795). Embracing the commitment of Black feminist approaches to intersectionality to shine a light on the impact of systemic racisms,[5] I build on such approaches to reveal the ways the vectors of power and institutions that undergird systemic racisms are saturated with beliefs, values, and practices concerning ecosystems and all their inhabitants—animals, plants, rivers, oceans, mountains, and the like.

Too often accounts of harms to environments are viewed as separate from the impacts and effects of social inequalities. While it is often acknowledged that harms to environments, such as those we see from hydraulic gold mining, frequently cause greater harms to groups of people and communities who also suffer from social oppressions, the two phenomena are treated as separate and, at best, additive. Racism, for example, even when it is conceived as systemic, is typically seen as separate from environmental degradation or the two are seen as additive—for example, racism results in Blacks living in more toxic environments. Here a component of environmental racism is acknowledged; Blacks are more likely to be exposed to environmental harms. However, what this approach can obscure is the fact that systemic injustices and environmental degradation are at times and in complex ways interfused. The particular ways in which they blend are geographically and historically specific, hence the need for ecointersectional analyses that aim to identify the complex beliefs, practices, and institutions that give rise to indifference and injustice. Ecointersectional analyses must be carefully situated and historically informed in order to understand the lineages and institutions that link the disposability of some groups of humans and the disposability of other lifeforms and ecosystems. As Devon Carbado explained, "all intersectional moves are necessarily particularized and therefore provisional and incomplete" as each such analysis "must necessarily limit itself to specific structures of power" (Carbado et al. 2013, 304).

It is crucial, however, that ecointersectional analyses do not reiterate or reinforce problematic ontological divides so common in Western sensibilities, such as those between humans and nature, or life and nonlife, and the various permutations thereof, which are often at the ontological heart of the links between environmental exploitation and the exploitation of groups of animals, including humans. The preface "eco-," in my usage, is an inclusive, gathering word that refers to the ways things happen together. Ecointersectional analyses include attention to ecosystems, those complex interactions between lifeforms, which of course include human lifeforms, and between lifeforms and life places, the physical, abiotic conditions in which lifeforms exist. An ecointersectional lens is particularly helpful in efforts to question and undo the various human/environment, bios/geos divides; just as race is not separate or separable from gender—does not constitute an ontological divide—so too we begin to appreciate that geos is not separate or separable from bios; they infuse in complex ways. Given this we need to shift sensibilities from a human/nature divide to worldings of the more-than-human;[6] and, as part of such a shift, remove the divide between bioethics and geoethics.

Ecointersectional analyses provide resources for attending to ecological indifference. But such analyses also reveal why pushing back against ecological indifference *by itself* is insufficient to address issues of injustice. Proponents of ecological justice, for example, argue for expanding the domain of moral considerability to "nature" and emphasize the interdependence of all species (e.g., Baxter 2005; Garner 2013; Nussbaum 2006; Schlosberg 2014). What is too often overlooked by such accounts is a recognition of the ways systemic oppressions and views about the environment are entangled. No merging of bioethics and geoethics will be adequate that does not understand and attempt to address the ways systemic racisms and ecological indifference are co-constituted.

As with any intersectional analysis, my ecointersectional analysis of the infusion of systemic racisms and environmental destruction in the California Gold Rush is not designed to erase other dimensions, but rather to attend to what can be seen when the focus is through this particular facet of the prism and attend to its intersections with other facets. In the words of Kara Thompson, who is speaking to issues of climate injustice, we need to see that "racism and climate change are genealogical and scalar. They belong to the procession of anthropogenic histories premised on white supremacy over black and brown bodies and nonhuman worlds, and on making these two at times indistinguishable" (Thompson 2017, 93).

Despite a number of calls for the field of bioethics to appreciate that climate change is, as Cheryl Cox Macpherson phrases it, "a bioethics problem," the health that climate change harms is too often focused on human health. Even when so-called planetary health is a focus, attention often returns to human well-being: "The concept of planetary health is based on the understanding that human health and human civilization depend on flourishing natural systems and the wise stewardship of those natural systems. However, natural systems are being degraded to an extent unprecedented in human history" (Whitmee, et al. 2015, 1974). Key for any effort to fuse bioethics and geoethics, to develop links between bioethics and environmental ethics, or to cultivate attention to environmental racism in bioethics, is to avoid reinscribing the very divisions—human/less than fully human/nonhuman—that are woven tightly into environmental exploitation and entwined inexorably with the exploitation of certain groups of people.

I am not claiming that this will be easy to do. In Western cultures, these divisions are bred-in-the-bone, so to speak. We inherit a language, sensibility, affective disposition that animates and is animated by these divides. Perhaps at a time when we understand all too well that human-environment interactions are transforming us all—changing the climate, impacting flora and fauna ranges, altering the acidity of surface ocean waters—perhaps we can become open to other sensibilities, other ways of worlding that are not grounded on a racialized human/environment divide. Perhaps we could attend to what Macarena Gómez-Barris refers to as "cataloging life otherwise," namely, "the emergent and heterogeneous forms of living that are not about destruction or mere survival within the extractive zone, but about the creation of emergent alternatives" (Gómez-Barris 2017, 4). Perhaps an attention to the many locations and innumerable ways systemic oppressions and ecological indifference have been infused will be a path forward.

Let us begin anew.

Notes

1 Following the practice of Jen Deerinwater, rather than referring to members of nations such as Maidu, Chumash, Tolowa, Miwok, Nisenan, Hupa, and Paiute, all communities in what is now known as California, as Native American or American Indians, I use the more general term, Indigenous. Deerinwater argues against the use of terms that include "American" as a category that signals the theft of land and resources, as well as rejecting the term "Indian," which "reinforces the idea that we are loinclothed savages whom Columbus

'discovered'" (2020, 47). I nonetheless recognize the risk of any term that homogenizes a group of people. It risks a "flattening [that] ignores that Indigenous people are not a race but rather hundreds of distinct nations with tribal sovereignty" (2020, 48).

2 Val Plumwood developed the conception of the "backgrounding of nature" to refer to this phenomenon of nature being relegated to a role that allowed usefulness without entailing moral considerability. For Plumwood, it was the backgrounding of nature that blocked efforts toward sustainability. "Dominant western culture has systematically inferiorised, backgrounded, and denied dependency on the whole sphere of reproduction and subsistence. This denial of dependency is a major factor in the perpetuation of the non-sustainable modes of using nature which loom as such a threat to the future of western society" (1993, 21).

3 I am not claiming that ecological indifference is a universal sensibility. I am saying that it is the dominant sensibility in the current global economy (Moore 2015, 2016). There are a number of cultures and communities that embrace sensibilities grounded in the relationality of things (Simpson 2017; Burkhart 2019; Harris 2017; Cadena 2019). The problem is that these are not the sensibilities that have the most power or impact in our current globalized world.

4 Three of the twenty-five Indian boarding schools run by the US government were located on land now known as California.

5 The distinction between individual racism and institutional or systemic racism was introduced in 1967 by Stokely Carmichael (Kwame Ture) and Charles V. Hamilton in *Black Power: The Politics of Liberation*. I modify Carmichael and Hamilton's original term to systemic racisms as a reminder that racism is not the same in all regions or in all time periods. Racializations are complex phenomena that are neither unified nor unchanging.

6 David Abram introduced the term "more-than-human" in his book *The Spell of the Sensuous* (1996). It is imperative in adopting the term to avoid the tendency to continue the very divide this term is designed to undo—human/more-than-human. We need to appreciate that the more-than-human both includes and exceeds the human. I realize that by retaining the term "human" within the locution, I and Abram risk reinforcing the ontological priority of homo sapiens, a priority afforded only to some people. While not minimizing these risks, I believe the locution has the potential to disrupt ontological habits of separation, attune us to the risks and possibilities of efforts to collapse dichotomies, as well as to seek ways of worlding that do not impose what Val Plumwood referred to as a hyperseparation of humans from the rest of nature (1993). My aspiration is that the term can become, as Penny Harvey, Christian Krohn-Hansen, and Knut G. Nustad phrase it, a "way of keeping open an unsettled space that allows us to remain attentive to a multiplicity that does not settle, and to uncertainties that are never simply resolved" (Harvey, Krohn-Hansen, and Nustad 2019, 4).

Bibliography

Abram, David. 1996. *The Spell of the Sensuous: Perception and Language in a More-Than-Human World*. Pantheon Books.

Alpers, Charles N., Michael P. Hunerlach, Jason T. May, and Roger L. Hotthem. 2005. "Mercury Contamination from Historical Gold Mining in California." USGS, Fact Sheet 2005–3014, Version 1.1. https://pubs.usgs.gov/fs/2005/3014/.

Baxter, Brian. 2005. *A Theory of Ecological Justice*. Taylor and Francis.

Beal, Frances M. 1969. "Black Women's Manifesto; Double Jeopardy: To Be Black and Female, from Third World Women's Alliance." http://www.hartford-hwp.com/archives/45a/196.html

Blakemore, Erin. 2023. "California's Little-Known Genocide." https://www.history.com/news/californias-little-known-genocide

Bowles, Samuel. 1869. *Our New West: Records of Travel Between the Mississippi River and the Pacific Ocean*. Hartford Publishing Company.

Burkhart, Brian. 2019. *Indigenizing Philosophy through the Land: A Trickster Methodology for Decolonizing Environmental Ethics and Indigenous Futures*. Michigan State University Press.

Burnett, Peter. 1851. "State of the State Address." Delivered January 6. https://governors.library.ca.gov/addresses/s_01-Burnett2.html

Cadena, Marisol de la. 2019. "Uncommoning Nature: Stories from the Anthropo-Not-Seen." In Penny Harvey, Christian Krohn-Hansen, and Knut G. Nustad (eds.), *Anthropos and the Material*. Duke University Press.

Carbado, Devon, Kimberlé Crenshaw, Vicki Mays and Barbara Tomlinson. "INTERSECTIONALITY: Mapping the Movements of a Theory," *10 DU BOIS REV*. 303 (2013). Available at: https://scholarship.law.columbia.edu/faculty_scholarship/2779

Carmichael, Stokely, and Charles V. Hamilton. 1967. *Black Power: The Politics of Liberation*. Vintage Books.

Cho, Sumi, Kimberlé Williams Crenshaw, and Leslie McCall. 2013. "Toward a Field of Intersectionality Studies: Theory, Applications, and Praxis." *Signs*, 38 (4): 785–810.

Collins, Patricia Hill. 2019. *Intersectionality as Critical Social Theory*. Duke University Press.

Collins, Patricia Hill. 1990. *Black Feminist Thought: Knowledge, Consciousness, and the Politics of Empowerment*. Unwin Hyman.

Combahee River Collective. 1979. "The Combahee River Collective Statement." In Zillah Eisenstein (ed.), Capitalist *Patriarchy and the Case for Socialist Feminism*. Monthly Review Press.

Cooper, Anna Julia. 1892. *A Voice from the South*. The Aldine Printing Company.

Cultural Survival. 2004. "California Indians Balance Toxics and Traditions." June 25. https://www.culturalsurvival.org/news/california-indians-balance-toxics-and-traditions.

Crenshaw, Kimberlé. 1989. "Demarginalizing the Intersection of Race and Sex: A Black Feminist Critique of Antidiscrimination Doctrine, Feminist Theory and Antiracist Politics." *University of Chicago Legal Forum*, 1 (8): 139–68.

Crenshaw, Kimberlé. 1991. "Mapping the Margins: Intersectionality, Identity Politics, and Violence against Women of Color." *Stanford Law Review*, 43 (6): 1244–99.

Deerinwater, Jen. 2020. "The Erasure of Indigenous People in Chronic Illness." In Alice Wong (ed.), *Disability Visibility: First-Person Stories from the Twenty-First Century*. Vintage Books

Feather River Tribal Health. n.d. "The History of the Maidu Indians." https://frth.org/history-of-the-maidu/

Garner, Robert. 2013. *A Theory of Justice for Animals: Animal Rights in a Nonideal World*. Oxford University Press.

Gómez-Barris, Macarena. 2017. *The Extractive Zone: Social Ecologies and Decolonial Perspectives.* Duke University Press.
Harris, Melanie L. 2017. *Ecowomanism: African American Women and Earth-Honoring Faiths.* Orbis Books.
Harvey, Penny, Christian Krohn-Hansen, and Kunt G. Nustad, eds. 2019. *Anthropos and the Material.* Duke University Press.
Hightower Jane M., Ann O'Hare, and German T. Hernandez. 2006. "Blood Mercury Reporting in NHANES: Identifying Asian, Pacific Islander, Native American, and Multiracial Groups." *Environmental Health Perspectives*, 114 (2): 173–5.
Hong, Young-Seoub, Yu-Mi Kim, and Kung-Eun Lee. 2012. "Methylmercury Exposure and Health Effects." *Journal of Preventive Medicine and Public Health*, 45 (6): 353–63.
Hopkins, Hop. 2020. "Racism is Killing the Planet." *Sierra Club*. https://www.sierraclub.org/sierra/racism-killing-planet
Lerner, Steve. 2010. *Sacrifice Zone: The Front Lines of Toxic Chemical Exposure in the United States.* MIT Press.
Macpherson, Cheryl Cox. 2013. "Climate Change is a Bioethics Problem." *Bioethics*, 27(6): 305–8.
Madley, Benjamin. 2016. *An American Genocide: The United States and the California Indian Catastrophe, 1846–1873.* Yale University Press.
Melosi, Martin V. 2022. *Water in North American Environmental History*. Routledge.
Moore, Jason W. 2015. *Capitalism in the Web of Life: Ecology and the Accumulation of Capital.* Verso.
Moore, Jason W. 2016. "The Rise of Cheap Nature." In Jason W. Moore (ed.), *Anthropocene or Capitalocene?: Nature, History, and the Crisis of Capitalism*. PM Press.
Nussbaum, Martha. C. 2006. *Frontiers of Justice: Disability, Nationality, Species Membership.* Belknap Press.
Plumwood, Val. 1993. *Feminism and the Mastery of Nature*. Routledge.
Ray, Keisha, and Jane Fallis Cooper. 2023. "The Bioethics of Environmental Injustice: Ethical, Legal, and Clinical Implications of Unhealthy Environments." *The American Journal of Bioethics*, 24 (3): 9–17.
Schlosberg, David. 2014. "Ecological Justice for the Anthropocene." In Marcel Wissenburg and David Schlosber (eds.), *Political Animals and Animal Politics*. Palgrave Macmillan.
Simpson, Leanne Betasamosake. 2017. *As We Have Always Done: Indigenous Freedom through Radical Resistance.* University of Minnesota Press.
Thompson, Kara. 2017. "Traffic Stops, Stopping Traffic: Race and Climate Change in the Age of Automobility." *ISLE: Interdisciplinary Studies in Literature and Environment*, 24 (1): 92–112.
Tuana, Nancy. 2023. *Racial Climates, Ecological Indifference: An Ecointersectional Approach.* Oxford University Press.
Whitmee, Sarah, Andy Haines, Chris Beyrer, et al. 2015. "Safeguarding Human Health in the Anthropocene Epoch: Report of The Rockefeller Foundation– Lancet Commission on Planetary Health." *The Lancet*, 386 (10007): 1973–2028.
World Health Organization. 2022–2023. "Midterm Results Report." https://www.who.int/about/accountability/results/who-results-report-2022-mtr/outcome/2022/healthy-environments-to-promote-health-and-sustainable-societies.

New Tools and Visions for Bioethics

13

The Science and Skill of Facing Change

Implications for Bioethicists

Marion Danis and Hollen N. Reischer

A great many bioethicists—be they clinical ethics consultants or academic scholars—often address ethical challenges that arise as a result of some substantial change that has occurred or is about to occur. Thus, many of these challenges require knowledge about coping with change. Consider calls for consultative advice from clinicians serving patients facing life-altering circumstances—a new illness, disability, or death—or calls from patients and families themselves. Even a change in circumstances that does not involve loss may require adjustment to change—a new life stage, a new child, a new treatment option. Other ethics consultation requests may pertain to changes in circumstances for individual health care providers and for organizations as a whole. Consider the need to help hospital leadership adjust to a drastic change in circumstances such as a major budget cut; an influx of new immigrants in the surrounding community; a request from clinicians for extremely expensive, innovative medical equipment. Yet, the competencies that ethics consultants are expected to possess do not explicitly include any knowledge or skill in coping with change or thinking about the ethics of change management (ASBH 2011).

Academic bioethicists are similarly likely to focus their scholarship on challenges posed by developments such as new scientific methodologies, technologies, or biological threats. The application of their theoretical analyses to more practical policy recommendations will require some attention to the way in which individuals and organizations cope with change.

The premise of this chapter is that an understanding of how individuals and organizations tend to react to change and what is required to effectively cope with change might be useful to bioethicists in their efforts to facilitate ethically informed adjustment to change. This premise dovetails with Lisa Parker's assertion in the first chapter of this book that attention to feelings and emotions is essential for effective bioethics practice.

Our suggestions come with the proviso that not all change is inevitable, necessary, or useful (Goodall 2024). The most skilled bioethicists will be aware not only of how people react to change but will also help them to evaluate it critically.

Integrating Perspectives on the Human Response to Change

Perspectives on Biological Response to Change

In his 2023 book, *Master of Change: How to Excel When Everything is Changing – Including You*, Brad Stulberg, a faculty member in the School of Public Health at the University of Michigan, points out how committed contemporary culture is to stability, and how problematic this commitment is in the face of the reality that change is inescapable. He describes recent evidence from psychology, biology, sociology, and neuroscience on the human response to change (Stulberg 2023).

Stulberg points out that Claude Bernard, the seventeenth-century French physiologist, proposed a model of physiology that considered change to be disruptive and threatening to health. Bernard's work was consistent with the subsequent concept proposed by Walter Cannon, the nineteenth- to-twentieth-century American physiologist, of *homeostasis*—the tendency of living systems to resist change in order to maintain stable, relatively constant internal environments. Stability, according to this conception, is maintained through a response to change that involves returning to the prior stable state. Externally imposed change is viewed as an undesirable challenge that must be overcome by an effort to regain the status quo.

In contrast, more recent neuroscience has shown that healthy biological systems adapt to change rather than rigidly resisting it. Joseph Eyer, a biologist, and Peter Sterling, a neuroscientist, proposed the concept of *allostasis* to reflect a sequence involving order, disorder, and *re*order (Eyer and Sterling 1988). Rather than returning to the same order or state of being after a disruption, organisms return to a stable state that is new and different from the prior state (as exemplified by the neuroplasticity of the human brain in response to new stimuli).

In summary, the homeostatic view of response to change assumes that humans avoid or refuse to acknowledge change, try to resist and stop change, give up resistance to change, or try to return to the way things were before change. In contrast, an allostatic response to change entails flexibility and enables preservation of a strong core of one's identity while at the same time adapting, evolving, and growing (Stulberg 2023). Accordingly, resistance and denial tend to be accompanied by a physiological stress response, whereas acceptance of the inevitability of change tends to be less physiologically stressful and less psychologically disturbing (Brick et al. 2019). Stulberg labels a mindset that allows a person to effectively proceed forward in the face of impermanence by turning their energy to acceptance and accommodation "rugged flexibility."

Philosophical and Psychological Perspectives on Impermanence and Equanimity

In line with physiological theories of change, several philosophical traditions have long recognized the pervasiveness of change and the cyclical nature of reality. For example, the attentiveness of Buddhist philosophy to the inevitability of suffering comes with encouragement to differentiate between what one can and cannot control, and to act on what one can control and accept or accommodate what one cannot. This is also central to late Roman Stoicism, particularly the basic teaching of Epictetus (Epictetus 1994). This approach might be thought of as pursuing wise hope and wise action in contradistinction to the extremes of either excessive optimism and denial or hopelessness and despair (Stulberg 2023).

Psychologists suggest that the development of this sort of wise resilience can be cultivated to prepare individuals to respond effectively to change. They recommend such behaviors as building connections through trustworthy, empathic relationships and joining groups; promoting wellness by exercising self-care, practicing mindfulness, and avoiding masking pain through the use of substances; finding purpose by being proactive, helping others, and setting realistic goals; accepting challenges as opportunities for growth; embracing healthy thoughts by keeping obstacles in perspective, accepting change, maintaining a hopeful perspective, and looking back on prior successes; and seeking help when feeling stuck or helpless (Palmiter et al. 2023).

Research on evidence-based psychotherapies such as Dialectical Behavior Therapy and Acceptance and Commitment Therapy, which are consistent with Buddhist thought on the nature of change and scientific evidence on human response to change, demonstrates that shifting cognitive and behavioral patterns in favor of greater reality acceptance and more flexible thinking leads to greater psychological health. Hallmark strategies of these approaches include practicing "radical acceptance"—accepting the reality of one's situation with neither positive nor negative judgment (Linehan 1993)—and willingness to "defuse" from thoughts and beliefs about how life should be, was, or might be in the future, and instead experiencing the reality of the present moment (Hayes, Strosahl, and Wilson 2002).

While impermanence may cause pain, if one expects change to occur, it is nonetheless possible to find life satisfaction and meaning. Importantly, even if one's overall life satisfaction may suffer from adverse change, it may be the case that well-being borne out of a meaningful, purposeful life may be particularly resilient or even increase. Psychiatrist and neurologist Victor Frankl introduced the idea of "tragic optimism"—the capacity to avoid running away from hardships, losses, and negative emotions, and instead accept them as opportunities to gain a sense of meaning and purpose. Frankl was a Holocaust survivor who had seen the worst of humanity in his own life—and believed that his ability to look for meaning in life under even the harshest of conditions had kept him alive (Frankl 1946).

Evidence for tragic optimism can be found in a study that revealed the mindset of people who were emotionally resilient after the terrorist attack on September 11, 2001. While nearly all participants reported feeling fear, despair, and other negative emotions, these feelings were less debilitating in those individuals who were able to make room for positive emotions of love and gratitude (Fredrickson et al. 2003). In another study, individuals with spinal cord injuries were found to have higher psychological well-being when they rated themselves as having and achieving clear life goals and believing their daily activities and overall lives were worthwhile, coherent, and meaningful (deRoon-Cassini et al. 2009).

The Psychological Meaning of Change in Narrative

There is mixed research about the typical course of accommodating to negative life-altering events such as losing a spouse or becoming disabled, with some evidence that life satisfaction eventually returns to baseline (Costa, McCrae, and Zonderman 1987) and other evidence that there are permanent losses in mean happiness (Lucas 2007). As it relates to the clinical ethicist, we highlight the role of psychological meaning-making in these contexts.

Research on the way people describe coping with life challenges demonstrates that the manner in which people make sense of and narrate stories of significant challenges is associated with their well-being, independent of the severity of the hardship itself. For example, parents of children with Down Syndrome (King et al. 2000) and highly stressed parents of children with autism spectrum disorder (Mason et al. 2019) have been found to have better physiological and psychological outcomes when the stories they tell integrate their challenging experiences into a fulfilling or meaningful life story.

In a somewhat similar vein, recent research shows that although adults with severe mental illness may narrate their pasts with a more negative tone than those without severe mental illness, their stories about the *future* tend to be no less positive—in other words, they demonstrate an openness to accommodation and acceptance which suggests a path forward (Jensen et al. 2020). For the clinical ethicist, this finding also highlights that the focus of a discussion (e.g., the past vs. the future) may strongly inform the perspectives elicited by stakeholders.

Knowledge of such "narrative outcomes" may be useful to a clinical ethicist. Elaborating on the above examples, a hypothetical ethics consultation might arise in the context of tension around whether a family opts in to early intervention for a child recently diagnosed with autism spectrum disorder. In this hypothetical example, the child's parents may view intervention as thwarting a potential positive future through accommodation to a "negative past," whereas the clinician may see early intervention as increasing the likelihood of a positive future. (Conversely, perhaps the parents advocate for early intervention due to their hope for a positive future, whereas they may be met with a provider's preference to take a "wait-and-see approach" informed by previous cases.) A clinical ethicist tuned in to the role of psychological meaning-making around complex change may be more apt to provide effective emotional validation and offer narrative reframing that may facilitate stakeholders in finding common ground. Here again we emphasize that the role of the clinical ethicist is not to push one party toward specific outcomes, but rather to help those they are consulting with make more ethical decisions by removing barriers to ethical thinking and behavior.

Further, a clinical ethicist might find it useful to understand how narrative meaning-making is tightly linked to personal identity. Imagine, for instance, that when a patient is facing a life-altering, chronic illness and is struggling with tough treatment decisions, a clinical ethicist might anticipate that part of what the patient is experiencing might include an initial resistance to their altered self. A conversation with the explicit aim of helping the patient weigh their treatment options might be most useful if it did not simply engage the patient in discussing their values and preferences, but also made room for discussing the patient's reactions to their changed circumstances and perceptions of self. This would mean getting to know the patient and something of their story. This might mean hearing their reactions not as denial—too often an implicit value judgment—but perhaps as puzzlement and anxiety about who the new self can be. This might also mean eliciting stories in which the patient describes instances of their resilient self, building the narrative scaffolding for identifying treatment decisions aligned with their core values and acting in accordance with the resilient, enduring features of their personal identity.

Interpersonal Psychological Processes

A consultant's consideration of their own thoughts and feelings about the change at hand and its subsequent implications for selfhood may stimulate both their empathy and a greater ability to view their personal responses through a neutral, rather than preferential, lens. Such an awareness guards against what has sometimes been referred to as "the psychologist's fallacy" (James 1983/1890), or the tendency to assume that others share the same point of view as themselves. In contemporary psychological research, the cultivation of nonjudgmental analysis to reduce such bias is referred to as "reflexivity," referring to the process of maintaining awareness that the researcher's (or in this case, the bioethicist's) own humanity is part and parcel of the analytic (consultative) process. Simply put, such considerations relate to recognizing the role of the bioethicist as a person involved in an inherently interpersonal process, rather than an objective tool somehow sitting outside of the human process.

We also note that individual patients' adjustments and choices they may face in response to change might or might not entail a morally charged balancing of personal interests. Individual patients who face illness or other life-changing events might need to take only their own preferences into account, but they might also need to consider the needs and preferences of significant others in their lives. For example, if an ethics consultant is to be cognizant of psychological recommendations to cope with change through building resilience through activities such as building relationships, joining groups, setting goals, finding a new sense of purpose, and so on, the consultant might encourage a patient to invite significant others to the conversation in an effort to understand the feasibility of decisions, reduce distress, and support ethical decision-making. The consultant might also encourage a patient to communicate and engage in dialogue with others in the patient's close social circle both prior to and following decision-making to broaden perspectives and enhance critical thinking.

In summary, the overall suggestion proposed in this section is not that ethics consultants should provide the kind of advice or intervention that a person with psychological expertise would provide, but rather that the advice that an ethics consultant offers should be compatible with advice informed by psychological science and its foundations. And at times, ethics consultants might consider inviting a professional with psychological expertise, just as other types of experts are often invited to engage in the care of a patient facing a complicated situation.

We suggest that clinical ethicists would do well to maintain awareness of the nuance inherent in individuals' responses to change, including their own. Reactions are likely to be complex, dynamic, and informed by individual meaning-making processes as well as interpersonal processes. Responses to change are also themselves subject to change. Such awareness of the psychological nature of change and psychologically supportive responses to change may enable ethicists to select appropriate and realistic goals and provide more effective consultation.

Organizational and Corporate Behavior and Policies in the Face of Change

Shifting to the experience of change in organizations, we begin by attending to the extent to which organizational experts have theorized and studied organizational change. Several theories about resistance to change have been prominent. First, a theory about cognitive dissonance emphasizes that people try to be consistent in their attitudes and behavior (Festinger 1957). When they encounter inconsistency between attitudes or between attitudes and behavior, they become uncomfortable and attempt to reduce distress by realigning the inconsistencies. If an organization pursues a change that is inconsistent with the attitudes of organizational members, it will encounter resistance.

A second theoretical approach to change management (Burnes 2015) relates to the magnitude of the psychological impact of change on individuals. The greater the anticipated psychological impact, the greater the need for affected parties to be actively involved in the change process for the change to be successful. Guest and colleagues (2010) contribute the idea of a social contract, which implies that there are unwritten expectations that individuals have about reciprocal roles that individuals and the organization are responsible for fulfilling. Finally, Oreg (2003) observes that individuals vary in the extent to which they are psychologically disposed to resist change.

What may be of particular interest to ethics consultants about the literature on business ethics and organizational change is the debate in that literature about the best approach to achieving ethically sound practice. Bernard Burnes, professor of Organizational Change and head of the Organizational Psychology Group at the Manchester Business School at the University of Manchester, writes:

> Since the early 1980s, the management of change has become focused on approaches that emphasize the deployment of power and politics in order to win compliance (Hendry 1996; Collins 1998). Instead of attempting to change behavior by imposition and coercion, what is required is an approach to change which promotes ethical behavior and allows those concerned to change of their

> own free will. . . . This will mean . . . returning to the ethically based approach of Kurt Lewin. (Burnes 2009, 361)

Kurt Lewin, one of the most influential social scientists of the twentieth century, believed that the improvement of human welfare required the resolution of social conflict. Social conflict, in turn, required the facilitation of learning that helped individuals to understand and restructure the world around as well as to learn about themselves to prepare for voluntarily changing their behavior. His views were based in part on his research on the influence of autocratic and democratic atmospheres on children (Lewin, 1939; Lippett and White 1960). Children operating under a democratic atmosphere where they could make their own decisions were more productive, quarreled less, and were friendlier than those in an autocratic atmosphere. He extended this research to studies of adults in the industrial setting and found that change occurred more successfully in environments that empower employees to act, create openness in communications, facilitate ownership of the change process and its outcomes, facilitate a culture of collaboration; and encourage continuous learning (Burnes 2009).

Burnes (2023) builds on these ideas, proposing that organizations ask some key questions to create conditions for successful management:

1. Why do we want to change?
2. Should we focus on individual, group, or system change?
3. Will there be resistance, and if so, from where?
4. Are we ready for change?
5. Who will manage the change process?
6. What are the frequency and magnitude of the changes required in order for us to survive?

While much of the attention to organizational change has been in the business ethics literature, organizational ethics has generated parallel interest in health care ethics (Spencer et al. 2000), with a focus on promoting a healthy organizational culture—an environment where employees feel empowered to speak up when they have ethical concerns.

Empowerment to speak up brings the necessity to attend to speech, whether expressions of ethical concern related to change, resistance to change, and even enthusiastic adoption of change. Weinfurt (2013) points out the human tendency to understand individual utterances from a solely descriptive perspective—that is, interpreting utterances at the level of their direct lexical meaning. It may be beneficial to also consider the meaning of utterances in context—that is, exploring the idiosyncratic function of the utterance, which may vary according to the individual's mental state or functional goals. Consulting at the organizational level may involve engaging with organizational communication and dialogues at multiple levels of interpretation.

Consider the application of the insights in this section to the case of an influx of new refugees or immigrants to a healthcare setting. For example, staff and providers' implicit and explicit biases or beliefs about fair resource allocation or political and moral responsibility may give rise to interprofessional conflicts or resistance to new organizational demands. In such a case, synthesizing the above theories suggests that individuals will vary in their level of resistance to serving these new patients, that this behavior may be unpredictable, that "speaking up" (or falling in line) may serve functions not immediately apparent, and constructive, empowering involvement of individuals in the process of adaptation can make the process more successful. In particular, a clinical ethics consultant might work with such a healthcare organization to help elicit providers' attitudes and values and dissonance (e.g., appeal to shared values of beneficence) rather than focusing on the factors that may increase resistance due to cognitive dissonance or individual dispositions.

Responding to Global Change

Consideration of change and how people respond to it would be incomplete without reflection on more widespread change—change occurring at a national or even global level. As several authors in this book point out, climate change is a case in point. Of relevance to the discussion in this chapter is the gap between what is required to respond to climate change and the response that is occurring. The UN panel report of 2023 describes the extent of climate change and what is required to address it (IPCC 2023). Numerous, complicated factors are involved in mitigating and adapting to climate change and barriers to adaptation are complex, including "limited resources, lack of private sector and citizen engagement, insufficient mobilization of finance (including for research), low climate literacy, lack of political commitment, limited research and/or slow and low uptake of adaptation science, and low sense of urgency" (IPCC 2023, 62).

Climate change poses overwhelming difficulties that defy adequate description, and the response to it must be multifaceted—it exemplifies drastic change that leaves no one untouched. It occupies everyone, ranging from international organizations to individuals and from those who welcome a leadership role to those who lag in their acknowledgment and act reluctantly. If we glean from what is known about responses to change, as alluded to above, we might extrapolate that the reactions to change on the part of individuals and organizations depend on their roles, their dispositions, and what is at stake for them—what's to be gained or lost from either accepting or rejecting the need to respond and adapt. What might be gained if bioethicists bear in mind the evidence about the human response to change as they consider the ethical concerns raised by climate change? The contribution of bioethics scholars to addressing the challenge of climate change has predominantly been to provide ethical analysis. Yet there is an urgent need to translate ethical analysis into action, and bioethicists could more effectively serve their important role when informed about the attitudes and behaviors engendered by climate change.

Given the need to translate ethical analysis into motivated action, as suggested earlier, consider the American Psychological Association's recommendations about the ways in which psychological science can contribute to addressing climate change (American Psychological Association n.d.). They point out that Americans tend to imagine climate change as distant and uncertain (Ballew et al. 2019) to avoid dealing with impending change and maintain privileged ways of living (Feygina, Jost, and Goldsmith 2010). Therefore, when climate change leads to major, unavoidable instability such as forced migration, in-group ideological thinking and radicalism tend to be activated and lead to violence and unrest. Drawing on this knowledge, practitioners are urged to leverage this same "need to belong in order to create a shared vision for action and a set of social norms that guide behavior" (American Psychological Association n.d.; see also Fielding and Hornsey 2016; Santos and Feygina 2017). Bioethicists can use this knowledge of how individuals and groups tend to react to disruptive change, whether they are working on problems such as resource distribution within a strained healthcare system or the use of limited natural resources for producing medical tests and devices.

The Role of Bioethicists When Change Is Afoot

Bioethics as a whole will play an unduly peripheral and less significant role than it could otherwise if it does not consider how to engage with others in addressing ethically charged issues (Danis 2022). Bioethicists' traditional approaches, which emphasize an analytical role regarding values and goals, are important, but bioethicists must also include stakeholders in deliberations and consider how to translate urgent goals such as the mitigation of climate change into policy and practice.

How might the insights gained from understanding the way individuals, organizations, and huge global entities respond to change be incorporated into the work of bioethics scholars and clinical ethicists? There is a long history of debate about the role of emotions in ethical analysis. Canadian philosopher Paul Thagard has written (2010, paragraphs 3–5):

> Ethical judgments are often highly emotional, when people express their strong approval or disapproval of various acts. Whether they are also rational depends on whether the cognitive appraisal that is part of emotion is done well or badly. Emotional judgments can be flawed by many factors, such as ignorance about the actual consequences of actions and neglect of relevant goals, such as taking into account the needs and interests of all people affected. Adam Smith is sometimes taken as preaching a gospel of self-interest, but his work on moral sentiments emphasized the need for ethics to be based on sympathy for other people. Hence the emotions involved in ethical thinking can be rational when they are based on careful consideration of a full range of appropriate goals, including altruistic ones. Ideally, this consideration should mesh with a visceral reaction that provides a

> motivation to act well and correct injustices. Being good requires both thinking and feeling.

Thagard offers a solidly plausible foundation for finding our way. Bioethics scholars and ethics consultants are well advised to acknowledge the emotions of those who are facing profound change and to help them reason about the best solution, including understanding reasoning about the meaning made of the emotions as well as the ethical implications of behaviors associated with the emotions. In so doing, the ethics consultant will be acting on the basis of sound scientific understanding to help others reach well-considered and fair resolutions of their ethical concerns. For example, acceptance of, accommodation to, and even pursuit of certain changes may be possible but may take significant time. Individuals and organizations—constituted of individuals—may need to process grief and other difficult emotions in order to reach eventual positive or ethical outcomes.

We have argued here that bioethicists will be more successful in contributing to the resolution of ethical concerns that arise from changing circumstances if they are attentive to the human response to change. The work of ethics consultants involves addressing value-laden concerns through "ethics facilitation," a process of respectfully helping others to confront and make decisions through conversation, careful listening, and inclusive deliberation. For their part, bioethics scholars who go beyond theoretical analysis to make policy recommendations should take into account how humans respond to change in order to make their recommendations feasible. The most successful bioethicists will combine this psychological understanding with their ability to engage with others in thoughtful consideration of change: How is the situation affecting relevant parties? Is the impending change inevitable or modifiable? In the face of change, should previously established goals be maintained or not? Should means of achieving goals be revised or not? Will the way we adapt to change be fair to all who are affected? When drastic change is afoot, bioethicists who are prepared to facilitate ethical deliberation can be useful partners in considering how to respond.

Bibliography

American Psychological Association. n.d. "Psychological Contributions to Addressing the Climate Crisis." https://www.apa.org/international/resources/psychological-contributions-climate-change-crisis.pdf.

ASBH. 2011. *Core Competencies for Healthcare Ethics Consultation*, 2nd ed. American Society for Bioethics and Humanities.

Ballew, M. T., A. Leiserowitz, C. Roser-Renouf, et al. 2019. "Climate Change in the American Mind: Data, Tools, and Trends." *Environment: Science and Policy for Sustainable Development*, 61 (3): 4–18.

Brick, N. E., B. L. Fitzpatrick, R. Turkington, and J. C. Mallett. 2019. "Anticipated Task Difficulty Provokes Pace Conservation and Slower Running Performance." *Medicine & Science in Sports and Exercise*, 51 (4): 734–43.

Burnes, B. 2009. "Reflections: Ethics and Organizational Change – Time For a Return to Lewinian Values." *Journal of Change Management*, 9 (4): 359–81.
Burnes, B. 2015. "Understanding Resistance to Change – Building a Coch and French." *Journal of Change Management*, 15 (2): 92–116.
Burzynski, M., C. Deuster, F. Docquier, and J. de Melo. 2022. "Climate Change, Inequality, and Human Migration." *Journal of the European Economic Association*, 20 (3): 1145–97.
By, R. T., B. Burnes, and M. Hughes. 2023. *Organizational Change, Leadership and Ethics*, 2nd ed. Routledge, Taylor and Francis.
Costa, P. T., R. R. McCrae, and A. B. Zonderman.1987. "Environmental and Dispositional Influences on Well-being: Longitudinal Follow-up of an American National Sample." *British Journal of Psychology*, 78 (3): 299–306.
Danis, M. 2022. "A Translational Role for Bioethics: Looking Back and Moving Forward." *Perspectives in Biology and Medicine*, 65 (4): 596–603.
deRoon-Cassini, T. A., E. de St. Aubin, A. Valvano, et al. 2009. "Psychological Well-being After Spinal Cord Injury: Perception of Loss and Meaning Making." *Rehabilitation Psychology*, 54 (3): 306–14.
Epictetus. 1994. *The Art of Living: The Classic Manual on Virtue, Happiness and Effectiveness*. A New Interpretation by Sharon Lebell. Harper San Francisco.
Frankl, V. 1946. *Man's Search for Meaning*. Beacon Press.
Festinger, L. 1957. *The Theory of Cognitive Dissonance*. Stanford University Press.
Feygina, Irina, John T. Jost, and Rachel E. Goldsmith. 2010. "System Justification, the Denial of Global Warming, and the Possibility of 'System-Sanctioned Change.'" *Personality and Social Psychology Bulletin*, 36 (3): 326–38.
Fielding, Kelly S., and Matthew J. Hornsey. 2016. "A Social Identity Analysis of Climate Change and Environmental Attitudes and Behaviors: Insights and Opportunities." *Frontiers in Psychology*, 7 (121): 1–12.
Fredrickson, B. L., Michele M. Tugade, Christian E. Waugh, and Gregory R. Larkin 2003. "What Good are Positive Emotions in Crises? A Prospective Study of Resilience and Emotions Following the Terrorist Attacks on the United States on September 11th, 2001." *Journal of Personality and Social Psychology*, 84 (2): 365–76.
Gardiner, S. M., and L. Hartzell-Nichols. 2012. "Ethics and Global Climate Change." *Nature Education Knowledge*, 3 (10): 5.
Guest, D. E., K. Isaksson, and H. De Witte, eds. 2010. *Employment Contracts, Psychological Contracts, and Employee Well-Being: An International Study*. Oxford University Press.
Goodall, A. 2024. "Mass Tech Layoffs? Just Another Day in the Corporate Blender." *New York Times*, March 21, 2024.
Hayes, S. C., K. D. Strosahl, and K. G. Wilson. 2002. *Acceptance and Commitment Therapy: The Process and Practice of Mindful Change*, 2nd ed. The Guilford Press.
Hendry, Chris. 1996. "Understanding and Creating Whole Organizational Change Through Learning Theory." *Human Relations* 49 (5).
IPCC. 2023. "Summary for Policymakers." In *Climate Change 2023: Synthesis Report. Contribution of Working Groups I, II and III to the Sixth Assessment Report of the Intergovernmental Panel on Climate Change* [Core Writing Team, H. Lee and J. Romero (eds.)]. IPCC, Geneva, Switzerland.
James, W. 1983 [1890]. *The Principles of Psychology*. Harvard University Press.
Jamieson, D. 1996. "Ethics and Intentional Climate Change." *Climatic Change*, 33: 323–36.
Jamieson, D., ed. 2003. *A Companion to Environmental Philosophy*. Blackwell Publishing.

Jensen, R. A. A., D. K. Thomsen, V. F. Bliksted, and N. Ladegaard. 2020. "Narrative Identity in Psychopathology: A Negative Past and a Bright but Foreshortened Future." *Psychiatry Research*, 290: 113103.
King, L. A., C. K. Scollon, C. Ramsey, and T. Williams. 2000. "Stories of Life Transition: Subjective Well-Being and Ego Development in Parents of Children with Down Syndrome." *Journal of Personality in Research*, 34 (4): 509–36.
Lewin, K., R. Lippitt, and R. White. 1939. "Patterns of Aggressive Behavior in Experimentally Created 'Social Climates.'" *Journal of Social Psychology*, 10: 271–99.
Linehan, M. M. 1993. *Cognitive-Behavioral Treatment of Borderline Personality Disorder.* Guilford Press.
Lippitt, R., and R. White. 1960. *Autocracy and Democracy: An Experimental Inquiry.* Harper and Row.
Lucas, R. E. 2007. "Adaptation and the Set-Point Model of Subjective Well-Being: Does Happiness Change After Major Life Events?" *Current Directions in Psychological Science*, 16 (2): 75–9.
Macedo, J. C. 2023. "Climate Change: A Bioethical Emergency and Health Priority." *Ethics, Medicine and Public Health*, 27: 100872.
Mason, A. E., J. M. Adler, E. Puterman, et al. 2019. "Stress Resilience: Narrative Identity May Buffer the Longitudinal Effects of Chronic Caregiving Stress on Mental Health and Telomere Shortening." *Brain, Behavior, and Immunity*, 77: 101–9.
Nolt, J. 2011. "How Harmful Are the Average American's Greenhouse Gas Emissions?" *Ethics, Policy & Environment*, 14: 3–10.
Oreg, S. 2003. "Resistance to Change: Developing an Individual Difference Measure." *Journal of Applied Psychology*, 88 (4): 680–93.
Palmer, C. 2011. "Does Nature Matter? The Place of the Nonhuman in the Ethics of Climate Change." In D. G. Arnold (ed.), *The Ethics of Global Climate Change.* Cambridge University Press.
Palmiter, D., M. Alvord, R. Dorlen, et al. 2023. "Building Your Resilience." *American Psychological Association.* Available at: www.apa.org/topics/resilience/building-your-resilience (accessed November 27, 2023).
Santos, Jessica, and Irina Feygina. 2017. "Responding to Climate Change Skepticism and the Ideological Divide." *Michigan Journal of Sustainability*, 5 (1): 5–23.
Spencer, E. M., A. E. Mills, M. V. Rorty, and P. H. Werhane. 2000. *Organization Ethics in Health Care.* Oxford University Press.
Sterling, P., and J. Eyer. 1988. "Allostasis: A New Paradigm to Explain Arousal Pathology." In S. Fisher and J. Reason (ed.), *Handbook of Life Stress, Cognition and Health.* John Wiley & Sons.
Stulberg, B. 2023. *Master of Change: How to Excel When Everything is Changing--Including You,* 1st ed., HarperOne.
Thagard, P. 2010. "Ethical Thinking Should be Rational AND Emotional: Morality Requires Both Thinking and Feeling." *Psychology Today*, June 18, 2010. Available at https://www.psychologytoday.com/us/blog/hot-thought/201006/ethical-thinking-should-be-rational-and-emtional.
UNESCO. 2024. "The Ethical Principles of Climate Change." January 18, 2024. Available at https://www.unesco.org/en/articles/ethical-principles-climate-change-0.
Weinfurt, K. 2013. "Understanding What Participants in Empirical Bioethical Studies Mean: Historical Cautions From William James and Ludwig Wittgenstein." *AJOB Primary Research*, 4 (3): 49–54.

14

Probing the Social Determinants of Health

Where Bioethics Is Heading

Gail E. Henderson

Since the beginning of the Covid-19 pandemic in 2020, we have been deluged with reports of its disproportionate impact on people by age, gender, race/ethnicity, underlying health conditions, geographic location, and access to health care. The United States Centers for Disease Control and Prevention (CDC) tracked Covid-19 cases, hospitalization, and death rates by race/ethnicity and gender, controlling for age, reporting significant differences. At first, explanations were linked to different comorbidities, or serious immune system deficits, or individuals who wouldn't be expected to do well when confronted with a severe respiratory infection. Yet for decades, CDC reports have typically revealed unequal morbidity and mortality statistics for the distribution of all major health problems in the United States by race/ethnicity, and studies have shown that these distributions often persist after "controlling" for known medical risk factors.

Social Factors in Health and Health Care

Echoing calls by bioethicists (Ray 2023) and health equity researchers (NASEM 2024) for rethinking what is needed to address disparities in health and health care, this chapter focuses on neglected, underlying themes that should be considered before we, as a society, are able to move forward with a deeper appreciation of the social and ethical roots of those disparities. Although focusing specifically on the essential background context for understanding health inequality in the United States, this analysis lends itself to adaptability to be applied elsewhere and to creating an agenda for change. It is grounded in the understanding that disparities reflect unjust conditions—better described as inequities in health outcomes. This essay is primarily based in the field of social epidemiology, defined as "investigations of social etiology of disease, systematically examining variations in the incidence of particular diseases among people differentially located in the social structure and attempts to explore the ways in which their position in the social structure tends to make them more vulnerable, or less, to a particular disease" (Berkman and Kawachi 2014). This reflects almost two centuries of observations about social conditions and health and changing historical and methodological approaches to social epidemiology. It also reflects very recent changes in the political landscape defining health inequities as well as efforts to understand the meaning of race terms employed in such work. Each resounds with ethical implications.

There is much about our current era that recalls the history of social medicine, long before the advent of the germ theory drew us away from focus on the social causes of disease. In the mid-1800s, social and political activists like Rudolf Virchow (the father of modern cellular pathology and of the field of social medicine), and Friedrich Engels (political theorist and revolutionary socialist), published data demonstrating that poverty, poor sanitation, and working conditions were related to greater illness and death. Investigating the 1847–8 typhus epidemic in Upper Silesia, Prussia, Virchow famously wrote, "Medical statistics will be our standard of measurement: we will weigh life for life and see where the dead lie thicker, among the workers or among the privileged" (Taylor and Rieger 1985). Numerous public health researchers of the time confirmed observations of the social causes of disease (e.g., Chadwick 1965). Despite these important descriptive and normative investigations, by the late nineteenth century, with the advent of the germ theory of disease, medicine turned away from addressing poverty and social ills to promote better health and toward growing faith in a single, necessary cause of infectious diseases, namely microbes. This dominant view prevailed, and by the mid-twentieth century, medicine's successes in diagnosis and treatment eclipsed scholarly and public attention to social causes of disease and strengthened focus on the individual in identifying the causes of and cures for ill health.

At the same time, advances in the methods of statistics and epidemiology made it possible to support causal claims that relied on knowledge of specific infectious or other agents. This was a major analytic transition. One of its best-known examples was in the mid-twentieth century, when Richard Doll and Bradford Hill's case-control study of smoking and lung cancer demonstrated a relationship, though without identifying a causal agent (Doll and Hill 1950). As Nancy Krieger (1994) described, this "spiderless" web of causation, otherwise known as "black box epidemiology," became the dominant approach. Researchers identified criteria that supported a relationship between a presumed cause (e.g., smoking) and an observed effect (e.g., lung cancer) and developed criteria that bolstered inference of cause and effect. By the 1970s, multivariate analysis employed newly available computational capability and the language of "risk factors." At the same time, while such techniques in epidemiology proliferated, researchers also began to look into the root causes of behaviors such as cigarette smoking. This meant exploring the science of individual nicotine addiction versus focusing on the social context of a host of unhealthy practices of which smoking was only one.

These trends set the stage for what has been called the "epidemiology wars," pitting attention to individual-level factors against societal-level causes and consequent preventive interventions (Poole and Rothman 1998). Methodological advances focused on developing multilevel (community, neighborhood, individual) and multi-method (quantitative and qualitative data) approaches. Those factors closest to the diseased or "at risk" individual were labeled proximate. Social factors such as education level or neighborhood characteristics, measured at neighborhood or community levels, were more distant or distal, and perhaps less amenable to change. At the same time, social scientists focused on demonstrating that social class is a "fundamental cause," meaning it influences multiple disease outcomes through multiple risk factors and access to resources. While specific measurements might differ across time and cultural contexts, these associations with health are reproduced no matter what the intervening or proximate variables, and no matter what the disease outcome, because they are embedded in the structure of society (Phelan, Link, and Tehranifar 2010).

The work of infectious disease researcher and visionary health justice advocate, Dr. Adaora (Ada) Adimora,[1] illustrates the epidemiology wars and the ways that mixed methods and multilevel models can be applied to understanding biological, behavioral, and demographic risk factors predicting disease, in her case, HIV incidence in the US South. In 2001, Adimora and her team began to explore contextual factors that might explain high rates of HIV and sexually transmitted infections. Results from focus groups with Black participants in rural North Carolina counties found "pervasive economic and racial oppression, lack of community recreation, boredom, and resultant substance abuse; many perceived a shortage of Black men because of their higher mortality and incarceration rates compared with whites, and believed this male shortage to be partly responsible for the concurrent sexual partnerships that they perceived as widespread among unmarried persons" (Adimora et al. 2001, 69). In a subsequent commentary, Adimora and epidemiologist colleague Victor Schoenbach asserted, "[g]iven the importance of contextual factors and the sharply contrasting social contexts for Blacks and Whites, *exclusive emphasis on individual risk factors and determinants is unlikely to produce solutions that will significantly decrease HIV rates among Blacks*" (Adimora and Schoenbach 2005, S115). In 2006, Adimora and colleagues conducted a case-control study of Black men and women, aged 18–61 years, with recent HIV diagnosis and age- and gender-matched controls in North Carolina. Although factors predicting HIV were high risk sexual and drug use behaviors, 27 percent of case subjects (and 69 percent of control subjects) did not exhibit such risk factors. This result was corroborated by a national study that found that while white young adults in the United States who engage in high-risk behaviors have increased risk of sexually transmitted disease and HIV, "Black young adults are at high risk even when their behaviors are normative" (Hallfors et al. 2007, 125).

Adimora's team then embarked on a multilevel analysis of sex ratio, poverty, and concurrent partnerships among men and women in the United States (Adimora et al. 2013). They found that counties with low sex ratios (i.e., more women than men), more poverty, and higher crime rates had greater concurrency. Perhaps most surprising, the great majority of whites and Hispanics, but only 7.85 percent of Blacks lived in balanced sex ratio counties. They concluded that such striking findings likely explain the profound Black-white differences in HIV infection. To isolate factors specific to the South, the team undertook a case-control study comparing neighborhood and state contexts for women living with and without HIV (Ludema et al. 2018). They identified a number of contextual differences, including eligibility for Medicaid, other income-related factors, access to HIV care, and incarceration rates. Southern neighborhoods all ranked lower on these factors than non-Southern locations. Building on the puzzle of individual-level risk for HIV, the team concluded that in order to address racial and geographic HIV disparities, structural barriers must be addressed. In 2020, Adimora gave a named Lectureship to the Infectious Diseases Society of America, titled "All Policy is Health Policy," in which she contextualized HIV among people of color with data on incarceration, voter suppression, and social justice; and that same year, with daughter Bria Godley and colleague Schoenbach, Adimora published, "Racial Justice and HIV in the United States: Now is the Time."

Race

Like social class, race has figured prominently in health outcomes research for decades, but unlike social class, race and ethnicity classifications are routinely collected by the US Census and the CDC for birth and death records, as well as accounts of hospitalization or disease outbreaks. Given the lack of representation in health research data, in 1990, NIH began to require grant awardees to demonstrate fair recruitment of individuals by race/ethnicity. Thus, these categories are embedded in administrative, health, and research data in the United States, underscoring the belief that race and ethnicity are biological.

There is, however, general agreement that race is a social—not biological—construct, a category created to support colonial subjugation of people of color. As historian Dorothy Roberts stated simply, "[r]ace was invented to support racism" (Roberts 2022; see also her 2011 book, *Fatal Invention: How Science, Politics, and Big Business Recreate Race in the 21st Century*). Sociologist David Williams and colleagues (Williams et al. 2019), along with many others (e.g., journalist Villarosa 2022; bioethicist Ray 2024, 2023), have argued that much of what "race" is measuring in models predicting health disparities is in fact "racism." They propose three dimensions of systemic racism: structural racism, cultural racism, and individual discrimination. Because racism is deeply embedded in the social structure, with links to mental and physical health outcomes, they argue that much like social class, racism in the United States is a fundamental cause of adverse health outcomes and inequities in health care.

Building on this assertion, in a 2022 special issue of *Health Affairs* devoted to "Racism and Health," health equity researcher Rachel Hardeman and colleagues ask, "[g]iven that structural racism is a system of interconnected institutions that operates with a set of racialized rules that maintain White supremacy, how can anyone accurately measure its insidiousness?" (Hardeman et al. 2022, 179). To advance the goal of incorporating valid measurement into health disparities research, their article identifies "three key areas that require scholarly attention: historical context, geographical context, and theory-based novel quantitative and qualitative methods that capture the multifaceted and systemic properties of structural racism as well as other systems of oppression"

(Hardeman et al. 2022, 179). In 2020, the American Medical Association (AMA) adopted the following policy to "acknowledge that although the primary drivers of racial health inequity are systemic and structural racism, racism and unconscious bias within medical research and health care delivery have caused and continue to cause harm to marginalized communities and society as a whole" (O'Reilly 2020). In 2021, CDC director Rochelle Walensky (2021) made a similar statement, calling racism a serious threat to public health. Both organizations developed health equity strategies to combat racism.

There are many researchers and advocates concerned with how race and ethnicity are understood and used in research. This includes public intellectuals whose mission is to debunk misunderstandings about race and genetics (e.g., Rutherford's highly readable 2021 book *How to Argue with a Racist: What Our Genes Do (and Don't) Say about Human Difference*). It also includes efforts by journals to harmonize reporting of race and ethnicity. For example, the AMA guidance on how to report race/ethnicity in medical journals states unequivocally: "Race and ethnicity are social constructs, without scientific or biological meaning" (Flanagin et al. 2021). In 2023, the National Academies' 200-page report offered a definitive account of the "Use of Race, Ethnicity, and Ancestry as Population Descriptors in Genomics Research" and offers thirteen recommendations, arguing against the use of these population descriptors in most genetic/genomic research. Although its mandate was to focus on genomic research, the committee recognized that their conclusions might well have implications for clinical medicine.

According to Recommendation 1, "the Typological categories, such as the racial and ethnic categories established by the U.S. Office of Management and Budget (OMB), are a poor fit for capturing human biological diversity. The committee cautioned against their use for many analytical purposes in genetics research. Specifically, *researchers should not use race as a proxy for human genetic variation*." Recommendation 6 argues, "researchers should tailor their use of population descriptors to the type and purpose of the study and explain how and why they used those descriptors." For only one ("health disparities research") of the six types of genetic/genomic studies does the report support using race, because it is deployed as a social variable. (The other five are gene discovery, trait prediction, cellular and physiological mechanisms, and human evolutionary history.)

In the eyes of the public, direct-to-consumer genetic analysis companies like 23andMe or AncestryDNA might foster the notion that genetic or continental ancestry is a likely candidate to replace race. The NASEM report considered genetic ancestry, defined as "encompassing a person's origin or descent, lineage, 'roots,' or heritage, including kinship" (NASEM 2024,12) and concluded it was flawed in ways similar to the use of race (instead recommending "genetic similarity" which is a much more complex approach). As a group of multidisciplinary colleagues argued (Lewis et al. 2022, 2), "the use of ancestry categories has technical limitations, fails to adequately capture human genetic diversity and demographic history, and risks retaining one of the most problematic aspects of race—an essentialist link to biology—by allowing genetic ancestry categories to stand in its place." Their abstract consists of one sentence:

"We must embrace a multidimensional, continuous view of ancestry and move away from continental ancestry categories."

Race in Medicine

Another important implication of recent scholarship has been to consider the continued use of race in medical care. As recalled by Vyas and colleagues (2020), in 2003 the *New England Journal of Medicine* hosted two Sounding Board articles on the use of race in medicine, asking authors to address whether it should continue to be used (Burchard et al. 2003) or not (Cooper et al. 2003), followed by a "perspective" from the journal deputy editor (Phimister 2003). While much has transpired since then, the nature of these arguments sounds surprisingly similar to current scholarship. Burchard and colleagues argued that there are considerable data that demonstrate the utility of race for understanding causality and effective treatments in medicine, while Cooper and colleagues argued that "[genetic] variation is continuous and discordant with race, systematic variation according to continent is very limited, and there is no evidence that the units of interest for medical genetics correspond to what we call races" (Cooper et al. 2003, 1167). Phimister concluded her essay with cautious equivocation:

> The goal of personalized medicine is the prediction of risk and the treatment of disease on the basis of a person's genetic profile—which would render biologic consideration of race obsolete. But it seems unwise to abandon the practice of recording race when we have barely begun to understand the architecture of the human genome and its implications for new strategies for the identification of gene variants that protect against, or confer susceptibility to, common diseases and modify the effects of drugs. (Phimister 2003, 1082)

Since the 2003 debate, medical researchers and clinicians (and NIH, CDC, and OMB) have continued to collect patient and research participant data by race and ethnicity—despite recommendations to the contrary. Thus, an important area of controversy continues to be the meaning of race in clinical medicine, emerging in debates regarding diagnostic algorithms and the advent of artificial intelligence and machine learning.

Bias in Algorithms

Bias in medical algorithm use is a popular concern. As Tipton and colleagues (2023) explain, race and ethnicity are often used as input variables in algorithms used to guide clinical decision-making and resource allocation and healthcare management. They observe, however, that "because race and ethnicity are socially constructed and thereby poor proxies for biological markers or genetic predisposition, when used in algorithms to guide clinical care their inclusion may introduce or exacerbate inappropriate, unequal treatment (healthcare disparities) and thereby contribute to or exacerbate unequal health outcomes (health disparities)" (Tipton et al. 2023, ES-2). In a seminal review, Vyas and colleagues described algorithms in cardiology, nephrology, obstetrics, and urology, featuring those that demonstrated bias against non-white patients. They concluded that "when clinicians insert race into their tools, they risk interpreting racial disparities as immutable facts rather than as injustices that require intervention" (Vyas 2020, 880).

To address the algorithm bias question across a much wider range of medical conditions and algorithms, and using a more robust methodology, Tipton and colleagues (2023) conducted a systematic review for the Agency for Healthcare Research and Quality, "Impact of Healthcare Algorithms on Racial and Ethnic Disparities in Health and Healthcare." They selected studies from 2011 to 2023. Out of 11,500 citations, 58 studies qualified for analysis, including those with algorithms that incorporated race and ethnicity and those that did not. Their results were complex, defying stereotypical conclusions that might be drawn from single case studies.

They observed that "[a]lgorithms have been shown to potentially perpetuate, exacerbate, and sometimes reduce racial and ethnic disparities." Specifically, "disparities were reduced when race and ethnicity were incorporated into an algorithm to intentionally tackle known racial and ethnic disparities in resource allocation (e.g., kidney transplant allocation) or disparities in care (e.g., prostate cancer screening that historically led to Black men receiving more low-yield biopsies)." Importantly,

> [i]n such cases the rationale for using race and ethnicity was clearly delineated and did not conflate race and ethnicity with ancestry and/or genetic predisposition. . . . However, when algorithms include race and ethnicity without clear rationale, they may perpetuate the incorrect notion that race is a biologic construct and contribute to disparities. Finally, some algorithms may reduce or perpetuate disparities without containing race and ethnicity as an input. (Tipton et al. 2023, ES-10)

Complexities in Measurement

Measurement within systems of structured inequalities faces other complex and challenging problems in how social variables are used. The concept of intersectionality is a key example. It was introduced in 1989 by feminist legal theorist Kimberlé Crenshaw, who famously argued that the combined identities of being female and Black were greater than the sum of racism and sexism. The concept of intersectionality "provides a framework for understanding the experiences of populations situated within multiple systems of oppression, particularly in relation to anti-discrimination law and gender-based violence" and which reveals "interlocking, cumulative effects of different social structures on health" (Fehrenbacher and Patel 2020, 145–6).

Although this theory is appealing in health disparities research, there are significant methodological challenges to incorporating intersectionality theory into quantitative population health research, improving its capacity to reflect the complex realities of how social context, behaviors, and life processes are biologically embodied (Bauer 2014, 17). In a recent advance, Homan and colleagues (2021) describe an empirical application of "structural intersectionality" in health disparities research, using state-level administrative data linked to individual data from the Behavioral Risk Factor Surveillance System to estimate multilevel models of how intersecting dimensions of structural oppression shape health.

As scholars take on these challenges, they focus on how the individual and social affect and are affected by each other, and how power is implicated in unequal systems. In 1999, A. J. McMichael wrote persuasively about epidemiology's preoccupation with individual-level risk factors (vs. population-level influences) in models that predict health outcomes, in an article memorably titled, "Prisoners of the proximate: Loosening the constraints on epidemiology in an age of social change." Similarly, social theorist and epidemiologist, Nancy Krieger, criticized the foundational use of "distal" and "proximate" in her 2008 article "Proximal, Distal, and the Politics of Causation: What's Level Got to Do with It?" She offers two key arguments: First, proximal/distal is a misleading distinction since social factors are thoroughly conjoined with biological ones, writing, "societal patterns of disease represent the biological consequences of the ways of living and working differentially afforded to different social groups." Second, "understanding of the societal distributions of health cannot be divorced from considerations of political economy and political ecology. . . . Driving health inequities are how power . . . structures people's engagement with the world and their exposures to material and psychosocial health hazards" (Krieger 2008, 223–4).

These also build on the influential work of Geoffrey Rose (1985), who proposed that the causes of disease incidence (occurrence in populations) are different from the causes of disease cases (in individuals). Invoking a Durkheimian perspective (Schwartz and Diez Roux 2001), he wrote that "although populations are comprised of individuals, the population has characteristics that are distinct from the mere summation of the characteristics of the individuals in the population" (2001, 436).

A key implication of Rose's work is that social facts cannot merely be translated into individual-level factors, with the assumption that they are the same. For example, living in a high unemployment area is not the same as an individual being unemployed. At the individual level, those without jobs are "exposed" (potentially to undesirable health outcomes), and those with jobs are "unexposed," but at a societal level, living in a high unemployment area has adverse effects on both groups (Schwartz and Diez Roux 2001, 437).

Throughout the history of social epidemiology, methods have evolved to take better account of these lived realities. Ethical issues are often reflected in this history. For example, if individual traits of risky behavior, poor habits, or failure to adhere to prescribed medicines are found to put people at risk for disease, then the fault is theirs and the solution lies in targeting individuals. If, on the other hand, community-level factors are the key determinants, then social responsibility should be pursued. Thus, the ways that epidemiologists and health researchers took up these evolving sets of knowledge about disease causation had political and philosophical implications.

One might also conclude that the political and philosophical ought to shape the way researchers initially frame the target of their questions about the causes of health and relevant interventions. The trend toward nuance in understanding individual and social, proximate and distal, and how they are interrelated is at odds with traditional methods, but not irreconcilable. The epidemiology wars can be resolved through more sophisticated, thoughtful modeling and measurement, as demonstrated above, by the work of Dr. Adaora Adimora.

Other important implicit or explicit normative issues are raised in studies of health disparities. For example, the selection of comparison or "reference" groups reflects ethical and value judgments (Harper and Lynch 2006, 139). Outcome variables selected to measure health inequalities "may inherently reveal what aspects of health inequality are important to capture" (Harper and Lynch 2006, 135). Similarly, in a 2018 essay on scholarship about Black communities, and habitual comparison with whites as the reference group, sociologist Robyn Autry writes that "sociology's race problem is bigger than the faulty lens that transforms some of us into social others, or social problems. There's a larger issue about the ongoing default status of whiteness as the standard used to define social difference and what is considered solid academic work in the first place" (Autry 2020, 10–11).

In Summary

We conclude in the first chapter of our book on health justice (King, Henderson, and Churchill 2022, 31–2) that the activism of Virchow in 1848 is just as important now, two hundred years after his birth. As social epidemiologist Jay Kaufman observed, "Typhus in Silesia is no different from Covid-19 in the U.S. Both are social diseases, where infection and death are entirely patterned by occupation, social relations, resources and discrimination. Nothing has changed, it's the same story." In a *New York Times* Guest Essay, he wrote, "the same social pathology that exacerbates the pandemic also debilitates our scientific response to it. . . . The real problem is simply that sick societies have sick institutions." This echoes the observations of physician-anthropologist Paul Farmer, treating TB and HIV in Haiti, the poorest country in the western hemisphere, who wrote, "inequality itself constitutes our modern plague" (Farmer 2001). This and the recent "discovery" of inequalities of Covid-19 constitute a wake-up call for everyone concerned with human health.

Initially, this chapter forecasts a discussion of themes that frame health inequality, and that should be understood before we, as a society, are able to move forward. This means that we must work together to understand the root causes of inequality and the nature of the data that generate our knowledge—including its implicit normative framings—before we are able to address those sources of inequality. As we describe in our concluding chapter (King, Henderson, and Churchill 2022, 137–41), "we cannot really understand health justice without appreciating the social determinants of health and reframing health in this way means recognizing that we have been working with an individualized and truncated notion of justice" (King, Henderson, and Churchill 2022, 138).

While the Covid-19 epidemic unveiled profound health inequities, it also revealed the importance of collaboration between bioethics and social epidemiology, beginning with how research questions are framed in the broadest sense and how results are translated into findings about "unequal treatment" (The IOM 2003 book by that name included multilevel attention to patient, provider, and system factors that lead to unequal outcomes; the updated version (NASEM 2024) addresses sources of continuing inequities; see also Burke et al. 2011). These collaborative projects must examine the variables and studies that are used to present results. How are individual and societal level variables presented? Are there biases or measurement questions? Is the structure of society identified and analyzed as a fundamental cause of inequities? Are different dimensions of racism being measured? At the same time, we must consider how to address inequities that are revealed.

Some authors reframe accepted wisdom to offer new insights, as when Dorothy Roberts (2022) states that race was invented to support racism, or taken-for-granted medical algorithms must be examined for harmful race/ethnicity biases that are baked in. Oxford University Press inaugurated a new series on "Bioethics for Social Justice" with Keisha Ray's 2023 book, *Black Health*. For some contentious issues, debate is essential. For example, given controversy over the role of race in medical care and research, what role should "color blindness" play to improve patient treatment and health outcomes? A 2024 TED talk as part of a program called "Open to Debate" featured Jamelle Bouie and Coleman Hughes debating "color blindness" in which: "One argues the term has been used to undermine policies that can address systemic racism, and thus reinforces it. The other argues that taking a colorblind approach by replacing race-based policies with class-based ones could reduce inequality." The answers are far from simple, and as we sort through such important questions, the ethical implications are profound.

Note

1 Dr. Adimora passed away on January 1, 2024, leaving a profound legacy in scholarship, clinical care, and advocacy.

Bibliography

Adimora, A. A., C. Ramirez, V. J. Schoenbach, and M. S. Cohen. 2014. "Politics and Policies that Promote HIV." *AIDS*, 28 (10): 1393–7.

Adimora, V. J., and V. J. Schoenbach. 2005. "Social Context, Sexual Networks, and Racial Disparities in Rates of Sexually Transmitted Infections." *Journal of Infectious Diseases*, 191: S115–22

Adimora, A. A., V. J. Schoenbach, F. E. A. Martinson, T. R. Coyne-Beasley, I. Doherty, T. R. Stancil, and R. E. Fullilove. 2006. "Heterosexually transmitted HIV infection among African Americans in North Carolina." *JAIDS*, 41 (5): 616–23.
Adimora, A. A., V. J. Schoenbach, F. E. A. Martinson, K. H. Donaldson, R. E. Fullilove, and S. O. Aral. 2001. "Social Context of Sexual Relationships among Rural African Americans." *Sexually Transmitted Diseases*, 28 (2): 69–76.
Adimora, A. A., V. J. Schoenbach, E. M. Taylor, M. R. Khan, R. J. Schwartz, and W. C. Miller. 2013. "Sex Ratio, Poverty, and Concurrent Partnerships Among Men and Women in the United States: A Multilevel Analysis." *Annals of Epidemiology*, 23 (11): 716–9.
Autry, Robyn. 2020. "Sociology's Race Problem: Urban Ethnographers Do More Harm than Good in Speaking for Black Communities." *Aeon*, November 26, 2020. https://aeon.co/essays/urban-ethnographers-do-harm-in-speaking-for-black-communities.
Bauer, G. R. 2014. "Incorporating Intersectionality Theory into Population Health Research Methodology: Challenges and the Potential to Advance Health Equity." *Social Science and Medicine*, 110: 10–17.
Berkman, L., and I. Kawachi. 2014. "Historical Framework for Social Epidemiology." In L. Berkman, I. Kawachi, and M. M. Glymour (eds.), *Social Epidemiology*, 2nd ed. Oxford University Press.
Burchard, E. G., E. Ziv, N. Coyle et al. 2003. "The Importance of Race and Ethnic Background in Biomedical Research and Clinical Practice." *New England Journal of Medicine*, 348: 1170–5.
Burke, W., K. A. Edwards, S. Goering, S. Holland, and S. B. Trinidad, eds. 2011. *Achieving Justice in Genomic Translation: Re-Thinking the Pathway to Benefit.* Oxford University Press.
Chadwick, Edwin. 1965. *1842 Report on the Sanitary Conditions of the Labouring Populations of Great Britain.* Edinburgh University Press.
Cooper, R. S., J. S. Kaufman, and R. Ward. 2003. "Race and Genomics." *New England Journal of Medicine*, 348: 1166–70.
Crenshaw, Kimberlé. 1989. "Demarginalizing the Intersection of Race and Sex: A Black Feminist Critique of Antidiscrimination Doctrine, Feminist Theory and Antiracist Politics." *University of Chicago Legal Forum*, 1 (8): 139–68.
Doll R., and A. B. Hill. 1950. "Smoking and Carcinoma of the Lung: Preliminary Report." *British Medical Journal*, 2: 739–48.
Farmer, Paul. 2001. *Infections and Inequalities: The Modern Plagues*. University of California Press.
Fehrenbacher, Anne E., and Dhara Patel. 2020. "Translating the Theory of Intersectionality into Quantitative and Mixed Methods for Empirical Gender Transformative Research on Health." *Culture, Health & Sexuality*, 22 (1 supplement): 145–60.
Flanagin, A., T. Frey, and S. L. Christiansen. 2021. "AMA Manual of Style Committee. Updated Guidance on the Reporting of Race and Ethnicity in Medical and Science Journals." *JAMA*, 326 (7): 621–7.
Godley, B. A., V. J. Schoenbach, and A. A. Adimora. 2020. "Racial Justice and HIV in the United States: Now is the Time." *Journal of the International AIDS Society*, 23: 10.
Giuste, F. O., L. He, P. Lais, W. et al. 2023. "Early and Fair COVID-19 Outcome Risk Assessment Using Robust Feature Selection." *Scientific Reports*, 13 (1): 18981.

Hallfors, D. D., B. J. Iritani, W. C. Miller, and D. J. Bauer. 2007. "Sexual and Drug Behavior Patterns and HIV and STD Racial Disparities: The Need for New Directions." *American Journal of Public Health*, 97 (1): 125–32.

Hao, B., Y. Hu, S. Sotudian, et al. 2022. "Development and Validation of Predictive Models for COVID-19 Outcomes in a Safety-Net Hospital Population." *Journal of the American Medical Informatics Association*, 29 (7): 1253–62.

Hardeman, R. R., P. A. Homan, T. Chantarat, B. A. Davis, and T. H. Brown. 2022. "Improving the Measurement Of Structural Racism To Achieve Antiracist Health Policy." *Health Affairs*, 41 (2): 179–86.

Harper, S. and J. W. Lynch. 2006. "Measuring Health Inequalities." In J. M. Oakes and J. S. Kaufman (eds.), *Methods in Social Epidemiology*. Wiley: Jossey-Bass.

Health Affairs. 2022. "Racism and Health." *Health Affairs*, 41 (2): 157.

Homan, P., T. H. Brown, and B. King. 2021. "Structural Intersectionality as a New Direction for Health Disparities Research." *Journal of Health and Social Behavior*, 62 (3): 350–70.

Institute of Medicine. 2003. *Unequal Treatment: Confronting Racial and Ethnic Disparities in Health Care*. The National Academies Press.

Kaufman, J. 2021. "Opinion: Science Alone Can't Heal a Sick Society." *New York Times*, September 10, 2021.

Kaufman, J. S., and R. S. Cooper. 2008. "Race in Epidemiology: New Tools, Old Problems." *Annals of Epidemiology*, 18 (2): 119–23.

King, N. M. P., G. E. Henderson, and L. R. Churchill. 2022. *Bioethics Reenvisioned: A Path toward Health Justice*. University of North Carolina Press.

Kramer, M. R., N. C. Black, S. A. Matthews, and S. A. James. 2017. "The Legacy of Slavery and Contemporary Declines in Heart Disease Mortality in the U.S. South." *SSM Population Health*, 3: 609–17.

Krieger, N. 1994. "Epidemiology and the Web of Causation: Has Anyone Seen the Spider?" *Social Science & Medicine*, 39 (7): 887–903.

Krieger, N. 2008. "Proximal, Distal, and the Politics of Causation: What's Level Got to Do with It?" *American Journal of Public Health*, 98 (2): 221–30.

Lewis, A. C. F., S. J. Molina, P. S. Appelbaum, et al. 2022. "Getting Genetic Ancestry Right for Science and Society." *Science*, 376: 250–2.

Ludema, C., A. Edmonds, S. R. Cole, et al. 2018. "Comparing Neighborhood and State Contexts for Women Living With and Without HIV: Understanding the Southern HIV Epidemic." *AIDS Care*, 11: 1360–7.

McCoy, D., W. Mgbara, N. Horvitz, W. M. Getz, and A. Hubbard. 2021. "Ensemble Machine Learning of Factors Influencing COVID-19 Across US Counties." *Scientific Reports*, 11 (1): 11777.

McMichael, A. J. 1999. "Prisoners of the Proximate: Loosening the Constraints on Epidemiology in an Age of Change." *American Journal of Epidemiology*, 149 (10): 887–97.

National Academies of Sciences, Engineering, and Medicine (NASEM). 2023. *Using Population Descriptors in Genetics and Genomics Research: A New Framework for an Evolving Field*. The National Academies Press.

National Academies of Sciences, Engineering, and Medicine (NASEM). 2024. *Ending Unequal Treatment: Strategies to Achieve Equitable Health Care and Optimal Health for All*. The National Academies Press.

O'Reilly, Kevin B. 2020. "AMA: Racism is a Threat to Public Health." *American Medical Association*, November 16, 2020. https://www.ama-assn.org/delivering-care/health-equity/ama-racism-threat-public-health.

Phelan, J. C., B. G. Link, and P. Tehranifar. 2010. "Social Conditions as Fundamental Causes of Health Inequalities: Theory, Evidence, and Policy Implications." *Journal of Health and Social Behavior*, 51 (Supplement): S28–40.

Phimister, E. G. 2003. "Medicine and the Racial Divide." *New England Journal of Medicine*, 348: 1081–2.

Popejoy, A. B., and S. M. Fullerton. 2016. "Genomics is Failing on Diversity." *Nature*, 538: 161–4.

Poole, C., and K. J. Rothman. 1998. "Our Conscientious Objection to the Epidemiology Wars." *Journal of Epidemiology and Community Health*, 52 (10): 613.

Ray, Keisha. 2023. *Black Health: The Social, Political, and Cultural Determinants of Black People's Health*. Oxford University Press.

Ray, Keisha. 2024. "Narrating the Black Body in 'Under the Skin.'" *Cambridge Quarterly Healthcare Ethics*, 33 (2): 275–79.

Roberts, Dorothy. 2011. *Fatal Invention: How Science, Politics, and Big Business Re-Create Race in the Twenty-First Century*. The New Press.

Roberts, Dorothy. 2022. "The Past and Future of Race, Health, and Justice." *National Academies of Science, Engineering, and Medicine (NASEM) Webinar on the Use of Race/Ethnicity in Biomedical Research*, December 14, 2022.

Rose, G. 1985. "Sick Individuals and Sick Populations." *International Journal of Epidemiology*, 14: 32–8.

Rutherford, A. 2021. *How to Argue with a Racist: What Our Genes Do (and Don't) Say About Human Difference*. The Experiment.

Schwartz, S., and R. Diez Roux. 2001. "Commentary: Causes of Cases and Causes of Incidence—a Durkheimian Perspective on Rose." *International Journal of Epidemiology*, 30 (3): 435–9.

Taylor, R., and A. Rieger. 1985. "Medicine as Social Science: Rudolf Virchow on the Typhus Epidemic in Upper Silesia." *International Journal of Health Services*, 15 (4): 547–59.

Tipton K., B. F. Leas, E. Flores, et al. 2023. "Impact of Healthcare Algorithms on Racial and Ethnic Disparities in Health and Healthcare." *Comparative Effectiveness Review* No. 268. (Prepared by the ECRI-Penn Medicine Evidence-based Practice Center under Contract No. 75Q80120D00002.) AHRQ Publication No. 24-EHC004. Rockville, MD: Agency for Healthcare Research and Quality.

Villarosa, Linda. 2022. *Under the Skin: The Hidden Toll of Racism on American Lives and on the Health of Our Nation*. Doubleday.

Vyas, D. A., L. G. Eisenstein, and D. S. Jones. 2020. "Hidden in Plain Sight — Reconsidering the Use of Race Correction in Clinical Algorithms." *New England Journal of Medicine*, 383: 874–82.

Walensky, Rochelle P. 2021. "Media Statement from CDC Director Rochelle P. Walensky, MD, MPH, on Racism and Health." *CDC Archive*, April 8, 2021. https://archive.cdc.gov/#/details?url=https://www.cdc.gov/media/releases/2021/s0408-racism-health.html.

Williams, D. R., J. A. Lawrence, and B. A. Davis. 2019. "Racism and Health: Evidence and Needed Research." *Annual Review of Public Health*, 40: 105–25.

Yudell, M., D. Roberts, R. DeSalle, S. Tishkoff., and 70 Signatories. 2020. "NIH Must Confront the Use of Race in Science." *Science*, 369: 1313–14.

15

The Citational Tyranny of Bioethics

Johnathan Flowers

In her text *Living a Feminist Life*, Sara Ahmed describes citation as "bricks" or "the materials through which, from which we create our dwellings" (Ahmed 2017, 16). Here, "dwellings" are the disciplinary spaces where we can take up residence, and citations, as "bricks," function to structure our disciplinary homes, providing essential organization to the academic field through how they not only enable the circulation of expertise but establish the authority of members of a field. Moreover, citations also establish a history of citation practices which are reproduced through instruction in the field. These citational practices, or "habits," allow academics to be identified as members of a field through how they structure their research. Thus, for Ahmed (2013), it is not simply citational practices that are reproduced, but also ways of doing scholarship in an academic field and the borders of the academic field itself. This chapter will apply Sara Ahmed's work to the field of bioethics to demonstrate how Bioethics serves to exclude disabled persons, disabled scholars, and knowledge of the lived experience of disability.

The word "reproduced" is crucial here because citation can be thought of as a form of reproductive technology, working to reproduce a world that takes some bodies, some ways of being, as central (Ahmed 2013). Technology should be understood not just as a physical artifact, but as a technique, method, or more specifically, habitual action as indicated above. As a habit, citation serves to provide the field with its form; as Ahmed (2006) notes, spaces are shaped by the habitual actions of the bodies that inhabit them, and insofar as a technique of citation is also a screening technique, one that selects appropriate bodies for inclusion within a field or a space, a citational politics is also a politics of exclusion. Thus, in the context of Bioethics, it is important to consider not just how citations are used as bricks to structure the field, but also how citations function to include or exclude forms of knowledge and ways of knowing specific to disability from the field. Put another way, we should consider which people and experiences are represented in the bricks upon which Bioethics is built.

Still further, as Ahmed (2019) notes, "[t]o be trained within a discipline is to learn to follow a citational path: certain work does not have to be regarded because it does not come into view if you follow a path, which means work can be discarded without deliberation." By "citational path," Ahmed is indicating the ways that training in an academic field requires following the "path" laid out by scholars which are taken to be foundational to that field. As an example, in philosophy, it is often claimed that "philosophy is a series of footnotes to Aristotle," which presumes an unbroken path from Aristotle and Western philosophy generally to modernity. On this view training in a discipline like philosophy is to inherit the path laid out by such citation. As fields which emerge as products of citation, which are also practices of selection, learning to work in an academic field is to inherit the mechanisms of selection within that field through one's training.

For Ahmed, this inheritance shapes how scholarship is produced. As good work is demonstrated through the expertise in a field which is established by citing the "important figures" within the field in one's research, scholarship is forced to follow the path laid out by citation within a field. Moreover, a citational practice within a field becomes a moral injunction: to cite correctly, to produce "good work," is to make oneself legible as participating in the field, as extending the line of the field through one's research. In contrast, "bad work" is work that does not choose to follow the citational path laid out. In the context of fields organized around white men, fields like philosophy and bioethics, as Ahmed (2019) notes, "Good habits in citation are about extending a line: you have to show how much you know of a field by citing those deemed to have shaped that field. To extend a line is to reproduce an inheritance." Further, by following the logics of the field, the citational practices of the field, Ahmed (2019) recognizes that we might bring ourselves into existence through our relationship to these "important figures," but in doing so, we may also eliminate other ways of explaining our existence. This is an issue that is particularly pressing for attempts to engage with the concerns of marginalized populations through bioethics and the citational politics of the field.

In the foregoing, "citational politics" describes the politics surrounding who is and is not cited as an authority, or a legitimate participant within an academic discipline. For academics, the citational politics of a discipline determines how one is perceived as a "serious scholar" through whom one cites and how one cites them in their work. To this end, the citational politics of academic disciplines are often leveraged against marginalized scholars within academic fields, including bioethics. We might describe the ways in which the citational politics of exclusion, or the ways that scholarship and the boundaries of a field are reproduced to exclude some scholars and not others, as "citational tyranny," or a citational politics that maintains structures and systems of oppression through exclusion. Here, "tyranny" is not exercised by a singular "tyrant," as might be the case with broader political structures; rather, it is the description of a field whose citational structure exercises oppressive power over who can and cannot participate within it as a knower and producer of knowledge.

Citational Tyranny and the Reproduction of Bioethics from the Dominant Position

A principal example of the ways that the citational politics of bioethics is leveraged against marginalized subjects is presented by Kiesha Ray (2021), in her blog post "We

Are Not Here to Save Bioethics: Amplifying Diverse Voices in Bioethics Today," which states the following regarding her experience as a woman of color and a bioethicist whose work focuses on the intersection of bioethics and race:

> One roadblock that I have encountered that I know is common is the "what you do is not bioethics" roadblock. I have encountered this roadblock many times in the bioethics job market. I've had to defend my work beyond the normal academic criticism and defend the necessity of my work, that it belongs in bioethics, and that it is not better suited in public health or sociology, or another discipline. I have had to prove that I have something worthwhile to say that is beneficial to the profession.

In Ray's examples above, it is the addition of race that serves to push it out of the purview of an "objective" field like bioethics. Work that focuses on the ways that race and bioethics intersect, and offers recommendations that proceed from this intersection, belongs in public health where such recommendations can be actualized as policy. In contrast, work at the intersection of bioethics and race belongs in sociology because the work isn't truly bioethical: it is an engagement with health issues proceeding from the intersection of race and society. Moreover, we should consider the ways in which Ray has had to prove that she has "something worthwhile to say that is beneficial to the profession." That is, even though Ray is extending the line of bioethics through her research, she is not doing so in ways that align with the direction of the field. Again, following Ahmed (2006, 2013) we might note that the shape of a field emerges as an effect, or *affect*, of how bodies tend in the same direction. In the context of academic fields, this tendency is maintained by citational practices and habits that center some bodies and not others.

Ray is not sanguine about the sources of this exclusion in the kinds of bodies that predominate the field of bioethics, stating, "We know that most of bioethicists are White and arguable because of this much of the academic work we produce centers whiteness, White privilege, and a misunderstanding of the far-reaching effects of racism on health" (Ray 2021). That is, because the majority of the participants in the field of bioethics are white, their research proceeds as if their white subject position is a universal position. As a universal position, the whiteness of bioethics is a result of the whiteness of the persons producing the knowledge that gives rise to the field of bioethics, and whose citation forms the boundaries of the field. Insofar as academic fields come to take the shape of the individuals who are most often cited and circulated within them and thereby take on a likeness to those individuals, citation serves to screen and limit those who participate in the field to only those who align with the image of the field as produced by the citational habits of the field. As Ray (2020) states:

> Topics like social justice, racial justice, disability ethics, LGBTQ ethics, topics specific to immigrants, Latinx populations, and Black populations are much less commonplace. This is partly due to bioethics programs' poor job of recruiting and retaining diverse bioethicists. And from my own experience, it is partly due to established bioethicists making it clear that these kinds of topics are not "real bioethics."

The above is critical for understanding the tyranny of the citational politics of bioethics as it connects the idea of "real bioethics" with not simply whiteness, but heteronormativity, ableism, and xenophobia. Heteronormativity, here, is valuable to note as, following Ahmed (2013), compulsory heterosexuality itself produces the world as a field of objects toward which we can reach. Like whiteness, compulsory heterosexuality emerges as a result of the ways in which the actions of heterosexual bodies serve to organize social and cultural space in line with the repeated citation of their actions. For Ahmed, this organization of space runs ahead of subjects before they emerge into it: the orientation of the field, of heterosexuality, is something that we are presumed to inherit upon arrival. It is naturalized into social spaces, including institutional spaces, and thus serves to orient subjects toward reachable objects. "Real bioethics," or bioethics that proceeds from the dominant subject position, a position that is treated as objective, is that toward which the field aspires through its citational practices.

In more specific terms, this tyranny functions as an example of what Derek Anderson (2017) calls "conceptual competence injustice," wherein members of a marginalized group make a conceptual claim and are then treated as if they have less credibility to make the claim while simultaneously being treated as if they have a lower degree of competence in the relevant domain of inquiry. In the context of bioethics and philosophy of disability, Licia Carlson (2021) argues that the proximity of some philosophers of disability to the subject of disability violates the prescribed norm that philosophers must approach the subjects of their inquiry from an affective or personal distance. Inasmuch as bioethics is a domain of philosophy, I would extend this distance to disabled bioethicists themselves who, by virtue of their disability, might be "too close" to the subject to engage in true philosophical discourse on the matter. Put simply, the argument that any ethical consideration of a subject must be done from an emotional distance to the subject such that the philosophical rigor of the work is not put into question by the affective attachment to that work. Disabled scholars working in bioethics might therefore be afforded less competence within bioethics by their very embodiment.

We can extend this critique to account for race by considering the ways in which Ray argues that she must demonstrate that she has something valuable to contribute to the profession. On this view, we might follow Ahmed (2016, 29) who states, "To be treated as a being who needs to provide evidence of being is also to be treated as an adverse party. The word adverse implies opposing. But it is often used to create a stronger impression, to convey a sense of hostility or harmfulness." While we will address Ahmed's consideration of "threat" in the following section, what we might take from this is the demand to not only justify her scholarship, but to justify her presence in the field as a *Black woman* working on questions of race in Bioethics. Following Carlson, we might also argue that the whiteness of Bioethics established by its citational tyranny also establishes a condition wherein Ray's competence, and the competence of her work, will be placed in question by her embodiment. Thus, as "conceptual competence injustice involves taking a marginalized person to be less credible than their epistemic peers" (Anderson 2017, 214), it is unsurprising that

Ray would have to "defend her work beyond the normal academic criticism," as the citational politics of the field is not oriented toward Ray as a legitimate knower.

To this end, Ahmed's (2019) observation that "[n]ot to cite white men is not to exist; or at least not to exist within this or that field. When you exercise these logics, you might come to exist, by writing out another history, another way of explaining your existence," applies directly to the situation of bioethics insofar as most bioethicists are white and able-bodied and thus their texts proceed from whiteness as a starting point. If participating in the field requires demonstrating knowledge of the important figures of the field, white men, then to participate or exist in the field of bioethics is to cite the work of white men which therefore extends that line. To this end, for bioethics to be white, for it to consider bioethics work that does not proceed from whiteness as "not bioethics," is to point to who is not cited and how the field maintains its whiteness, it's shape. Thus, as "institutions become given, as an effect of the repetition of decisions made over time, which shapes the surface of institutional spaces" (Ahmed 2013, 157), the institution of bioethics *becomes white* through the repeated decisions of who to cite, how to cite, and in what way. Hence, citation in bioethics confers or passes down legitimacy through citational practices. That is, it confers legitimacy upon only that work which subjects itself to the conformity to the image of *appropriate scholarship.* Within this context, work only *becomes bioethics* when it engages with the appropriate subjects of the field.

Ray's observation of the whiteness and masculinity of bioethics also applies to disability: insofar as the majority of participants in the field of bioethics are themselves neurotypical, able-bodied, or do not identify themselves as disabled, the issues of ableism in addition to racism and other axes of marginalization persist because the scholars that are most directly involved in the reproduction and production of the field of bioethics are those bodies that most closely approximate an assumed norm. To this end, bioethical work that deviates from this norm, or even asks that the broader field engage with experiences that deviate from this norm, is to be rendered as "not bioethics" or "activism" by the field, positions which enable the field to ignore the critiques made. In the context of disability advocacy, that scholarship advocating on behalf of disabled persons is treated as activism, rather than genuine inquiry, indicates how the citational politics of the field of bioethics serves to structure it as treating the neurotypical, the able bodied, the sane as the universal position. In treating disability scholarship as "activism" or scholarship on race as "not bioethics," the field may exclude this knowledge and the scholars that produce it, from participation, a point addressed in the next section.

How Mislabeling Disability Scholarship as Activism Maintains Ableism

The above characterizes the citational tyranny of bioethics as the domination of the field by the narrow perspective of the neurotypical, able-bodied subject and the knowledge that follows from it. In the above, the declaration that work that does not proceed from the dominant subject position is "not bioethics" also carries with it the implication that such work has no *benefit* to bioethics unless it can demonstrate its benefit through the structures of legitimization provided by the citational politics of bioethics, a citational politics that organizes the subject perspective from which bioethics must proceed as "objective" by virtue of its dominant social position. To this end, any Bioethical work that focuses on bioethical issues that affect a marginalized group is not true scholarship: it is partisanship or advocacy. As described by Peter Singer (2005, 55):

> Bioethics, as a field or discipline, should not dedicate itself to advocacy for anyone. Its only commitment, as a field, is to pursue knowledge and understanding with integrity and respect for the views of other scholars in the field. It should serve neither those with money and power nor those without it—or rather, it serves all of us best by preserving its independence and freedom of opinion, encouraging open debate and the free exchange of ideas.

In Singer's view, the distinction between the mere partisan or propagandist and the philosopher or scholar is the willingness to be moved by "good argument" and not dismiss out of hand arguments that do not engage in advocacy for those who an individual bioethicist might view as having been wronged. For Singer, advocates for disabled persons, and we might also extend this to racial minorities, in bioethics are engaged in exactly this behavior, and it is on this ground that Singer rejects Kuzewski's call for bioethics to grow a conscience and engage in advocacy on behalf of disabled persons, advocacy which Singer rejects as within the purview of the field of bioethics, much less "good scholarship."

Here, we might draw parallels between the accusation that Ray's work is not bioethics and the argument that work in bioethics that advocates on behalf of disabled people is "not bioethics." Peter Singer makes this clear when he states, "For the entire field to take up an advocacy stance would imply that bioethicists who do not share the party line should be excluded or dismissed from the field" (Singer 2001, 55), which is to say that the bioethicist who engages in advocacy, who asks that the field itself consider the merits of arguments that fall under Singer's wide umbrella of "advocacy," polarizes the field and prevents genuine discourse from occurring. Thus, for Singer, the demands from disability bioethicists and disabled persons that bioethics engage with the arguments against the current practice of bioethics are not simply calls for further engagement, "Taken together, they amount to a concerted attack, not just on a particular ethical position, but on the very possibility of pursuing applied ethics as a free and critical inquiry" (Singer 2001, 85).

As an attack on the freedom of bioethics to engage in inquiry, work that advocates on behalf of a marginalized group is a *threat* to the practice of bioethics which, for Singer, is characterized by "independence and freedom of opinion" and the "free exchange of ideas." On this point, we might return to Ahmed's statement in the previous section: "To be treated as a being who needs to provide evidence of being is also to be treated as an adverse party. The word adverse implies opposing. But it is often used to create a stronger impression, to convey a sense of hostility or harmfulness." This sense of hostility is articulated in Singer's concern that an "advocacy stance" would risk pushing out those scholars who did not share in the advocacy stance. In other words, Singer is concerned that those scholars who did not reproduce the "line" of advocacy would be consequently excluded from the field for their failure to do so. This concern is ironic, given the previous section's articulation of the citational tyranny of bioethics: insofar as scholarship that "advocates" on behalf of marginalized groups by engaging with the bioethical implications of their marginalization fails to reproduce the line of "good scholarship," scholars who engage in this work are excluded from the field. Singer's fear, therefore, may be read as a fear that the citational tyranny of bioethics will itself be turned upon him and those who share his views.

In keeping with the above, for Ahmed, independence and freedom of inquiry embody a moral order that maintains the sanctity of bioethics as an objective discipline. Singer locates this in the impartiality of the field of ethics, of which Bioethics is a subdiscipline, stating: "Ethics goes beyond 'I' and 'you' to the universal law, the universalizable judgment, the standpoint of the impartial spectator or ideal observer, or whatever we choose to call it" (Singer 2011, 11). Put simply, ethics requires that we suspend our situated perspectives and adopt a universalist perspective such that we may only act upon judgments that we may universalize (Singer 2011, 279). In doing so, we suspend our subjective position to consider issues from an impartial standpoint such that our own interests do not color the inquiry. To allow our interests to color our inquiry would, in Singer's view, fail to take seriously the commitment of ethics and bioethics to the "integrity and respect of other scholars in the field," because a failure to share in the valuing of our interests is, on Singer's view, tantamount to failing to respect the scholar as engaged in a legitimate project of inquiry.

Here, we see the slide from responsible academic and intellectual conduct into appropriate *moral conduct* as determined by the citational politics of the discipline. The practice of bioethics becomes a moral practice with moral ends that terminate in "appropriate scholarship," through engaging in appropriate habits of scholarship which include maintaining the appropriate distance from the object of inquiry. However, as indicated in the second section, the citational politics of bioethics organizes the field such that marginalized scholars working on issues of oppression in bioethics are treated as inherently closer to their subject. This organization results in the questioning of objectivity and, as Ray shows us, the value of the scholarship to the field of bioethics. In short, marginalized scholars, and work by marginalized scholars within bioethics, face additional obstacles because it is not taken as "objective" or "neutral" by virtue of the position of the scholar and the subject matter they are engaged with. To turn back to citational tyranny, the citational practice of objectivity as reproduced through the whiteness and ability status of the dominant scholars within the field of bioethics serves to organize and delimit what is and is not bioethics to that which aligns with the "neutral" position as it emerges from the scholastic activities of the power majority.

Nondisabled Ignorance as Bioethical Citational Practice

Christine Wieseler (2021) describes the above organization of bioethics around an "objective" or "neutral" subject position as "objectivity as neutrality," which allows bioethicists to dismiss the credibility of disabled scholars and the scholarship they produce. This dismissal consequently leads to what Wieseler calls "non-disabled ignorance," or the ways in which bioethics treats social position and ability in specific as irrelevant to epistemic inquiries. On this view, "non-disabled ignorance" allows bioethicists to reject outright or deem as less credible even empirical studies, such as assessments of quality of life for disabled persons, that threaten their ongoing belief that to live a disabled life is to live a life that is of less worth than that of an able-bodied person. Following Wieseler, it is this commitment of bioethicists to "objectivity as neutrality," shaped by "non-disabled ignorance," which reinforces the perspective of disability as inherently negative as the "objective" position and enables the persistence of ableism within bioethics. To this end, any argument that threatens this "objective" position does not proceed from an objective position that is, purportedly, free of bias; it is a position with an agenda or an aim, and consequently, not the purview of "objective" scholarship like bioethics.

It is this commitment to objectivity as neutrality that allows bioethicists to reject evidence that contradicts the prevailing opinion that disabled lives are less fulfilling than those of nondisabled persons in two ways: first, by denying that disabled people are credible sources upon their own experience, and second by assuming that a bodily impairment presumes a diminished or impaired quality of life. Wieseler, citing Singer, describes his position as justifying the former through arguing that if disabled people state that they have similar or better quality of life than nondisabled persons, then their definition of "quality of life" must be different than the accepted definition for it cannot be possible that disabled persons have a similar quality of life to nondisabled persons. The latter bioethicists justify by treating impairment and an *impaired life* as functionally identical, which is not the case.

Understood from a perspective of citational politics, since it cannot be possible that disabled persons can reproduce the "line" of a good life due to their impairment because an impairment necessarily means an impaired quality of life, any work that holds this position is suspect. Work that claims that disabled persons may live fulfilling lives despite their impairment is either mistaken or proceeds from a subject position that is neither objective nor neutral and can consequently be ignored. Further, any scholar who advances such a claim, or relies on work that advances such a claim, may also be treated as not reproducing the "line" of good scholarship because their work does not conform to a citational practice that privileges objectivity and neutrality. In short, "objectivity as neutrality," as a citational politics of bioethics, exercises tyranny by rejecting any work that does not align with its supposedly neutral, and ableist, subject position as unworthy of inclusion within the field.

In the foregoing, we can see the way in which objectivity as neutrality functions as a citational habit that guides who or *what* can be cited in the discipline: because disabled persons cannot be trusted to be objective reporters on their own quality of life; and because a disability *must necessarily* result in a lower quality of life, bioethicists can exclude from the citational history critical elements of disabled experience by virtue of its lack of objectivity. Moreover, this lack of objectivity enables one to level questions regarding the quality of work that proceeds from these subject positions. Insofar as objectivity may be taken as a mark of the "purity" of an inquiry, work that focuses on subjective experiences may be taken as less "pure," less universalizable, to follow Singer, and thus less valuable. Anderson describes this in terms of prestige bias within the discipline of philosophy:

> Feminist philosophy and critical philosophy of race, for example, are perceived to be popular areas of study for marginalized philosophers. Conceptual competence injustice encourages the thought that these "specialty" areas are the domains of the less conceptually competent, that they are less difficult areas to work in than "purer" forms of philosophy such as mainstream metaphysics and epistemology. (Anderson 2017, 221)

Insofar as we can take the ways that philosophy encourages the belief that subdisciplines that focus on marginalized philosophy, and we might include Philosophy of Disability in this list, are less pure by virtue of being the domain of the less culturally competent, it is also the case that bioethics inherits this belief. After all, as Singer suggests, bioethics is a sub-domain of ethics, which itself is part of the field of philosophy, and thereby inherits all the rigorous structures of its parent discipline, including a commitment to objectivity. If this is the case, we can follow Wieseler and take "purity" to be synonymous with "objectivity as neutrality," and thus the question of the conceptual difficulty of subdisciplines that focus on marginalized experiences is that they are seen as less "pure" and "less difficult" because they are less objective. Insofar as these fields are taken as the domain of the less conceptually competent, we can see the way in which conceptual competence requires objectivity from this view.

The foregoing accounts for Shelley Tremain's (2017) observation that disabled philosophers confront enormous challenges to their work on the basis of their status as knowers. Again, following Carlson and Wieseler above, the citational politics of bioethics is exercised in the mode of citational tyranny, which polices the ways in which disabled philosophers and other marginalized subjects participate within philosophy broadly, and bioethics specifically. Because disabled philosophers and bioethicists are treated as if they are not as conceptually competent as their colleagues by virtue of their embodiment and focus of their scholarship, disabled philosophers and bioethicists are routinely challenged by the citational politics of the field to justify their inclusion and their value. Put another way, it becomes the habit of the field of bioethics to view work that proceeds from a marginalized subject position with skepticism, a habit that is reinforced by citational practices that maintain the field of bioethics in a state of citational tyranny.

In keeping with the above, we could also position bioethics' rejection of Ray's work as the consequence of objectivity as neutrality as a citational practice which renders her work "not objective" and Ray herself "too close" to the subject matter. Further, her work is better described as either "policy" or "sociology," but not "bioethics" because its unique focus on advocacy and the application of bioethical methodologies to the concerns of a marginalized population means that her work falls short of the standards established by objectivity as neutrality as a citational practice. Further, it means that it lacks the objective rigor demanded by the citational politics of bioethics as inherited from the broader field of philosophy. That is, Ray's work, like the work of philosophers of disability, fails to extend the line of bioethics through its refusal to reproduce the ends of "objectivity" toward which the field aspires. By not participating in a citational politics that reproduces "objectivity as neutrality," Ray is viewed as less conceptually competent, and her work is treated as less "pure" within the discipline.

This accounts for Ray's experience of encountering "roadblocks" doing her work in bioethics, as the citational tyranny of bioethics generates an institutional context wherein Ray is constantly subjected to conceptual competence injustice by virtue of her embodiment and her work. To this end, Ahmed uses the term "brick wall" to describe the concretization of habits, including citational habits, that gives shape to institutions. In as much as academic fields come to be through their citational practices, these "brick walls" will be visible to participants depending on how they align with the citational practices of the field. Insofar as for Ahmed, the form that an institution takes is the result of the mechanisms of social order that govern the behavior of those within the institution, it is also the result of the repeated actions of the bodies that dominate the institution. Thus, to white, able-bodied bioethicists, these "brick walls" serve to organize the boundaries of the field in ways that are "objective" and "neutral." However, to those subjected to this position, these "brick walls" have been erected through citational tyranny to prevent the circulation of nonnormative work through the field. However, is it by means of disrupting the citational practices and disciplinary norms of bioethics that this citational tyranny can be ended.

Conclusion: Black, Brown, and Queer Resistance in Bioethics

In *What's the Use? On the Uses of Use*, Ahmed (2019) states: "Sometimes in order to survive institutions we need to transform them" (189). Applied to the wave of bioethical fields like Queer Bioethics, LGBTQIA Bioethics, Latinx Bioethics, Disability Bioethics, and even Feminist Bioethics, we might position these fields as responses to mainstream or dominant bioethics by individuals who need to transform the institution of bioethics in order to survive. To be clear, survival is at stake in the transformation of the field of bioethics as the remit of bioethics serves to shape the health outcomes of countless people. Moreover, as the ongoing Covid-19 pandemic has indicated, marginalized persons routinely receive prejudicial or substandard health care treatment, treatment that is often enabled by existing approaches to bioethics. That is, the need to transform bioethics is not just a necessity from an academic perspective, it is an imperative given the ways that work in bioethics, and bioethics itself, is taken up beyond the boundaries of the field to make policy decisions.

To this end, the transformation of the field of bioethics requires the decentering of the dominant subject position and the citational practices that take it as the point from which the field unfolds, instituting new citational practices in their places. This reinstitution is implicit in the very definition of new fields of bioethics like Black bioethics, which Ray (2020) defines it in the following:

> In many ways, Black Bioethics can be explained very simply as the exploration and interrogation of any event, ideal, technological advancement, person, or institution that directly or indirectly affects the health or well-being of Black (loosely defined) individuals or the Black population. Black bioethics is taking what we do in bioethics and specifically applying it to Black people. But in other ways Black bioethics is more than this; it is a rebellion against bioethics.

In contrast, Cristina Richie draws on Halberstam's "Queer Art of Failure" to set forth a vision of Queer bioethics as "a field that fundamentally opposes categorization" (Richie 2016, 365). In principle, Halberstam's "Queer Art of Failure" seeks to decenter traditional understandings of success, specifically that a queer politic might mean "embracing the incoherent, the lonely, the defeated, and the melancholic formulations of selfhood" (Halberstam 2011, 148), as well as those political orientations that themselves are not representative of the "heroic" queer narrative of overcoming. Taken up through Queer bioethics, the "Queer Art of Failure" enables Queer bioethics to reject concepts like "heterofuturity," the idea that contributing to the future requires heterosexual reproduction; heteronormativity, and cisnormativity or the normalization of cisgender existence is the "normal" or default experience of gender. In light of this, Cristina Richie defines queer bioethics in the following:

> Queer bioethics itself is a failure to the medical community—both in that it represents a nontraditional approach to bioethics and that many of the sensibilities are distasteful to conventional LGBT bioethics. And yet, there could not be a Queer bioethic without failure and rejection. (Richie 2016, 371)

The latter is important as, for Richie, the objectives of Queer bioethics are firmly grounded in the overturning of the status quo. In doing so, Queer bioethics seeks to disrupt the default assumptions of bioethics, such as reproduction as an end goal, as well as centering the less powerful, challenging the legitimacy of normative ideas of health and sexuality, and challenging the ways in which the field of bioethics has become complacent in the face of injustice and discrimination embedded in the medical system, in the encounters with medical apparatus, and in our very conceptions of health (Whalert and Fiester 2012). Put simply, by centering the Queer body and queer experience as the point from which citational practices unfold, Richie's Queer bioethics acts as a practice of rebellion against the citational tyranny of mainstream bioethics through its disruption of citational practice.

Here, Ray's description of Black bioethics as a "rebellion against bioethics" also applies to Queer bioethics, insofar as both are rebelling against the citational tyranny of the field of bioethics, which is important as it indicates precisely what is necessary to end the citational tyranny of bioethics: rebellion against the extant citational practices and politics of the field. Ahmed describes this as creating a "we" from an absence:

> To make a "we" from a not requires being willing to be that "we." So I call upon "not white men" to be rebels, not to keep citing white men, or not to cite just them or not to enlist their help to become them or not to aim to become as like them as you can be given the body you have. (Ahmed 2014)

It is the act of not following the citational practices of bioethics, not citing white men, or the experiences of the white subject, that enables both Queer and Black bioethics to create a space, a "we" that enables bioethical inquiry into the experiences of marginalized people.

Doing so not only transforms the scholar into a rebel, as Ahmed notes, and allows for the creation of citational practices that resist the citational tyranny of mainstream bioethics, it also allows for the revaluation of "not-bioethics" in the process. Once more, Ahmed is valuable here:

> To be doing *not philosophy* is a way of framing one's relation to philosophy albeit in apparently negative terms. *Not philosophy* is practiced by those who are not philosophers, and aims to create room within philosophy for others who are not philosophers. . . . Not philosophy aims not to reproduce the body of philosophy by a willful citational practice: if philosophers are cited (and in this book many philosophers are cited) they are not only cited alongside those who are not philosophers but are not given any priority over those who are not. (Ahmed 2017, 15)

Insofar as bioethics is a subdiscipline of philosophy, held to the same citational practices of philosophy, and is taken by its dominant members as engaged in the same "objective" project as mainstream philosophy, we might treat Ray's Black bioethics and Richie's Queer bioethics as forms of "not-philosophy" or, more specifically, forms of "not-bioethics" which intentionally seek to make room within bioethics for people who are not bioethicists. In the context of this piece, we might say that Queer and Black bioethics follows in the path laid forth by Ahmed (2017), as making room in bioethics for those who are judged as not meeting the criteria for human, where that criteria "is often attached to other nots, not human as not being: not being white, not being male, not being straight, not being able-bodied" (Ahmed 2017, 15). In essence, Black and Queer bioethics engage in a willful citational practice that disrupts the citational tyranny of bioethics to create room for those persons deemed not able to participate in the field, or in projects that proceed from their lived experience, due to not meeting the criteria for humanity, not being able to "fit" into the space of bioethics.

To this end, Ray's description of the citational practices of Black bioethics, which reference "articles, podcasts, blogs, graphic art, and other materials that reference black people's health or black bioethicists working in the field" (Ray 2020), serves as an example of the ways that Black bioethics serves to rebel against the citational tyranny of traditional bioethics. That is, even in its choice of materials, Black bioethics seeks to rebel against the normative ways in which Bioethics is done. It is, as Ahmed might describe, a "bioethics of the not," or bioethics that willfully seeks not to reproduce the "line" of bioethics that proceeds from "objectivity as neutrality" and holds itself to the norms of justification of the field of philosophy. It is bioethics that, like Queer and Disability bioethics, responds to Ahmed's (2019) recognition that "To build an alternative university requires crafting different routes from what is behind us: the fainter trails, the less used paths. I think crafting is a good word for this work: it takes willed work not to reproduce an inheritance, not to create the same old shape."

Bibliography

Ahmed, Sara. 2006. *Queer Phenomenology: Orientations, Objects, Others*. Duke University Press.
Ahmed, Sara. 2007. "A Phenomenology of Whiteness." *Feminist Theory*, 8 (2): 149–68.
Ahmed, Sara. 2013. "Making Feminist Points." *Feministkilljoys*. https://feministkilljoys.com/2013/09/11/making-feminist-points/.
Ahmed, Sara. 2014. "White Men." *Feministkilljoys*. https://feministkilljoys.com/2014/11/04/white-men/.
Ahmed, Sara. 2016. "An Affinity of Hammers." *Transgender Studies Quarterly*, 3 (2): 22–35.
Ahmed, Sara. 2017. *Living A Feminist Life*. Duke University Press.
Ahmed, Sara. 2019. *What's the Use? On the Uses of Use*. Duke University Press.
Anderson, Derek Egan. 2017. "Conceptual Competence Injustice." *Social Epistemology*, 31 (2): 210–23.
Carlson, Licia. 2021. "Why Does Intellectual Disability Matter to Philosophy?: Toward a Transformative Pedagogy." *Philosophical Inquiry in Education*, 23 (2): 72–82.
Dotson, Kristie. 2011. "Concrete Flowers: Contemplating the Profession of Philosophy." *Hypatia*, 26 (2): 403–9.
Dotson, Kristie. 2012. "How Is This Paper Philosophy?" *Comparative Philosophy*, 3 (1): 3–29.
Halberstam, Jack. 2011. *The Queer Art of Failure*. Duke University Press.
Ray, Keisha. 2020. "Black Bioethics and How the Failures of the Profession Paved the Way for Its Existence." *Bioethics Today*. https://bioethicstoday.org/blog/black-bioethics-and-how-the-failures-of-the-profession-paved-the-way-for-its-existence/
Ray, Keisha. 2021. "We Are Not Here to Save Bioethics: Amplifying Diverse Voices in Bioethics." *Bioethics Today*. https://bioethicstoday.org/blog/we-are-not-here-to-save-bioethics-amplifying-diverse-voices-in-bioethics/
Richie, Cristina. 2016. "Lessons from Queer Bioethics: A Response to Timothy F. Murphy." *Bioethics*, 30 (5): 365–71.
Singer, Peter. 2001. "Response to Mark Kuczewski." *The American Journal of Bioethics*, 1 (3): 55–6.

Singer, Peter. 2005. "Ethics and Disability: A Response to Koch." *Journal of Disability Policy Studies*, 16 (2): 130–3.
Singer, Peter. 2011. *Practical Ethics*. Cambridge University Press.
Tremain, Shelley. *Foucault and Feminist Philosophy of Disability*. Cambridge Univ. Press, 2017.
Whalert, Lance, and Autumn Fiester. 2012. "Queer Bioethics: Why Its Time Has Come." *Bioethics*, 26: ii–iv.
Wieseler, Christine. 2021. "Objectivity as Neutrality, Nondisabled Ignorance, and Strong Objectivity." *Social Philosophy Today*, 32: 85–106.

16

Visionary Bioethics

A Biopolitical Approach to Bioethical Inquiry

Leah Lomotey-Nakon

In this chapter, I propose visionary bioethics as a biopolitical approach to bioethical inquiry and decision-making. The chapter proceeds with a demystification of external and internal mechanisms within bioethics that have contributed to the separation of critical approaches within the field. I then move to investigate four approaches to placing visionary fiction in dialogue with bioethics to examine the usefulness of visionary fiction as an analytical model of inquiry for bioethics that invites generative examination and generous reimagination of biomedicine. I build on bioethics' shared history with speculative fiction to suggest that visionary bioethics can hold productive tensions in biomedicine that open generative spaces for critical ethical analysis that do not rely on ontological claims about race, class, ability, and gender.

Background

Western bioethics, like its corollary field of biomedicine, is the product of carefully disciplined disciplinary boundaries. The remarkably rapid rise of bioethics and coalescing of substantial authority and power in a relatively short period of time has largely contributed to its ability to constrain and align the discourse to the power structures within academia and biomedicine (Rothmann 1991). The managerial authority of bioethicists grew within academia (research ethics) and healthcare (clinical ethics), in part due to its effective scope narrowing and tone policing to position the field as a neutral, but largely uncritical arbiter of biomedical authority. Though there is a strong history of critical engagement with this positionality that was sustained within and outside of the field, until the Covid-19 pandemic, the traditional discourse within bioethics positioned social and political analyses as tangential to bioethics and in so doing, effectively ignored how race and class influenced both the subjects and methods of bioethical inquiry (Russell 2022).

The flattening and narrowing of the field collapse the scope of inquiry and critical engagement as tangential to scholarly inquiry and clinical practice (Ashby and Morell

2018). The prioritization of neutral engagement with biomedicine effectively cordons off critical analyses of health and healthcare and siloed discourses including ethics of care and feminist approaches to bioethics, public health ethics, cultural bioethics, Black bioethics, and organizational bioethics (Koch 2012). Ultimately, the prioritization of neutrality diminishes the analytical and methodological potential of bioethics, including clinical ethics, research ethics, and organizational healthcare ethics, to serve as checks on the epistemic and sociopolitical powers of biomedicine.

The structured inattentiveness to social and political analyses of healthcare and biomedicine is especially detrimental to the validity of bioethical inquiry, given that bioethics emerged to mitigate the worst effects of the technological and scientific management of biomedicine, which played out along racialized and classed axes. There is evidence that the careful trading of thick moral narrative inquiry for thin cases that are abstractions of bodies neutralized of their histories no longer provides an acceptable return on investment for the field. The disconcerting absence of bioethical discourse about growing birth and health injustices prior to the emergence of the Covid-19 pandemic is emblematic of this inattentiveness. Furthermore, the structured inattentiveness is noticeable to the larger industry. The inclusion of health equity and, though later reversed, exclusion of clinical ethics in the 2023 Joint Commission Standards can arguably be attributed to bioethics' narrowed scope of engagement (McLeod-Sordjan, Swidler, and Fins 2023).

In the wake of widespread attention to equity in healthcare and other institutions during the Covid-19 pandemic, the critical discourses within bioethics are gaining prominence and moving from marginality in relation to the larger bioethical discourse. Bioethics, in part due to its participation in the arbitration of "crisis standard of care" practices during the pandemic, is moving beyond the benign acknowledgment of biases and disparities in healthcare to investigate how biases and inequities shape bioethical inquiry and clinical decision-making (Annas 2021). Indeed, there are an impressive number of bioethicists and adjacent scholars who are working to remedy the structured inattentiveness of bioethics to biopolitical considerations, including but not limited to the contributors to the 2021 special issue of the *American Journal of Bioethics* on *Ethics, Medicine, and Racism*. Though these authors primarily look toward the contemporary impact of the disciplinary narrowing on the practices of bioethics, an older line of critique that reclaims the hidden disciplinary roots might serve as a more viable path to a biopolitically valid methodological approach within bioethics.

Bioethics as/in Science Fiction Imaginaries

Though somewhat disconnected, there is a growing field of inquiry connecting the fields of speculative fictions and bioethics. Strengthened by the public's rediscovery of Octavia Butler's *Parable of the Sower* series during the Covid-19 pandemic, scholars and activists began engaging speculative fiction to reimagine power relations in their respective spheres of influence. Science and technology scholars and literary critics such as Ruha Benjamin, Wendy Hui Kyong Chun, Alondra Nelson, and Sami Schalk have all suggested that speculative fiction provides platforms for bioethics to resist scientism and connect critical biomedical and sociopolitical imaginations.

The growing interest in connecting bioethics and science fiction is fascinating, given that the trajectory of bioethics mirrored that of speculative fiction, which rapidly expanded in the post-Second World War era as society wrestled with the social, cultural, and economic implications of the rapid advance of technoscience (Clayton 2013). The two fields similarly examine the implications of biotechnological advancement and the range of possibilities for human flourishing, and the disciplinary lines between speculative fiction and bioethics have long been blurred (Schick 2016). As British-based bioethicist Sarah Chan argued, the primary methodological tools of bioethics (case studies, thought experiments) might well be considered forms of speculative fiction (2009). Like bioethics, speculative fiction, especially the subgenre of science fiction, erased race through idealistic multiculturalism or replicated racial hierarchies uncritically. Bioethics as a discipline is a discursive field designed to develop intersubjective assumptions governing the boundaries of appropriate professional behavior. The supremacy and distinction of bioethics as a managerial authority are attributed to progenitors of bioethics, such as Daniel Callahan, and the significant investment of intellectual capital to distinguish bioethics from science fiction and establish the former as more than a scholarly genre of speculative fiction and navel gazing (Schick 2016).

Counter to Callahan's concern, it is this very overlap of discursive concern about the posthuman future and technological advancement that other scholars suggest invites generative engagement between the two fields. Bioethics and science fiction are parallel responses to existential fears about the posthuman future but have developed divergent modes of inquiry. The narrowing of bioethics has flattened space for multiple subjectivities to the "case," while the genre of science fiction provides a thick model of engaging multiple subjectivities and futures (Clayton 2013). While traditional science fiction overwhelmingly celebrates the possibilities of human transformation, bioethics maintains a pessimistic approach rooted in social science realism and moral philosophy (Clayton 2013). Finally, counter to the reliance on the scientific imagination and complicity with scientism that undergirds bioethical inquiry, science fiction provides a mechanism of engagement with critical theories of biopower. It is this final approach that provides the most generative model for bioethics to resist the ordering nature of scientism and more successfully mediate technoscientific advances toward the teleological ends of biomedical research and clinical decision-making (Clayton 2013).

Engaging bioethics as a speculative fiction also moves clinical and analytical bioethics toward thicker description of moral cases and exploration of ethical issues. As the rich fields of narrative medicine and medical humanities indicate, literary approaches to bioethics allow for immersion in different textual worlds. This immersion not only improves moral reasoning, but such an immersion eschews the illusion of clinical or philosophical analytical distance in favor of experiencing a narrative journey (Clayton 2013). By deploying tools of fiction, narrative bioethics can more effectively engage the moral concerns that emerge within biomedicine and biomedical technology in ways that democratically build methodological rigor and scholarly integrity by acknowledging the impossibility of neutrality within a field designed upon persuasive discourse (Chan 2009). Since speculative fictions are designed to "push the boundaries of our ethical imagination," engaging bioethics as a literary form acknowledges the situated nature of ethical knowledge and therefore avoids the temptation for bioethics to perform allegiance to scientism in exchange for biomedical legitimacy (Chan 2009, 225).

Analyzing the connections between speculative fiction and bioethics also illuminates how bioethics might provide greater insights to health and healthcare policy-making. Both science fiction and bioethics anticipate the moral problems of technologies, research methodologies, and biomedical treatment pathways (Schick 2016). Bioethics initially emerged with two distinct trajectories: *regulatory bioethics* focused on rights and choice led by legal and philosophical scholars, and *prophetic bioethics* focused on sociocultural meanings governed by theologians, social scientists, and nonanalytic philosophers. The development of the Human Genome Project and Ethical Legal and Social Implications research initiative paved the way for what Schick calls anticipatory bioethics, a mode of engagement that reifies the imagined dystopian/utopian future while eschewing moral obligations to the imagined future. The social and political institutions within the United States are saturated with sociotechnical imaginaries that turn speculative fiction from genre to a "cultural modality" (Schick 2016, 225). The danger of the ascendance of anticipatory bioethics is that it does not resist this larger societal temporal moral imagination and instead invites apocalyptic apathy regarding the agentic power of bioethics. Counter to Clayton and Chun's positive readings of the possibilities of science fiction, Schick warns that bioethics informed by the cultural modality of speculative and science fiction have tempted bioethicists into a form of moral bypassing that bounds responsibility and moral agency. In this reading, the critical engagement between bioethics and science fiction must lead to a demystification of the methodological connections toward a more politically engaged bioethical approach that effectively shifts policies and practices.

Finally, critically engaging the connections between bioethics and science fiction illuminates how both genres overwhelmingly rely on ontological claims about human nature rooted in eighteenth-century racial logics. While bioethics historically reifies scientism, science fiction historically deploys uncritical multiculturalism, subordinates dark-skinned species that replicate racialized hierarchies, or completely ignores race altogether. The traditional approaches within both genres naturalize oppression and marginalization based on race, gender, class, and ability in ways that conceal how suffering is sociopolitically constructed and maintained.

A New Imaginary

Within science fiction, counter to this epistemic violence, is the subgenre of visionary fiction, a field that actively engages in biopolitical inquiry, defies ontological claims of sociobiological inferiority, and reimagines the boundaries of liberation (Pasco, Anderson, and DasGupta 2016). Writers such as Octavia Butler model a way of resisting the sociotechnical imaginary by constructing new worlds unburdened by sociocultural constraints (Schalk 2018). These writers engage in social protest through conscious reimagining of disability, race, gender, and nonhuman relationships that effectively subvert the overall genre of speculative fiction (Dubey 2010). Their work both highlights the contemporary structure of society that marginalizes groups and constrains moral agency. Rather than sociopolitical escapism, visionary fiction invites readers to engage in biopolitical analysis and inhabit epistemic resistance by exposing the inner workings of our sociopolitical milieu (Schalk 2018).

Visionary fiction uses defamiliarization and denaturalization of the world to draw the reader's attention to the mutability of social constructions (Schalk 2018). Said differently, visionary fiction exposes how much of the current social world is created and sustained by conscious and unconscious decisions. Visionary fiction thus represents a praxis of rejecting the social and political "facts" and "rules" that seem naturally occurring and thereby shows the complicated interplay between individual and collective moral agency.

Most importantly, visionary fiction might be understood as a pedagogical project of consciousness-raising and moral reformation that is generative not only of a pedagogy of the oppressed but also of a pedagogy of the oppressor (Freire 1970). Indeed, medical humanists have suggested that visionary fiction is a powerful pedagogical tool that can leverage the praxis of narrative medicine to help clinical trainees expand their moral imagination concerning the relationship between the medical sciences and the persistence of social and racial inequities (Pasco, Anderson, and DasGupta 2016). For Pasco and colleagues, "visionary medicine" deploys visionary fiction to effectively help physicians-in-training develop a holistic understanding of the mechanisms of biopolitical suffering, how those mechanisms map onto the clinical setting, and the ways in which one can intervene to prevent limited notions of flourishing from prevailing in biomedical research and practice (Pasco, Anderson, and DasGupta 2016). Since visionary fiction effectively refashions the sociopolitical imaginary, visionary medicine is posited to help clinicians craft alternative notions of care and human flourishing in ways that actively resist epistemic violence and its material corollaries within biomedicine.

Visionary medicine counters the scientism embedded within biomedical research and practice and helps nurture critical engagement that expands the range of moral possibilities. Echoing the observations of Schick concerning the cultural saturation of sociotechnical imaginaries, Pasco, Anderson, and DasGupta (2016) suggest that physicians must develop skills that counter these imaginaries to equitably advance biomedical research and clinical practice. Visionary medicine also provides an avenue for biomedical researchers and clinicians to shift their imagination and perceptions of poor and non-white patients that move beyond individual to institutional and ideological changes that address the loci of power within biomedicine.

Visionary fiction provides entryways toward new imaginaries and helps readers to inhabit and reimagine their perceptions of nonwhiteness (Womack 2013). Visionary medicine pushes the boundaries of narrative medicine by helping researchers and practitioners with varying lived experiences move beyond merely sympathizing with the life worlds of those who experience sociopolitical and economic marginalization. Such efforts to "achieve" cultural competency treat marginalized people as rooted in static understandings of "diverse" cultural contexts. Even Johnathan Metzl's (2014) construction of structural competency, which recognizes the systems in which people are embedded, fails to fundamentally reshape or counter providers' imagination of justice outside of the contemporary or past structures of oppression. Engaging visionary fiction helps providers resist these logics and envision a more transformative practice of care and futurity for those *made* vulnerable by sociopolitical and economic marginalization and kept vulnerable by institutional policies and individual practices.

Toward a Visionary Bioethics

Following the constructive framework of visionary medicine as a pedagogical and analytical framework that contributes to institutional and ideological change within biomedicine, I advance that an analogous approach to bioethics can defamiliarize and denaturalize the sociopolitical imaginary that undergirds bioethics. Like biomedicine, the imaginary cultivated by bioethical discourse limits critical engagement with socioeconomic bias, medical realism, and neoliberalism behind the veil of objectivism and neutrality (Pasco, Anderson, and DasGupta 2016). A visionary approach to bioethical inquiry creates analytical space to critique the technoscientific imaginary while maintaining a generous and generative engagement with biomedicine. Like visionary fiction, visionary bioethics inhabits rather than avoids sociopolitical tensions toward a cocreated liberation in ways that resist epistemic violence, reveal mechanisms of injustice undergirding ethical decision-making, and reimagine the obligations of bioethics toward remedying the biopolitical injustices within biomedicine.

In addition to serving as an analytical approach, visionary bioethics has the potential to serve as a pedagogical tool for developing critical moral reflection and reflexive praxis within clinical ethics and healthcare organizational ethics. Engaging visionary fiction allows those administering and practicing medicine to expand their capacity for bioethical deliberation by exposing them to alternative imaginations of sociopolitical liberation and human flourishing. Furthermore, engaging visionary fictions within bioethical pedagogy provides liminal space to investigate personal and collective complicity with structures of oppression. It does so without reinforcing ontological beingness that suggests critical inquiry is liberative primarily to those who have been forced to navigate life within the folds of biopower and therefore their burden to resolve (Anderson 1995).

Just as Pasco and colleagues' construction of visionary medicine focuses on the pedagogical potential of engaging visionary fiction for medical trainees, I offer visionary bioethics as a pedagogical tool for all those who have moral agency within biomedicine, including, but not limited to, researchers, clinicians, allied health professionals, and hospital administrators. The managerial authority of traditional bioethics has led to a focus on the role of clinical providers and academic researchers within biomedicine; however, a visionary approach to bioethics acknowledges the situated nature of biomedicine within a larger healthcare industry. In the United States, physicians have constrained power within the medical industrial complex. Their work is shaped by the decisions of hospital administrators, insurance companies, health technology designers, and health policymakers. Visionary bioethics expands the scope of interest and responsibility to assert bioethics education as critical for the next generation of business, technology, policy, and finance leaders. Furthermore, bioethical engagement using the tools of visionary fiction, as opposed to other methods of bioethical deliberation, might allow these leaders to engage in critical engagement with the sociotechnical imaginary in ways that invite new imaginations of socioecological flourishing within and beyond biomedicine.

Bibliography

Anderson, Victor. 1995. Beyond Ontological Blackness : An Essay On African American Religious and Cultural Criticism. Continuum.

Annas, George J., and Sondra S. Crosby. 2021. "Standard Racism: Trying to Use 'Crisis Standards of Care' in the COVID-19 Pandemic." *The American Journal of Bioethics*, 21 (8): 1–3.

Ashby, Michael A., and Bronwen Morrell. 2018. "To the Barricades or the Blackboard: Bioethical Activism and the 'Stance of Neutrality'." *Journal of Bioethical Inquiry : An Interdisciplinary Forum for Ethical and Legal Debate*, 15 (4): 479–82.

Chan, Sarah. 2009. "More than Cautionary Tales: The Role of Fiction in Bioethics." *Journal of Medical Ethics*, 35 (7): 398–9.

Clayton, Jay. 2013. "The Ridicule of Time: Science Fiction, Bioethics, and the Posthuman." *American Literary History*, 25 (2): 317–43.

Dubey, Madhu. 2010. "Speculative Fictions of Slavery." *American Literature*, 82 (4): 779–805.

Freire, Paulo, Donaldo P. Macedo, and Ira Shor. 2018. *Pedagogy of the Oppressed*, trans. Myra Bergman Ramos. 50th anniversary ed. Bloomsbury Academic.

Holloway, Karla F. C. 2011. *Private Bodies, Public Texts: Race, Gender, and a Cultural Bioethics*. Duke University Press.

Koch, Tom. 2012. *Thieves of Virtue: When Bioethics Stole Medicine*. MIT Press.

Metzl, Jonathan M., and Helena Hansen. 2014. "Structural Competency: Theorizing a New Medical Engagement with Stigma and Inequality." *Social Science & Medicine*, 103: 126–33.

Pasco, John Carlo, Camille Anderson, and Sayantani DasGupta. 2016. "Visionary Medicine: Speculative Fiction, Racial Justice and Octavia Butler's 'Bloodchild'." *Medical Humanities*, 42 (4): 246–51.

Renee McLeod-Sordjan, Robert Swidler and Joseph J. Fins. March 24, 2023. Where is Clinical Ethics in the Revised Hospital Accreditation Standards? The Hastings Center Bioethics Forum. https://www.thehastingscenter.org/where-is-clinical-ethics-in-the-revised-hospital-accreditation-standards.

Rothman, David J. 1991. Strangers at the Bedside : A History of How Law and Bioethics Transformed Medical Decision Making. BasicBooks.
Russell, Camisha. 2022. "Meeting the Moment: Bioethics in the Time of Black Lives Matter." *The American Journal of Bioethics*, 22 (3): 9–21.
Schalk, Sami. 2018. *Bodyminds Reimagined:(Dis)Ability, Race, and Gender in Black Women's Speculative Fiction.* Duke University Press.
Schick, Ari. 2016. "Whereto Speculative Bioethics? Technological Visions and Future Simulations in a Science Fictional Culture." *Medical Humanities*, 42 (4): 225–31.
Womack, Ytasha L. 2013. Afrofuturism: The World Of Black Sci-fi And Fantasy Culture (1st ed.). Lawrence Hill Books.

Index

Note: Page number with "n" refer to note numbers

About the Contributors

Howard A. Brody, a physician, philosopher, and pioneer in the field of medical ethics, died in July 2024, no more than a month after having completed his chapter for this book. He directed programs in medical ethics and humanities at Michigan State University in East Lansing and the Institute for Medical Humanities at the University of Texas Medical Branch at Galveston. He was a compassionate family physician as well as a distinguished contributor to medical ethics research and scholarship. He wrote pivotal essays and books on end-of-life care, medical placebos, moral conflicts within the pharmaceutical industry, and other topics. His books have been translated into six languages. Among his many accolades, Brody served as president of the Society for Health and Human Values, was the 2009 recipient of the Lifetime Achievement Award from the American Society for Bioethics and Humanities, and was elected to the National Academy of Medicine within the National Academies of Sciences, Engineering, and Medicine in 1995.

Virginia A. Brown serves as a research scholar in social justice and population health at The Hastings Center. Her work centers on protecting the autonomy of persons living with serious mental illness using psychiatric advance directives. She received a $1.5 million grant in August 2024 from PCORI to study organizational trustworthiness and community-engaged research. Her publications include "What Makes Palliative Mental Health Care Ethical Health Care?" in the *AMA Journal of Ethics* and "A Critical Moment in Bioethics: Reckoning with Anti-Black Racism through Intergenerational Dialogue" in the *Hastings Center Report*.

Larry R. Churchill is Professor of Medical Ethics Emeritus at Vanderbilt University Medical Center in Nashville. He played a major role in developing two bioethics programs, one at Vanderbilt and the other at the University of North Carolina, Chapel Hill, where he was Chair of the Department of Social Medicine. Professor Churchill has been cited for excellence in teaching at both Vanderbilt and UNC. He is a member of the National Academy of Medicine and a Fellow of The Hastings Center. He is the author of seven books, including most recently *Ethics for Everyone: A Skills-Based Approach* (2020), and with Nancy M. P. King and Gail E. Henderson, *Bioethics Reenvisioned: A Path toward Health Justice* (2022). Churchill's work has been featured in popular media such as *USA Today*, *The New York Times*, *Bill Moyers Journal*, and the Alex Gibney documentary *Money-Driven Medicine*.

Marion Danis is a physician and bioethicist. She served on the faculty at the University of North Carolina, Chapel Hill from 1978 to 1997. She subsequently served as Chief of the Bioethics Consultation Service at the National Institutes of Health from 1997 until 2023. She has chaired the Ethics Committee of the Society of Critical Care Medicine, has chaired the International Society on Priorities in Health Care, has served on the board of directors of the American Society for Bioethics and Humanities, and has chaired the Fellows Council of the Hastings Center. Her research has focused on patient treatment preferences, on finding strategies for fair resource allocation through public deliberation, on promoting strategies to reduce health disparities, and on ways to improve ethics consultation. Her publications include several books: *Ethical Dimensions of Health Policy*, *Research Ethics Consultation: A Casebook*, and *Fair Resource Allocation and Rationing at the Bedside.*

Johnathan Flowers is Assistant Professor of Philosophy at California State University, Northridge. Flowers's research areas include African American intellectual history, Japanese aesthetics, American pragmatism, philosophy of disability, and philosophy of technology. His first monograph, *Mono No Aware and Gender as Affect in Japanese Aesthetics and American Pragmatism*, was published in 2023.

Arthur W. Frank is Professor Emeritus at the University of Calgary, Canada. Since his retirement in 2013, he has been Professor II at VID Specialized University in Oslo and Visiting Professor in the Program in Narrative Medicine at Columbia University in the City of New York. In 2023, he was Francqui Fellow at the University of Ghent, Belgium, delivering a lecture series on humanities in medicine. His books on illness experience, ethics, clinical care, and narrative include *At the Will of the Body* (1991/2003), *The Wounded Storyteller* (1995/2013), *The Renewal of Generosity* (2004), *Letting Stories Breathe* (2010), and most recently, *King Lear: Shakespeare's Dark Consolations* (2022), in Oxford's "My Reading" series. He is an elected fellow of the Royal Society of Canada and winner of their medal in bioethics. His other recognitions include the lifetime achievement award from the Canadian Bioethics Society.

Stephen M. Gardiner is Professor of Philosophy and Ben Rabinowitz Professor of the Human Dimensions of the Environment at the University of Washington, Seattle, where he is also Director of the Program on Ethics. Steve is the author of *A Perfect Moral Storm: The Ethical Tragedy of Climate Change* (2011) and coauthor of *Debating Climate Ethics* (2016). His edited books include *The Ethics of "Geoengineering" the Global Climate* (2020), *The Oxford Handbook of Environmental Ethics* (2016), and *The Oxford Handbook of Intergenerational Ethics* (2025). His latest book, *Dialogues on Climate Justice* (coauthored with Arthur Obst), is written both for general readers and college students. It tells the story of Hope, a fictional protagonist whose life is shaped by climate change, through a series of conversations about ethics and justice in a climate-challenged world.

Gail E. Henderson is a social scientist in the Department of Social Medicine at UNC School of Medicine in Chapel Hill. Her research investigates responses to emerging technologies, including gene transfer research. While director of the UNC Center for Genomics and Society, she supported interdisciplinary projects addressing technological advances in genomics and bioinformatics. In 2022, she coauthored a book with Nancy M. P. King and Larry R. Churchill, *Bioethics Reenvisioned: A Path toward Health Justice.*

Gregory E. Kaebnick is a senior research scholar and director of research at The Hastings Center. He has also served as associate editor and editor and is now a coeditor of the *Hastings Center Report*. His research focuses on the development and use of biotechnology for nonhuman organisms and the use of deliberative public engagement for guiding policy decisions about biotechnology. He is the principal investigator of a project, The Ethics of Deliberate Extinction, funded by the National Science Foundation. He is the author of *Humans in Nature: The World as We Find It and the World as We Create It*, published in 2014.

Nancy M. P. King is Emeritus Professor of Social Sciences and Health Policy at Wake Forest University School of Medicine, Winston-Salem, and former codirector of the Wake Forest University Center for Bioethics, Health, and Society and Bioethics Graduate Program. She has published over 100 scholarly articles and book chapters and is coeditor of *The Social Medicine Reader* (2019) and *Bioethics, Public Moral Argument, and Social Responsibility* (2012). Her most recent book is *Bioethics Reenvisioned: A Path toward Health Justice*, coauthored with Larry R. Churchill and Gail E. Henderson (2022). Professor King is a Fellow of the Hastings Center and a member of the AAHRPP Board of Directors and has served on the NIH Recombinant DNA Advisory Committee and the DHHS Secretary's Advisory Committee for Human Research Protections.

Elizabeth Lanphier is a faculty member in the Ethics Center at Cincinnati Children's Hospital Medical Center and in the Department of Pediatrics at the University of Cincinnati College of Medicine. She also holds affiliations with the Philosophy and Women, Gender, and Sexuality Studies departments at the University of Cincinnati, the Center for Public Engagement with Science, the Institute for Philosophy and Public Policy, and is a lecturer in the Program in Narrative Medicine at Columbia University in the City of New York. As a philosopher and clinical ethicist, Elizabeth has published on topics including shared and collective responsibility for health, reproductive justice, narrative practices in healthcare and bioethics, and trauma-informed care.

Leah Lomotey-Nakon is a multidisciplinary trained researcher at Baylor University in Waco, committed to community-engaged mixed-method research to identify the root causes of health injustice and address wicked problems impacting human flourishing. Dr. Lomotey-Nakon's work focuses on health care and the healthcare industries in the Southern United States and West Africa. Her current research investigates the socioecological relationships between multigenerational faith formation and reproductive health outcomes, as well as the sociopolitical ramifications of health philanthropy on health outcomes.

Cheryl C. Macpherson is Professor in the Department of Clinical Skills at St George's University, Grenada, where she integrated climate change into a required medical school course on bioethics. She is Senior Research Fellow in the Windward Islands Research and Education Foundation (WINDREF); Principal Investigator on the Caribbean Research Ethics Education initiative (NIH-Fogarty Award # R25TW009731), the CREEi-Hastings Center Bioethics Scholars Program (2022), and the CREEi-Hastings Center Climate Bioethics Program (2023); and Joint Editor of *Global Bioethics*. With over eighty publications, her seminal bioethics publications on climate change include "Should Physicians or Health Organizations be Environmentally Active" in *Medical Professionalism: Theory, Education, and Practice*. She edited and contributed to the book *Bioethical Insights into Values and Policy: Climate Change and Health* (2016) and reviews for the NIH, Wellcome Trust, Wellcome Open Research, Oxford University Press, and numerous journals.

Takunda Matose is a philosopher and bioethicist at Cincinnati Children's Hospital Medical Center and the University of Cincinnati College of Medicine who researches the intersection of political philosophy, bioethics, and the philosophy of race. He is interested in racial health justice and has written about the racial dimension of pandemics, maternal health disparities, health care in carceral complexes, and public health in Africa.

Lisa S. Parker, a philosopher, is the Dickie, McCamey & Chilcote Professor of Bioethics and Director of the Center for Bioethics & Health Law at the University of Pittsburgh, where she directs the MA Program in Bioethics and is a faculty member in the Gender, Sexuality, and Women's Studies Program. Her research focuses on ethical issues in the design and conduct of research, particularly genetic and mental health research, as well as critical analysis of bioethics as a social practice and field of inquiry. She collaborates to study ethical, legal, and social issues (ELSI) related to medicine, public health, and emerging technologies. For the National Human Genome Research Institute of NIH, she has served on the Advisory Council, advised the ELSI Program, and chaired the Genomics and Society Working Group.

Hollen N. Reischer is a clinical psychologist and a faculty member in the Department of Psychology at the University at Buffalo, SUNY. She received her PhD at Northwestern University, in Evanston. She also serves on the ethics committee of the Erie County Medical Center. She uses mixed methods to study the psychological lives of mid- to late-life adults, particularly in the areas of narrative identity, ego integrity, and self-transcendence, and she has published this research in outlets such as the *American Journal of Bioethics* and the *Journal of Personality*. Her basic research seeks to explore the stories and values of individuals, families, and communities as they cope with personal challenges such as life-limiting illness and systemic problems such as lack of access to quality care. Her applied research seeks to investigate the possibilities of providers' and ethicists' engagement with lived experience and personal meaning-making as routes to promoting individual dignity as well as health equity in marginalized communities.

Travis N. Rieder is Director for Education Initiatives and Associate Research Professor at the Johns Hopkins Berman Institute of Bioethics in Baltimore. He also holds appointments in the Departments of Philosophy and Health Policy & Management at Johns Hopkins University. Travis has written on a wide variety of topics in bioethics and moral philosophy, ranging from ethical and policy issues surrounding pain, drugs, addiction, and North America's overdose crisis, to climate ethics and procreative ethics. His most recent book is *Catastrophe Ethics: How to Choose Well in a World of Tough Choices* (2024), which explores how to live a morally justifiable life when so many of our individual actions implicate us in massive structural harms and injustices.

David Schenck is the former director of the Ethics Program at the Medical University of South Carolina in Charleston, and was on the faculty of the Center for Biomedical Ethics and Society at Vanderbilt University Medical Center in Nashville. He is the lead author of *Into the Field of Suffering: Finding the Other Side of Burnout*, a book drawing on conversations with healthcare providers, patients, and families, that argues the caregiver's experience of suffering is not simply a trial to be endured but an opportunity for learning and transformation to be embraced. He is also coauthor of two books that approach ethics and healing in healthcare from an empirical perspective, *Healers: Extraordinary Clinicians at Work* and *What Patients Teach: Everyday Ethics of Healthcare*. Schenck taught philosophy and religion for twenty years and has published widely in bioethics, philosophy, and religious studies. He was founding executive director of a free medical clinic, healthcare advocate for the homeless, and a 25-year hospice volunteer.

Nancy Tuana is DuPont/Class of 1949 Professor of Philosophy and Women's, Gender, and Sexuality Studies at Penn State, University Park, and the founding director of the Penn State Rock Ethics Institute in State College. Her work on climate justice includes research on the topic of gender and climate change, and her recent book, *Racial Climates, Ecological Indifference: An Ecointersectional Approach*, focuses on the intertwinings of systemic racism and climate injustice. In the field of feminist philosophy, she is committed to approaches that bring together different lineages of liberatory thought, including Black feminist philosophy, Latin American theory, decolonial approaches, Indigenous thought, queer theory, and disability theory. Tuana is also committed to engaged philosophy. She has developed expertise in working as a member of scientific teams to address issues of adaptation to climate impacts that are attentive to the values and lifeways of those impacted. She is currently a member of the NSF-funded research collaboration, Megalopolitan Coastal Transformation Hub.

Paul Tubig is Assistant Professor of Philosophy at Georgia Southern University in Statesboro. He received his PhD in Philosophy from the University of Washington, Seattle. His main research interests lie in social and political philosophy, ethics, and the philosophy of disability, with special emphasis on issues related to global health justice and neurotechnology. His work has appeared in *Monash Bioethics Review*,

Cambridge Quarterly of Healthcare Ethics, *International Journal of Feminist Approaches in Bioethics*, and numerous edited collections.

Katharine Wright is a freelance ethics consultant and former assistant director of the Nuffield Council on Bioethics in the UK. She is an internationally recognized expert in bioethics and its intersection with policy and practice, with a particular interest in the ethics of global health research, and in concepts of vulnerability and inclusion/exclusion from research. She was responsible for the Nuffield Council's 2020 report on the ethical conduct of research in global health emergencies and is currently working with the WHO's Health Ethics and Governance Team on the ethical challenges in health and climate policy.

www.ingramcontent.com/pod-product-compliance
Ingram Content Group UK Ltd.
Pitfield, Milton Keynes, MK11 3LW, UK
UKHW020213290926
15470UKWH00001B/168

9 781666 959383